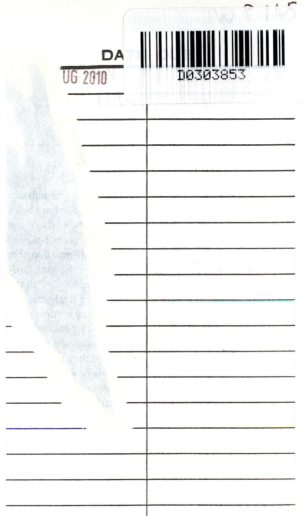

NOTICE

Medicine is an ever-changing science. As new research and clinical experience broaden our knowledge, changes in treatment and drug therapy are required. The authors and publisher of this work have checked with sources believed to be reliable in their efforts to provide information that is complete and generally in accord with the standards accepted at the time of publication. However, in view of the possibility of human error or changes in medical sciences, neither the authors nor the publisher nor any other party who has been involved in the preparation or publication of this work warrants that the information contained herein is in every respect accurate or complete, and they disclaim all responsibility for any errors or omissions or for the results obtained from use of the information contained in this work. Readers are encouraged to confirm the information contained herein with other sources. For example and in particular, readers are advised to check the product information sheet included in the package of each drug they plan to administer to be certain that the information contained in this work is accurate and that changes have not been made in the recommended dose or in the contraindications for administration. This recommendation is of particular importance in connection with new or infrequently used drugs.

GYN ONCOLOGY HANDBOOK

Edited by

Joseph T. Santoso, MD

Associate Professor and Director
Division of Gynecologic Oncology
Department of Obstetrics and Gynecology
The University of Tennessee
Memphis, Tennessee

Robert L. Coleman, MD

Associate Professor
Division of Gynecologic Oncology
Department of Obstetrics and Gynecology
The University of Texas Southwestern
Dallas, Texas

McGraw-Hill
Medical Publishing Division

New York / Chicago / San Francisco/ Lisbon
London / Madrid / Mexico City / Milan / New Delhi
San Juan / Seoul / Singapore / Sidney / Toronto

McGraw-Hill

A Division of The McGraw·Hill Companies

GYN ONCOLOGY HANDBOOK

1234567890   DOCDOC   09876543210

ISBN: 0-8385-3532-1 (Domestic)

This book was set in Times Roman by Atlis Graphics & Design.
The editors were Andrea Seils and Scott Kurtz.
The production supervisor was Catherine Saggese.
The cover designer was Mary McKeon.
The index was prepared by Patricia Perrier.
R.R. Donnelly/Crawfordsville was printer and binder.

This book is printed on acid-free paper.

Library of Congress Cataloging-in-Publication Data
Cataloging-in-publication data for this title is on file at the Library of Congress.

INTERNATIONAL EDITION ISBN 0-07-112458-6
Copyright © 2001. Exclusive rights by The McGraw-Hill Companies, Inc., for manufacture and export.
This book cannot be re-exported from the country to which it is consigned by McGraw-Hill, Inc. The International Edition is not available in North America.

CONTENTS

LIST OF CONTRIBUTORS

Robert L. Coleman, MD
Division of Gynecologic Oncology
Department of Obstetrics and Oncology
The University of Texas Southwestern
Dallas, Texas

Sara Crowder, MD
Division of Gynecologic Oncology
Department of Obstetrics & Gynecology
The University of Texas Medical Branch at Galveston
Galveston, Texas

Sandra Hatch, MD
Department of Radiation Oncology
The University of Texas Medical Branch
Galveston, Texas

Christine Lee, MD
Division of Gynecologic Oncology
Department of Obstetrics and Gynecology
The University of Texas Medical Branch at Galveston
Galveston, Texas

Joseph A. Lucci III, MD
Division of Gynecologic Oncology
Department of Obstetrics & Gynecology
The University of Texas Medical Branch at Galveston
Galveston, Texas

Joseph T. Santoso, MD
Division of Gynecologic Oncology
Department of Obstetrics and Gynecology
The University of Tennessee
Memphis, Tennessee

PREFACE

This handbook was initially written at the University of Texas Southwestern for medical students, residents, and fellows. With user feedback, it has evolved into a pocket handbook that helps house staff, nurses, and clinical practitioners take care of gynecologic oncology patients at the University of Texas Medical Branch. We are indebted to these clinicians, who have, in turn, become our teachers and improved the quality of this book.

Our aspiration is that readers will use this *GYN Oncology Handbook* as a guideline; it should not replace the standard textbooks and good clinical judgment. There is a tremendous amount of information that physicians and other health care professionals must know. This book provides concise and easy-to-use guidelines that should help clinicians take care of patients. It contains the standard chapters on disease sites followed by management of commonly encountered complications. An outline of procedures was written to help exhausted house staff in dictating surgical cases, and a synopsis of treatment modality was also provided in an outline form. Finally, the appendices provide concise information on relevant medical care.

This book could not have been written without the help of many people. From the University of Texas Medical Branch, Kristi Barrett, with the support of Mac McConnell, extensively edited and reformatted the original text. Amy Fenwick comprehensively reviewed it while studying for her board exams. Thanks to Sherry Bastien for her tremendous secretarial skills. At McGraw-Hill, Andrea Seils and Scott Kurtz continuously provided support that has made this book a reality.

Joseph T. Santoso
Memphis, Tennessee

Robert L. Coleman
Dallas, Texas

GYN ONCOLOGY HANDBOOK

I | DISEASE SITES

1 Preinvasive Disease—Cervical Dysplasia

Sara Crowder and Joseph T. Santoso

SCREENING

Who: any sexually active female.
When: initiation of intercourse or beginning at age 18, then
  yearly for life in patients with risk factors.
Purpose: screening for dysplasia (precancerous lesions).

RISK FACTORS

Human papillomavirus (HPV) infection, smoking, multiple
sexual partners, early coitarche.

CERVICAL ANATOMY

The cervix consists of ectocervix (squamous epithelium) and
endocervix (columnar epithelium). During menarche, estrogen
induces a process whereby the columnar epithelium undergoes
change to become squamous epithelium (metaplasia). The area
undergoing metaplasia is known as the transformation zone;
this is the site where dysplasia occurs.

BETHESDA CLASSIFICATION

The 1991 *Bethesda system* describes cellular findings from Pap
smear of the cervix and should be used as a screening tool.
Biopsies are required to direct treatment because the false-
negative rate for Pap smears can be up to 40%. The categories
are as follows:

A. Statement on the adequacy of the specimen for diagnostic
    evaluation:
    1. Satisfactory.
    2. Satisfactory but limited by . . . (specify reason).
    3. Unsatisfactory . . . (specify reason).

B. General categorization (optional, for possible clerical triage):
   1. Within normal limits.
   2. Infection or reactive/reparative changes (see descriptive diagnosis).
   3. Epithelial cell abnormality (see descriptive diagnosis).
C. Descriptive diagnosis:
   1. Infection: *Trichomonas, Candida,* coccobacilli, *Actinomyces,* herpes simplex virus.
   2. Reactive and reparative changes: atrophic, inflammation, radiation, chemotherapy, intrauterine device, other.
   3. Epithelial cell abnormalities.
      a. Squamous cell:
         (1) ASCUS (atypical squamous cells of undetermined significance): qualify.
         (2) SIL (squamous intraepithelial lesion).
             • Low-grade SIL, encompassing:
               —Mild dysplasia/cervical intraepithelial neoplasia (CIN) I.
             • High-grade SIL, encompassing:
               —Moderate dysplasia/CIN II.
               —Severe dysplasia/carcinoma in situ (CIS)/ CIN III.
         (3) Squamous cell carcinoma.
      b. Glandular cell:
         (1) Endometrial cells, cytologically benign, in a postmenopausal woman.
         (2) Atypical glandular cells of undetermined significance (AGUS): qualify.
         (3) Adenocarcinoma.
         (4) Endocervical, endometrial, extrauterine, not otherwise specified.
      c. Other epithelial malignant neoplasm (specify).
   4. Nonepithelial malignant neoplasms (specify).
   5. Hormonal evaluation (applies to vaginal smears only): compatible with age/history, not compatible with age/history, evaluation not possible due to . . . (specify).

MANAGEMENT OF SQUAMOUS DYSPLASIA

A. ASCUS
   1. Low-risk patient: repeat Pap smear in 3 to 4 months. If two subsequent Pap smears are normal, return to yearly testing. If repeat Pap smear is ASCUS, consider colposcopy (see Procedure section).
   2. High-risk patients (unreliable for follow-up, HIV+): perform colposcopy. Repeat Pap smear is not needed.
B. Low-grade SIL
   1. Repeat Pap smear (same as ASCUS).
   2. Perform colposcopy, cervical biopsies as needed, and endocervical curettage (ECC).
   3. If biopsy consistent with low-grade SIL and ECC is negative, consider cryotherapy versus observation.
C. High-grade SIL
   1. Consider loop electrosurgical excision procedure (LEEP).
   2. Perform colposcopy, cervical biopsies as needed, and ECC.
   3. If biopsy consistent with high-grade SIL and ECC is negative, consider LEEP, conization, or hysterectomy.
   4. If ECC positive, consider top hat LEEP or conization.

MANAGEMENT OF GLANDULAR DYSPLASIA

A. AGUS:
   1. Repeat Pap smear.
   2. Perform ECC, endometrial biopsy; consider hysteroscopy.
   3. AGUS can originate from the cervix, uterus, fallopian tube, or ovary. It is essential to work up a cause of this, especially in postmenopausal women, with appropriate biopsies as described earlier as well as a pelvic ultrasound and a CA-125 level.
   4. Results of AGUS workup:
      The glandular cells from an AGUS Pap smear may represent endocervical or endometrial cells. The significance of atypical endometrial cells on a Pap smear has

been studied: 20% have cancer, 10% endometrial hyperplasia, 10% polyps, 60% no pathological finding.[1]

TREATMENT

Colposcopy, cryotherapy, LEEP, conization, hysterectomy (see Chap. 24).

CONTROVERSIES/SPECIAL ISSUES

A. Pregnancy and cervical dysplasia[2]:
   1. Follow-up with Pap smear and colposcopy every 2 to 3 months.
   2. ECC should not be performed during pregnancy.
   3. Dysplastic lesions, including high-grade SIL, can be observed as the majority regress spontaneously.
   4. Obtain a cervical biopsy if suspicion for invasive cancer is high—higher blood flow during pregnancy causes more bleeding. A combination of Monsel's solution and pressure should stop majority of the bleeding episodes.
   5. Postpartum follow-up with biopsies and ECC is recommended at 6 weeks.
B. Positive margin on biopsies (LEEP) with high-grade SIL:
   1. In young women who want to preserve fertility, high-grade SIL with positive margins may be followed with Pap smears.
   2. If Pap smears continue to be abnormal, consider reconization. If fertility is not an issue, consider hysterectomy.
C. Lack of endocervical cells on Pap smear: Pap smear does not need to be repeated in a low-risk patient. If repeat Pap smear is desired, wait 6 weeks for epithelial repair.

REFERENCES

1. CHERKIS RC, PATTEN SF, DICKINSON JC, et al: Significance of atypical endometrial cells detected by cervical cytology. Obstet Gynecol 69:786, 1987.
2. YOST NP, SANTOSO JT, ILIYA FA, MCINTIRE DD: Postpartum regression rates of antepartum cervical intraepithelial neoplasia II and III lesions. Obstet Gynecol 93:359, 1999.

| Preinvasive Disease—Endometrial Hyperplasia

Sara Crowder and Joseph T. Santoso

GENERAL

A. Endometrial hyperplasia is a common entity; it accounts for about 5% of postmenopausal bleeding. Most cases are easily treated.
B. Definitions:
   1. *Hyperplasia:* thickened endometrium caused by an increase in the size and number of glands.
   2. *Simple hyperplasia:* crowded endometrial glands with densely cellular stroma. Foam cells may also be found in the stroma.
   3. *Complex hyperplasia:* back-to-back glands with irregular outlines and intraluminal papillae.
   4. *Atypia:* nuclear atypia, which is characterized by irregular shape and/or size, thickened nuclear membrane, prominent nucleoli, and coarse chromatin texture.
   Note: the term *carcinoma in situ* is not reproducible and should not be used in referring to this entity.

RISK FACTORS

Endometrial hyperplasia results from excess unopposed estrogen, and its risk factors are similar to those listed for endometrial cancer.

SIGNS AND SYMPTOMS

Most common are irregular or abnormal vaginal bleeding. In postmenopausal women, endometrial atrophy, not cancer or hyperplasia, is the most common cause of abnormal vaginal bleeding.[1] Vaginal bleeding from atrophy usually consists of spotting. In contrast, cancer produces persistent vaginal bleeding. Clinicians should obtain an endometrial biopsy in postmenopausal patients with vaginal bleeding.

DIAGNOSIS

Made by endometrial biopsy or D&C.

WORKUP

- Rule out other causes of uterine bleeding (i.e., pregnancy, dysfunctional uterine bleeding, cancer, polyps, exogenous estrogen, atrophy).
- Obtain a Pap smear to rule out cervical pathology. The Pap smear can only detect 30% of endometrial cancers.[2]

TREATMENT

A. Adolescent patients:
  1. Prescribe oral contraceptives for 6 months, then repeat endometrial biopsy.
  2. If repeat biopsy is benign, observe for normal ovulatory cycles. If cycles are irregular, cycle with medroxyprogesterone acetate (Provera) monthly until ovulatory cycles ensue or patient desires fertility.
B. Patients of reproductive age: prescribe oral contraceptives for 3 months, then repeat biopsy and, if benign, cycle with oral contraceptives or induce ovulation for fertility.
C. Perimenopausal patients: consider hysterectomy or progestin cycles, depending on the severity of hyperplasia, other indications, and the desire of patient. Can use Provera, 20 mg PO for 10 days each month for 6 months; Depo-Provera, 200 mg IM every 2 months for 3 doses; or megestrol acetate (Megace), 80 mg PO bid. Sampling should be performed every 3 months to rule out progression of hyperplasia.
D. Postmenopausal patients: hysterectomy and bilateral salpingo-oophorectomy (BSO) unless otherwise contraindicated.

PROGNOSTIC FACTORS

Endometrial hyperplasia may be a precursor lesion of endometrial carcinoma, as illustrated in Table 2–1.

TABLE 2–1. Progression of Endometrial Hyperplasia to Carcinoma[3]

Types	Patients (No.)	Progression to cancer in >1 yr of observation (%)
No atypia		
Simple (cystic)	93	1
Complex (adenomatous)	29	3
Atypical		
Simple with atypia	13	8
Complex with atypia	35	29

CONTROVERSIES/SPECIAL ISSUES

- Complex atypical hyperplasia in postmenopausal women should be treated with a hysterectomy and BSO unless compelling contraindications exist.
- BSO should be performed as metastases to adnexa from primary uterine cancer are common (found in 6% to 10% of patients with clinical stage I disease).
- In nonsurgical candidates, treatment options include radiation therapy or hormones. If grade 1 adenocarcinoma is found, an MRI can be obtained to rule out invasion. If adenocarcinoma is not invasive, give megestrol acetate, 80 mg b.i.d. for 3 months. Endometrial biopsy can be repeated at the end of 3 months; if the lesion has regressed, give a maintenance dose of megestrol acetate, 20 mg b.i.d. This treatment provides a 75% rate of remission and 25% rate of persistence or progression.[4,5]

REFERENCES

1. LIDOR A, ISMAJOVICH B, CONFINO E, DAVID MP: Histopathological findings in 226 women with post-menopausal uterine bleeding. Acta Obstet Gynecol Scand 65:41, 1986.
2. FUKUDA K, MORI M, UCHIYAMA M, IWAI K, IWASAKA T, SUGIMORI H, YAMASAKI F: Preoperative cervical cytology in endometrial carcinoma and its clinicopathologic relevance. Gynecol Oncol 72:273, 1999.

3. KURMAN RJ, KAMINSKI PF, NORRIS HJ: The behavior of endometrial hyperplasia. A long-term study of "untreated" hyperplasia in 170 patients. Cancer 56:403, 1985.
4. KIM YB, HOLSCHNEIDER CH, GHOSH K, NIEBERG RK, MONTZ FJ: Progestin alone as primary treatment of endometrial carcinoma in premenopausal women. Cancer 79:320, 1997.
5. RANDALL TC, KURMAN RJ: Progestin treatment of atypical hyperplasia and well-differentiated carcinoma of the endometrium in women under age 40. Obstet Gynecol 90:434, 1997.

3 | Vulvar Cancers

Sara Crowder, Robert L. Coleman, and Joseph T. Santoso

GENERAL

- Vulvar cancers are rare, comprising 5% of all gynecologic tumors.
- The incidence of vulvar intraepithelial neoplasia (VIN) is increasing, but the incidence of vulvar carcinoma is stable.
- Five-year survival rate for 611 treated patients with epidermoid invasive cancers[1] is as shown in Table 3–1.

TABLE 3–1.

Stage	Survival (%)
I	71
II	61
III	44
IV	8

RISK FACTORS

- Age: the average patient is about 70 years old, but 15% are less than 40 years old.
- Human papillomavirus (HPV): some studies have shown about 50% of vulvar cancers are HPV positive.
- VIN: this has a much longer transition time than cervical intraepithelial neoplasia (CIN). It may regress spontaneously.
- Diabetes mellitus, hypertension, atherosclerosis, and obesity are prevalent; however, these may be risk factors or simply due to the age of onset. Smoking, cervical carcinoma, immunosuppression, and chronic irritants have also been implicated.

SIGNS AND SYMPTOMS

- Common findings are pruritus, mass, pain, bleeding, or ulceration.
- Fifty percent of cases are asymptomatic and present only with vulvar lesions.

DIAGNOSIS

- Obtain a biopsy of any suspicious vulvar lesion.
- Delay of diagnosis by both patient and physician is common.
- Patients are frequently treated medically without histologic diagnosis, resulting in a delay of diagnosis. A repeat biopsy should be obtained of any vulvar lesion that is not responding medically.
- Because of the multifocal nature of VIN, about 20% of patients with an initial biopsy indicating VIN III were reported to have microinvasive cancer in their resected vulvar specimen.[2]

WORKUP

- Tissue diagnosis is made by biopsy (usually punch biopsy).
- Perform a physical examination, with attention to any involvement of the vagina, urethra, anus, and accurate measurement of the vulvar and inguinal lesions.
- Obtain a chest x-ray and pelvic CT scan for advanced disease to rule out pelvic inguinal and lymphadenopathy.
- Barium enema, cystoscopy, and proctoscopy should be performed, as directed by symptoms or clinical findings.

STAGING

Surgical staging is as follows:[3]

0: carcinoma in situ, intraepithelial carcinoma [T1S].
I: tumor of 2 cm or less and confined to vulva. No nodal metastases. [T1N0M0].
    IA: stromal invasion of 1 mm or less.
    IB: stromal invasion greater than 1 mm.
II: tumor greater than 2 cm and confined to vulva or perineum. No nodal metastases [T2N0M0].
III: tumor of any size that extends to lower urethra, vagina, anus, or unilateral node metastasis [T3N0M0 or T3N1M0 or T1N1M0 or T2N1M0].
IVA: tumor that extends to upper urethra, bladder mucosa, rectal mucosa, pelvic bone, or bilateral regional nodal

metastasis [T1N2M0 or T2N2M0 or T3N2M0 or T4 any N M0].

IVB: any distant metastases, including pelvic lymph nodes [any T, M1].

HISTOLOGY

- Squamous cell is the most common type (86%), followed by melanoma (4.8%), sarcoma (2.2%), basal cell, Bartholin's gland, adenocarcinoma, and undifferentiated (see the Controversies/Special Issues section at the end of the chapter for a discussion of treatment of nonsquamous vulvar cancer).
- Vulvar tumors are metastatic in origin about 8% of the time. Tumors that commonly metastasize to the vulva include those of the cervix, endometrium, ovary, bladder, urethra, vagina, breast, kidney, stomach, and lung, as well as melanoma, gestational choriocarcinoma, neuroblastoma, and lymphoma.

TREATMENT

Prior to any treatment, colposcopy of the cervix, vagina, and vulva should be performed to rule out synchronous preinvasive/invasive lesions. (*Note:* there is no need to perform colposcopy of the vulva if a patient has CIN.) In a study of 169 women with invasive vulvar cancer, 13% had a second squamous neoplasm of the genital tract.[4]

General Treatment Recommendations

The treatment is mainly surgery with postoperative radiation for poor prognostic factors. If the initial lesion is too large for surgery with clear margins, the treatment should be preoperative chemoradiation followed by surgery to remove residual tumor.

1. *Stage I:* wide local excision can be used for lesions with less than 1-mm invasion of surrounding tissue. Radical local excision with a 1-cm margin may be used instead of a radical vulvectomy with deeper lesions of 2 cm diameter or less; there is an absence of lymphatic vascular space inva-

sion (LVSI) and clinically normal nodes. Indications for groin lymph node dissection (LND) are determined by the depth of invasion (see Table 3–2).

If one positive microscopic node is found, the clinician may observe. If two or more positive nodes are found, radiate ipsilateral and contralateral groin, as well as pelvic nodes. Positive inguinal nodes confer a 25% risk of positive pelvic nodes.

2. *Stages II and III:* perform radical vulvectomy with bilateral inguinal lymphadenectomy. Use three separate incisions. A 1-cm fresh free margin (0.8-mm fixed) around the cancer has been shown to be a strong predictor of decreased recurrence.[7] If the lesion's size compromises the surgical margin to the rectal or urethral sphincter, consider preoperative chemoradiation therapy to reduce the size, followed by surgery to remove residual tumor.

TABLE 3–2

Depth of invasion	Treatment
< 1 mm	Nodal dissection is *not* necessary as there is a low incidence of metastases
> 1.0 mm but < 5.0 mm	Ipsilateral[a] superficial[b] inguinal lymph node dissection
> 5 mm	Perform radical local excision or radical vulvectomy with ipsilateral superficial inguinal LND, as outlined in preceding text

[a]Ipsilateral dissection is acceptable in lateral lesions (≥ 2 cm away from the midline), but bilateral dissection should be performed if the vulvar lesion is in the midline.

[b]Send the lymph nodes for a frozen section; if the superficial inguinal nodes are negative or if there is only one microscopic positive node, there is no need for further nodal dissection. If the frozen section is positive, perform a deep inguinal node dissection and contralateral inguinal node dissection. This tissue does not need to be sent for a frozen section because the residual tumor can be radiated. (*Note:* give adjuvant radiation to inguinal and pelvic nodes.[5]) Patients with positive deep inguinal nodes, however, have been shown to have better outcomes if nodes are removed (no relapses) rather than radiated (18.5% relapses).[6]

3. Advanced disease: treat with exenteration when possible. Chemoradiation therapy can be given preoperatively, postoperatively, or for palliation with unresectable disease.
4. Indications for ipsilateral inguinal lymphadenectomy: tumor size less than 2 cm, depth of invasion greater than 1 mm, nonmidline location, well differentiated (grade 1), nodes not clinically involved.

PROGNOSTIC FACTORS

A. Size of lesion, number of nodes with tumor, histology, stage, LVSI.
B. Independent risk factors for nodes with tumor:
   1. Clinically suspicious nodes, high grade, LVSI, deep invasion, older age.
   2. Groin node metastases are related to tumor thickness/invasion.[8] (See Table 3–3.)

TABLE 3–3

Tumor thickness	≤ 1 mm	2 mm	3 mm	4 mm	5 mm	> 5 mm
Positive groin nodes (%)	2.6	8.9	18.6	30.9	33.3	47.9
Number of patients	38	56	59	68	57	286

ROUTE OF SPREAD

- Direct extension to adjacent organs (vagina, rectum, urethra).
- Lymphatic: embolization to superficial inguinal to deep inguinal (femoral) to iliac (pelvic) nodes. Labium majus/minus drains ipsilaterally. Clitoris, urethra, perineum drain bilaterally. Although direct lymphatic channels from the clitoris to the pelvic nodes have been demonstrated, their clinical significance is unknown.
- Hematogenous spread to distant organs.

FOLLOW-UP

- Follow-up visits should be scheduled every 3 months for 2 years, then every 6 months for the next 3 years, then yearly after 5 years.
- Examination should focus on lymph node survey, vulvar examination ($\pm$ colposcopy), and any vulvar or other symptoms.
- There are no specific tumor markers or tests to follow, and imaging studies should be ordered based on symptoms. Especially watch for new vulvar lesions or symptoms.

RECURRENT DISEASE

Local recurrence of disease in the vulva has up to a 75% salvage rate if surgically resectable. Recurrent disease often occurs at sites other than the initial disease site, which suggests that many such instances are actually new primary tumors. Groin recurrences are almost always fatal but can be palliated with resection or radiation. Distant metastases can be palliated with cisplatin-based chemotherapy.

CONTROVERSIES/SPECIAL ISSUES

A. Management of VIN: the main goal is to identify invasive cancer. After careful colposcopic examination and biopsy of the most suspicious lesion, treatment of VIN includes observation, cavitronic ultrasound surgical aspirator (CUSA), laser, and wide local excision.
B. Nonsquamous histology in vulvar cancer:
   1. Verrucous carcinoma: exophytic growth resembling warts. Microscopically, well-differentiated epithelial cells are seen "pushing" the tumor-dermal border. Patients have an excellent prognosis as it rarely metastasizes. Because radiation may transform it into a more malignant form, the treatment is radical local excision.
   2. Adenocarcinoma (includes Bartholin): an enlarged Bartholin's gland in a woman older than 50 years of age

should be excised because of the risk of Bartholin's gland carcinoma. These can be either adenocarcinoma or squamous cell. Treatment is radical vulvectomy with inguinal node dissection.

3. Basal cell carcinoma "rodent ulcer": rare, seen mostly in the elderly. Treatment is radical local excision without nodal dissection.

4. Meckel cell tumor: neuroendocrine tumor of the skin, which has a poor prognosis.

5. Melanoma: the most common nonsquamous cell carcinoma (4.8% of all vulvar cancers). It may arise from pre-existing pigmented lesions or from normal-appearing skin. There are three types: acral lentiginous, nodular, and superficial spreading. Lesions may metastasize to the cervix, vagina, urethra, or rectum. Treatment is radical local excision with a 1- to 2-cm margin. A wider margin does not affect survival. Inguinal node dissection is useful mainly to determine prognosis. Consider using a sentinel node approach to reduce morbidity. A lesion with less than 0.76-mm invasion of surrounding tissue has little metastatic potential; therefore, it does not need node dissection. (See Table 3–4.)

6. Paget's disease: eczematoid, weeping red lesion. Fifteen percent of cases have underlying adenocarcinoma (in contrast to breast Paget's, which is associated with 100% ade-

TABLE 3–4. Staging: Cutaneous Melanoma Classification Adapted for Vulva

Level	Clark's level	Chung	Breslow
I	Intraepithelial	Intraepithelial	< 0.76 mm
II	Into papillary dermis	< 1 mm from granular layer	0.76–1.50 mm
III	Filling dermal papillae	1.1–2 mm from granular layer	1.51–2.25 mm
IV	Into reticular dermis	> 2 mm from granular layer	2.26–3 mm
V	Into subcutaneous fat	Into subcutaneous fat	> 3 mm

nocarcinoma). Histology shows a nest of large pale cells infiltrating upward toward epithelium and may be confused with malignant melanoma. However, Paget's disease will stain positive for carcinoembryonic antigen (CEA). Melanoma will stain positive for S-100 protein and melanoma antigen HMB45. Treatment is wide local excision (full skin thickness) with multiple frozen sections as Paget's is truly an intraepithelial neoplasia. Obtain a 2-cm margin. If disease recurs, perform wider excision. If there is an underlying adenocarcinoma (15% of cases), proceed with radical vulvectomy and bilateral lymphadenectomy.

C. Lymph node dissection in vulvar carcinoma:

1. *Superficial inguinal nodes:* eight to 10 nodes between Camper's fascia and the cribriform fascia; bordered by the inguinal (Poupart's) ligament superiorly, the sartorious muscle laterally, and the adductor longus muscle medially. Because superficial inguinal node dissection without tumor at the initial surgery is associated with a 5% inguinal node recurrent rate,[9] it has been suggested that routine inguinal node dissection should include both superficial and deep inguinal nodes. This approach causes significant leg edema, especially with postoperative radiation. An alternative approach is removal of superficial nodes and any deep nodes medial to the femoral vein while preserving the fascia lata; this method is reported to show no inguinal node recurrence.[10]

2. *Deep inguinal nodes (femoral nodes):* three to five nodes beneath the cribriform fascia (fascia lata) medial to the femoral vein. Cloquet's node is the last or uppermost node of the deep femoral group but may be absent in up to 54%. The deep femoral nodes are classically described as being located beneath the cribriform fascia. However, studies and experience have shown that the deep femoral nodes are always situated within the openings in the fascia at the fossa ovalis. Thus, a deep femoral lymphadenectomy does not require removal of the fascia lata (cribriform fascia).[11,12]

3. *Pelvic nodes:* these nodes receive drainage from the nodal chains located above them (i.e., from the superficial and deep inguinal nodes) and drain superiorly to the para-aortic nodes. It is easy to become confused because, historically, the pelvic nodes were referred to as the "deep" nodes. Typically the pattern of spread is predictable. There are not positive pelvic nodes without positive inguinal nodes. Similarly, there are not positive deep inguinal nodes without positive superficial inguinal nodes. This concept led to the theory of a "sentinel node," which historically was Cloquet's node—the uppermost deep inguinal node (between the superficial and deep inguinal nodal chains). Some reports contradicted the reliability of finding Cloquet's node and the predictability of its status.

4. *Intraoperative sentinel lymph node mapping:* the concept of ordered lymphatic drainage is being taken a step further to locate a "sentinel node" at which the tumor first drains. The mapping can be accomplished by injecting Isosulfan blue dye into the dermis at the vulvar lesion, exposing the superficial inguinal lymph nodes, and watching where the blue dye first drains. In theory, these first nodes should be at highest risk for metastasis, but if they are negative for cancer, no further dissection is needed. This method is still in the experimental phase (GOG 173).

5. *Drainage:* lateral structures drain ipsilaterally, and midline structures (clitoris, urethra, perineum) drain bilaterally. Patients rarely have positive contralateral nodes without positive ipsilateral nodes (about 2.5%).

D. Depth of invasion versus tumor thickness: the depth of invasion is measured from the epithelial-stromal junction of the most superficial adjacent dermal papillae. Tumor thickness is measured from either the surface in nonkeratinized tissue or from the bottom of the granular area when there is surface keratinization.

E. Vulvar dystrophy:
1. Nonmalignant vulvar lesions are usually accompanied by severe pruritus.
2. Squamous cell hyperplasia (previously known as hyperplastic dystrophy): pathology shows thickening and widening of rete ridges and a hyperkeratotic surface, with or without atypia. Obtain a biopsy prior to treatment. Treatment is corticosteroid cream topically, as noted in the following.
3. Lichen sclerosis: etiology unknown but has been recently associated with HLA DQ7 (class II HLA complex) and other autoimmune factors. The interleukin-1 receptor antagonist gene relates to lichen sclerosis severity. Pathology shows thinning and blunting of rete ridges. Treatment is clobetasol proprionate 0.05% b.i.d. for 2 to 3 months, with the dose gradually lowered and stopped, then as needed for symptoms (e.g., once a week). A widely used alternative is 2% testosterone cream (petroleum). Apply tid for 6 weeks, then one to two times a week. However, a recent randomized placebo-controlled trial showed symptoms were not improved over emollient base alone.[13] Another alternative is 400 mg progesterone-in-oil mixed with 40 oz Aquaphor; apply on the vulva twice daily until skin improvement is noted, then every other day. Prolonged use may result in masculinization. Steroid cream should be discontinued once pruritus resolves as continued use may cause additional atrophy. An alternative treatment is Merring neurectomy or ethyl alcohol injection to the vulva under local or general anesthesia.
4. Mixed dystrophy: follow a combination of the aforementioned treatment methods.

REFERENCES

1. SHEPERD J, SIDERI M, BENEDET J, MAISONNEUVE P, SEVERI G, PECORELLI S, ODICINO F, CREASMAN W: Carcinoma of the vulva. J Epidemiol Biostat 3:117, 1998.

2. Chafe W, Richards A, Morgan L, Wilkinson E: Unrecognized invasive carcinoma in vulvar intraepithelial neoplasia (VIN). Gynecol Oncol 31:154, 1988.

3. American Joint Committee on Cancer: Vulva, in *AJCC Cancer Staging Manual,* 5th ed. Philadelphia, Lippincott-Raven, 1997.

4. Mitchell MF, Prasad CJ, Silva EG, Rutledge FN, McArthur MC, Crum CP: Second genital primary squamous neoplasms in vulvar carcinoma: Viral and histopathologic correlates. Obstet Gynecol 81:13, 1993.

5. Homesley HD, Bundy BN, Sedlis A, Adcock L: Radiation therapy versus pelvic node resection for carcinoma of the vulva with positive groin nodes. Obstet Gynecol 68:733, 1986.

6. Stehman FB, Bundy BN, Thomas G, Varia M, Okagaki T, Roberts J, Bell J, Heller PB: Groin dissection versus groin radiation in carcinoma of the vulva: A Gynecologic Oncology Group study. Int J Rad Oncol Biol Physics 24:389, 1992.

7. Heaps JM, Fu YS, Montz FJ, Hacker NF, Berek JS: Surgical-pathologic variables predictive of local recurrence in squamous cell carcinoma of the vulva. Gynecol Oncol 38:309, 1990.

8. Homesley HD, Bundy BN, Sedlis A, Yordan E, Berek JS, Jahshan A, Mortel R: Prognostic factors for groin node metastasis in squamous cell carcinoma of the vulva. Gynecol Oncol 49:279, 1993.

9. Burke TW, Levenback C, Coleman RL, Morris M, Silva EG, Gershenson DM: Surgical therapy of T1 and T2 vulvar carcinoma: Further experience with radical wide excision and selective inguinal lymphadenectomy. Gynecol Oncol 57:215, 1995.

10. Bell JG, Lea JS, Reid GC: Complete groin lymphadenectomy with preservation of the fascia lata in the treatment of vulvar carcinoma. Gynecol Oncol 77:314, 2000.

11. Borgno G, Micheletti L, Barbero M: Topographic distribution of groin lymph nodes: a study of 50 female cadavars. J Reprod Med 35:1127, 1990.

12. Disaia PJ, Creasman WT: *Clinical Gynecologic Oncology.* 5th ed., St. Louis, Mosby Yearbook. 1997, p. 206.

13. Sideri M, Origoni W, Spinaci L, et al: Topical testosterone in the treatment of vulvar lichen sclerosus. Int J Gynecol Obstet 46:53, 1994.

| Vaginal Cancer

Christine Lee and Joseph T. Santoso

GENERAL

- Vaginal cancers are rare (1 to 2%) and usually occur in the upper half of the vagina.
- Most (80%) are metastases from the cervix or uterus. Staging protocols dictate that if tumor is present on either the cervix or vulva, the primary cancers are thought to be from these two places rather than from the vagina.

RISK FACTORS

Age, preinvasive disease, human papillomavirus (HPV), irradiation, known increase in vaginal adenocarcinoma with in utero diethylstilbestrol (DES) exposure.

SIGNS AND SYMPTOMS

Patients with early disease are usually not symptomatic. Advanced disease presents with bleeding, mass, foul-smelling discharge, and pain.

DIAGNOSIS

Confirmation is through colposcopic-directed biopsy or vaginal mucosa lesion resection.

WORKUP

- Complete history and physical examination.
- Chest x-ray to rule out distant metastases.
- Cytoscopy and proctoscopy to rule out bladder or bowel involvement.
- IVP or CT scan.

STAGING

Clinical staging is as follows:

I: limited to vaginal wall.

II: parametrial tissue (IIA and IIB—proposed substage).
    IIA: subvaginal infiltration, not into parametrium.
    IIB: extends to parametrium, but not pelvic wall.
III: extends to pelvic wall.
IV: extends beyond true pelvis, involves bladder/rectum, etc.

HISTOLOGY

- Primarily squamous cell (80% to 90%), adenocarcinoma (5%), and melanoma (3%).
- Other types include verrucous and clear cell.
- Most common in pediatric tumors: sarcoma botryoides (embryonal rhabdomyosarcoma).

TREATMENT

A. CIS (Stage 0):
    1. Intracavitary radiation: incapacitated or nonsurgical candidate.
    2. Surgery: partial or total vaginectomy (with split-thickness skin graft) is treatment of choice if invasion is suspected or if patient over 45 years. Patients at low risk for invasion (under 45 years old) may also undergo ablation with a cavitronic ultrasound surgical aspirator (CUSA) or a CO_2 laser (to 2 mm).
    3. 5-Fluorouracil (5-FU): 1.5 g (one-quarter applicator full) 5% 5-FU cream intravaginally for 1 night per week for 10 weeks. Repeat the course until CIS disappears. *Note:* the vulva should be covered with petroleum jelly to prevent irritation from 5-FU.
B. Stages I through IV: whole pelvic radiation therapy followed by tandem and ovoids in one to two applications.
C. Exceptions in treatment: if the tumor is in the upper third of the vagina, surgery may be performed (radical hysterectomy with pelvic lymphadenectomy and partial/complete radical vaginectomy).

D. For locally advanced vulvo-vaginal carcinoma, exenteration may be performed. An alternative to exenteration is to treat the pelvic (internal) disease with chemoradiation therapy and treat the external disease with a radical vulvectomy and bilateral inguinal lymphadenectomy.

E. Patients with recurrence after surgical therapy may receive radiation. Local recurrence after radiation may be treated with exenteration.

F. A select group of stage IV patients may be treated with exenteration.

G. Rhabdomyosarcoma is treated with surgery with radiation and chemotherapy.

PROGNOSTIC FACTORS

Stage most important (see Table 4–1); another factor is nonepithelial histology.

ROUTE OF SPREAD

A. Via lymph node drainage:
   1. Complex (a lesion can drain to any node). In general, a lesion in the distal vagina will drain like vulvar carcinoma (inguinal nodes); a lesion in the proximal vagina will drain like cervical carcinoma (obturator nodes).
   2. Direct extension to adjacent organs (bladder, rectum); similar to that of cervical cancer.

TABLE 4–1. Stage Predicts Survival[1]

Stage	Number of patients treated	Number of patients alive after 5 yr (%)
I	73	56 (77%)
II	110	49 (45%)
III	174	54 (31%)
IV	77	14 (18%)
Total	434	173 (40%)

FOLLOW-UP

Similar to that for cervical cancer.

RECURRENT DISEASE

- Central recurrence may be treated with exenteration.
- Chemotherapy: cisplatin has modest activity.

REFERENCE

1. KUCERA H, VAVRA N: Radiation management of primary carcinoma of the vagina: Clinical and histopathological variables associated with survival. Gynecol Oncol 40:12, 1991.

5 | Cervical Cancer

Sara Crowder, Christine Lee, and Joseph T. Santoso

GENERAL

- Cervical cancer accounts for about 15,000 new cases per year, 5,000 deaths per year, and 6% of all malignancies in women in the United States. Worldwide, it is the second most common cancer in women after breast cancer (> 470,000 new cases are cervical cancer annually).
- Five-year survival rate for 9964 patients with squamous carcinoma treated by all modalities[1] is as follows (Table 5–1):

TABLE 5–1.

Stage	Survival (%)
IA1	95
IA2	95
IB	80
IIA	69
IIB	65
IIIA	37
IIIB	40
IVA	18
IVB	8

- Five-year survival rate for 1121 patients with adenocarcinoma treated by all modalities[1] is as follows (Table 5–2):

TABLE 5–2.

Stage	Survival (%)
IB	83
IIA	50
IIB	59
IIIA	13
IIIB	31
IVA	6
IVB	6

RISK FACTORS

- Related to human papillomavirus (HPV) infection (especially types 16, 18, 31, and 45).
- Early initiation of intercourse, multiple sexual partners, multiparity, and smoking.

SIGNS AND SYMPTOMS

- Most common: vaginal bleeding (postcoital, intermenstrual) and vaginal discharge.
- In advanced cases: foul odor, pelvic pain, lumbosacral or gluteal pain, urinary frequency, and urinary or rectal pain.
- Classic triad of recurrence: sciatica, unilateral leg edema, and ureteral obstruction.

DIAGNOSIS

- The Pap smear is the best screening tool. Fifty percent of newly diagnosed women with cervical cancer never had a Pap smear.
- A Pap smear is recommended at onset of sexual activity or age 18. After three consecutive normal examinations, the screening interval may be increased. The American College of Obstetricians and Gynecologists recommends yearly examination for patients with any risk factor for cervical cancer (HPV infection, HIV, high-risk behavior).
- Confirmation of diagnosis requires a cervical tissue biopsy.

WORKUP

- Complete history and physical examination (especially careful evaluation of lymph nodes, as well as pelvic and rectal examinations).
- Biopsy-proven evidence of carcinoma (Pap and/or endocervical curettage is insufficient).
- Chest x-ray.
- Laboratory studies: CBC, chemistry panel, and liver function tests.
- Rule out ureteral obstruction with IVP or CT scan.

STAGING

A. Cervical cancer is staged clinically. FIGO staging requires a pelvic examination, cervical tissue (cone biopsy for stage IA and tissue biopsy for other stages), chest x-ray, IVP (may be substituted with CT scan). For more advanced cases, use cystoscopy, proctoscopy, and barium enema.

B. FIGO staging[2]:

   I: carcinoma confined to the cervix.

   IA: preclinical invasive carcinoma diagnosed by microscope only.

   IA1: stromal invasion of 3 mm or less in depth and lesion width less than 7 mm.

   IA2: stromal invasion of more than 3 mm, but 5 mm or less, and width less than 7 mm.

   IB: tumor larger than IA2 and confined to the cervix. All gross lesions, even with superficial invasion.

   IB1: tumor width of 4 cm or less.

   IB2: tumor width greater than 4 cm.

   II: invades beyond the uterus but does not involve the pelvic wall or the lower third of the vagina.

   IIA: without parametrial invasion.

   IIB: with parametrial invasion.

   III: disease involving lower vagina or pelvic wall.

   IIIA: involves lower third of the vagina, no extension to pelvic wall.

   IIIB: extends to pelvic wall (pelvic fixation is not required) or causes hydronephrosis (not hydroureter) or nonfunctioning kidneys.

   IV: metastatic diseases.

   IVA: spreads to bladder or rectum.

   IVB: spreads to distant organs.

C. Microinvasive disease (Society of Gynecologic Oncologist's definition): stromal invasion 3 mm or less in depth from the base of epithelium without lymphatic/vascular space involvement (LVSI) or confluent lesion in squamous carcinoma. *Note:* stage IA adenocarcinoma is controversial because measurement of depth of invasion in the endo-cervix is difficult and nonstandard. Successful conservative management of stage IA adenocarcinoma has been reported.[3]

HISTOLOGY

Eighty-five percent are squamous cell, 10% are adenocarcinoma, and 5% are adenosquamous, clear cell, small cell, verrucous, etc.

TREATMENT

A. Surgery: can be performed up to stage IIA with equivalent efficacy compared with radiation; has advantage of sparing ovarian function in premenopausal patients. Bulky (cervical diameter > 4 cm) cervical cancer is thought by some clinicians to be better treated with chemoradiation than surgery. Radical hysterectomy has mortality rate of less than 1%. Morbidity includes risk of fistula formation (1% to 2%), blood loss, and bladder atony requiring intermittent self-catheterization, anticholinergics, or α antagonists.
  1. Stage IA1 without LVSI:
     a. Cervical conization or simple hysterectomy cured virtually all patients.
     b. A 1% risk of nodal metastases/recurrent disease.
  2. Stage IA1 with LVSI, stage IA2:
     a Modified radical (type II) hysterectomy and pelvic lymphadenectomy.
     b. Stage IA1 with LVSI has a 5% risk of nodal metastases.
     c. Stage IA2 correlates with 4% to 10% risk of nodal involvement.
  3. Stage IB through stage IIA: Radical (type III) hysterectomy and pelvic and para-aortic lymphadenectomy.
  4. Adjuvant radiation may be given to postoperative patients with intermediate risk factors. This group is defined as stage IB with the features indicated in Table 5–3.

TABLE 5–3.

Capillary lymphatic/ vascular involvement	Stromal invasion	Tumor size
Present	Deep 1/3	Any
Present	Middle 1/3	> 2 cm
Present	Superficial 1/3	> 5 cm
Absence	Deep or middle 1/3	> 4 cm

Postoperative pelvic radiation reduces recurrence by 50%. In a recent study, 6% of patients who received postoperative radiation suffered grade 3–4 toxicity versus only 2% in the observation group.[4]

B. Radiotherapy: can be used for all stages. In the United States, radiation is mostly used in stages IIB through IV or for patients with earlier stages who are not surgical candidates. Recent studies show that adding cisplatin during whole pelvic radiation improves survival by 30% to 50%.[5]

C. The complications of radiation are mainly gastrointestinal, such as proctitis and colitis, and genitourinary, such as cystitis and vaginal stenosis.

1. *Teletherapy* with whole pelvis radiation therapy in a fraction of 180–200 cGy per day for 5 weeks (equal to a total dose of 4500–5000 cGy) is initially recommended. The goal is to treat the whole pelvis, parametria, iliac, and (if involved) periaortic lymph nodes.

2. Teletherapy is followed by *brachytherapy* with tandem and ovoid insertion (equal to total dose of 8500 cGy at point A and 6500 cGy at point B) over two applications, each lasting approximately 2 days (low-dose rate, or LDR). High-dose rate (HDR) therapy is similar but requires much less time to administer dose. Usually done as outpatient over a few minutes for three to five weekly applications. The goal is to deliver high doses to the uterus, cervix, vagina, and parametria.

3. *Point A* is defined as 2 cm superior to the external os and 2 cm lateral from the midpoint of the plane of the uterus. This represents the parametria.

   4. *Point B* is defined as 2 cm superior to the external os and 5 cm lateral from the midpoint of the plane of the body. This represents the pelvic side wall.
D. Adjuvant radiation may be given to postoperative patients with intermediate risk factors as previously mentioned.
E. Chemotherapy is mainly used in adjuvant radiation or for palliation in recurrence. The most active agent is cisplatin. Carboplatin has a similar activity to that of cisplatin.[6] Other chemotherapeutic agents with some activity: ifosfamide and paclitaxel (Taxol). Ineffective chemotherapeutic agents: etoposide, bryostatin, and topotecan.

PROGNOSTIC FACTORS

- Major factors for recurrence include LVSI, lymph node involvement, depth of invasion, status of resection margin, and tumor size. The chances of survival for patients with squamous and adenocarcinoma are about equal.
- Minor factors for recurrence include tumor DNA ploidy and expression of certain oncogenes (HER-2/neu).

ROUTE OF SPREAD

- Primarily by direct extension.
- Lymph node metastases (*pericervical → internal/external iliac, obturator → para-aortic → thoracic duct → left scalene*). Inguinal nodes are rarely involved (via round ligament).
- Hematogenous spread.

FOLLOW-UP

- Most recurrences appear within 2 years after diagnosis. For the first 2 years, patients should return for follow-up every 3 months. For the third through fifth years, schedule follow-up examinations every 6 months; thereafter, once a year.
- Each examination includes node survey, pelvic examination, guaiac test, and Pap smear.
- Obtain a chest x-ray or CT scan only if indicated from examination or symptoms.

RECURRENT DISEASE

- Classic triad: see section on Signs and Symptoms earlier.
- Common sites of recurrence (nonirradiated patients): vaginal cuff (25%), pelvic (25%), and outside the pelvis (50%).
- Evaluate for central recurrence (no distant metastases).
- Consider pelvic exenteration. Surgical mortality is 2%. Long-term morbidity is greater than 50%.
- Fifty percent of exenterations are aborted intraoperatively due to evidence of distant metastases on exploratory laparot-omy.
- If recurrence is noted distally, consider salvage chemotherapy (20% response rate).

CONTROVERSIES/SPECIAL ISSUES

- Cancer (greater than stage IA1) found after simple hysterectomy for presumed benign disease can be treated by postoperative radiation therapy or radical parametrectomy and lymphadenectomy.
- If grossly involved pelvic lymph nodes are detected at the time of radical hysterectomy, excision of the nodes may improve local control. Conflicting data exist on whether to remove the uterus or to leave it in place to assist brachytherapy.
- Choice of treatment of stages IB and IIA: most clinicians agree that patient survival is the same whether the treatment is surgery or radiation, but morbidity differs. A randomized clinical trial[7] concluded that surgery with postoperative radiation has greater complications than radiation alone.
- Enlarged fibroids are a challenge for dosimetry. Consider brachytherapy and hysterectomy after 6 weeks. Alternatively, consider leuprolide acetate (Lupron) to shrink fibroids, then radiate.
- For patients wishing to maintain fertility, consider Schauta's vaginal radical trachelectomy and laparoscopic lymphadenectomy followed by cerclage; these procedures may be performed in patients with selected stage I cancer.
- In patients who receive primary radiation teletherapy for bulky stage IB cervical cancer followed with postradiation

hysterectomy, the surgery increases cost and morbidity without clear improvement of local tumor control.

- Tumor marker measurement in cervical cancer is not standard of care.
- Estrogen replacement therapy may be safely prescribed to patients with invasive cervical cancer regardless of their histology and stage.
- Pregnant patients with cervical cancer have similar survival as nonpregnant patients. Patients with stage IA and small stage IB disease in the second trimester of pregnancy may have limited delays in therapy to allow fetal viability without seriously compromising patient survival. The safety of therapy delay for patients with bulky stage I lesions or more advanced stages is not established.

REFERENCES

1. BENEDET J, ODICINO F, MAISONNEUVE P, SEVERI G, CREASMAN W, SHEPHERD J, SIDERI M, PECORELLI S: Carcinoma of the cervix uteri. J Epid Biostat 3:28, 1998.
2. FLEMING ID, COOPER JS, HENSON DE, et al (eds): *AJCC Cancer Staging Manual,* 5th ed. Philadelphia, Lippincott-Raven, 1998, p 179.
3. SCHORGE JO, LEE KR, STEETS EE: Prospective management of stage IA cervical adenocarcinoma by conization alone to preserve fertility: a preliminary report. Gynecol Oncol 78:217, 2000.
4. SEDLIS A, BUNDY BN, ROTMAN MZ, LENTZ SS, MUDERSPACH LI, ZAINO RJ: A randomized trial of pelvic radiation therapy versus no further therapy in selected patients with stage IB carcinoma of the cervix after radical hysterectomy and pelvic lymphadenectomy: A gynecologic oncology group study [see comments]. Gynecol Oncol 73:177, 1999.
5. NCI clinical announcement, 2/1/99—National Cancer Institute PDQ treatment summary. Available: http://cancernet.nci.nih.gov/pdq/pdq_treatment.shtml.
6. WEISS GR, GREEN S, HANNIGAN EV, et al: A phase II trial of carboplatin for recurrent or metastatic squamous carcinoma of the uterine cervix: a Southwest Oncology Group study. Gynecol Oncol 39:332, 1990.
7. LANDONI F, MANEO A, COLOMBO A, PLACA F, MILANI R, PEREGO P, FAVINI G, FERRI L, MANGIONI C: Randomised study of radical surgery versus radiotherapy for stage IB-IIA cervical cancer. Lancet 350:535, 1997.

6 | Epithelial Uterine Cancer

Sara Crowder and Joseph T. Santoso

GENERAL

- Endometrial carcinoma is the most common gynecologic cancer, with 35,000 new cases per year in the United States.
- About 75% of the cases are found as stage I (survival about 75% or higher).
- Five-year survival[1] is as shown in Table 6–1.

TABLE 6–1.

Stage	Survival (%)
I	86
II	66
III	44
IV	16

RISK FACTORS

- Predisposing factors: obesity, unopposed estrogen, late menopause (> 52 years), nulliparity, anovulatory cycles, tamoxifen, and endometrial hyperplasia.
- Protective factors: oral contraceptives (relative risk [RR] = 0.5) with use for at least 12 months; protection can last 10 years. Smoking (RR = 0.7), especially in obese women.

SIGNS AND SYMPTOMS

Common findings are abnormal uterine bleeding and/or discharge.

DIAGNOSIS

Diagnosis is through endometrial biopsy or D&C. Negative endometrial biopsy in a symptomatic patient should be followed by a fractional curettage with hysteroscopic guidance, because endometrial biopsies have a false-negative rate of 5% to 10%.

WORKUP

A. Diagnosis should be definitively established by histologic sampling. Fractional D & C not required but may be helpful if suspected endocervical involvement.
B. Prior to surgery, workup should include:
   1. Chest x-ray to screen for lung metastasis.
   2. Pap smear to rule out cervical carcinoma.
   3. Routine screening laboratory studies (CBC, liver function tests, electrolytes) to rule out occult metastasis or medical disease.
   4. CA-125 level (see later Controversies/Special Issues section).
   5. Consider sigmoidoscopy or barium enema only in patients with disease palpable outside the uterus, with symptoms of bowel disease, or strong family history of colon cancer.
   6. CT scan may be obtained in some cases to identify the primary site of cancer.

STAGING

A. In 1988, FIGO assigned a surgical pathological staging classification. Patients deemed inoperable can have a clinical stage assigned.
B. Corpus cancer is *surgically* staged (FIGO, 1988); staging category must include grade (e.g., stage IBG2):

    IA: tumor is limited to the endometrium.
    IB: invasion of less than half of the myometrium.
    IC: invasion of more than half of the myometrium.
   IIA: endocervical glandular involvement only.
   IIB: cervical stromal invasion.
  IIIA: tumor invades serosa or adnexa or positive peritoneal cytology.
  IIIB: vaginal metastases.
  IIIC: metastases to pelvic or para-aortic lymph nodes.
  IVA: tumor invasion of bladder and/or bowel mucosa.
  IVB: distant metastases, including intra-abdominal and/or inguinal lymph nodes.

C. Grades of adenocarcinoma:

G1: well-differentiated adenomatous carcinoma ($\leq 5\%$ solid).

G2: differentiated adenomatous carcinoma with partial solid areas (5% to 50% solid).

G3: predominantly solid or entirely undifferentiated carcinoma ($> 50\%$ solid).

D. Corpus cancer clinical staging (FIGO, 1971)—for patients who do not have surgery (requires uterine sounding and a positive endocervical curettage [ECC] to evaluate cervical involvement):

I: the carcinoma is confined to the uterus.

IA: the length of the uterine cavity is less than 8 cm.

IB: the length of the uterine cavity is more than 8 cm.

II: the carcinoma involves the corpus and the cervix.

III: the carcinoma extends outside the uterus but not outside the true pelvis.

IV: the carcinoma extends outside the true pelvis or involves the bladder or rectum.

HISTOLOGY

- Primary: endometrioid adenocarcinoma (75%), adenosquamous (20%), and others (5%) (papillary serous, clear cells, etc.).
- Metastatic: the uterus can have metastases from ovary, breast, or stomach. Metastatic lesions to the endometrium are usually accompanied by disseminated disease.

TREATMENT

A. In contrast to patients with cervical carcinoma, those with endometrial carcinoma fare better with a hysterectomy or a hysterectomy and radiation than with radiation alone. The mainstay of therapy is therefore surgical, with or without adjuvant radiation. Several clinical trials have looked at hormone therapy and chemotherapy as adjuvant treatment in early-stage endometrial cancer, but none show a survival advantage over traditional surgery and radiation.

B. Surgical therapy:

1. Surgical staging includes vertical abdominal incision, peritoneal washings of pelvis and abdomen, exploration for palpable metastases, total abdominal hysterectomy and bilateral salpingo-oophorectomy (TAH-BSO), then opening and inspection of the uterus to determine depth of invasion. If depth is not grossly evident, obtain a frozen section. Pelvic and para-aortic lymph nodes and omental sampling are performed based on the following criteria in this high-risk group:
   a. Myometrial invasion of more than half.
   b. Isthmus/cervical extension.
   c. Extrauterine spread (including adnexa).
   d. Serous, clear cell, squamous, or undifferentiated cell types.
   e. Enlarged suspicious lymph nodes.
   f. Grade 3 carcinoma.
2. A pneumonic to remember the above six criteria is "Can't Go Home, Let's Do Sampling" for Cervix, Grade, Histology, Lymph nodes, Depth, and Spread.
3. Pelvic and para-aortic lymph node dissection (LND), not complete removal, is needed. However, all palpably enlarged nodes should be removed. Some clinicians may sample only the para-aortic nodes when the pelvis will receive adjuvant radiation anyway.
4. Negative pelvic nodes confer only 1.5% risk of positive para-aortic nodes. In contrast, positive pelvic nodes are associated with 50% positive para-aortic nodes.
5. Omentectomy should be performed on patients with stage I carcinoma having serous or clear cell histology or positive retroperitoneal nodes.[2]
6. Stages I and II occult positive ECC without other clinical evidence of cervical involvement: TAH-BSO and washings and/or LND, as outlined earlier. Radical hysterectomy does not improve survival.[3] Vaginal hysterectomy with laparoscopic LND may be performed on selected patients.
7. Stage II: three treatment options are available, as follows:
   a. Surgery:
      (1) Modified radical hysterectomy, BSO, pelvic lymph node dissection, washing, omental sam-

pling, peritoneal biopsy, and resection of para-aortic nodes, if suspicious.

(2) As previously, but using only extrafascial hysterectomy with pelvic and para-aortic node sampling.[4]

b. Combined surgery and radiation: preoperative external pelvic radiation plus intracavitary cesium; to be followed in 6 weeks (to decrease inflammation and edema) with a simple hysterectomy and bilateral salpingo-oophorectomy. There is no survival difference when performed between 0 and 10 weeks. This combination treatment has a high rate of rectovaginal/bowel obstruction complications.

8. Stage III and IV: surgery and/or radiation and/or chemotherapy. Removal of primary tumor is desirable in most situations, even with metastatic abdominal disease.

C. Radiotherapy:

1. Adjuvant pelvic radiation:

a. Low-risk patients (stage IA with grade 1 or 2) do not need postoperative radiation.

b. Intermediate risk patients (stages IB, IC; occult IIA and B, any grade; grade 3, any stage without nodal involvement): postoperative radiation decreases recurrence but does not affect survival.[5]

c. High-risk patients (tumor invading nodes and distant organs) may receive individualized radiation. Whole abdominal radiation versus adjuvant cisplatin *plus* doxorubicin is being studied (see Gynecologic Oncology Group [GOG] 122).

d. May extend radiation field to para-aortic nodes in the following situations:

(1) Biopsy-proven para-aortic nodal metastasis. Radiation to the para-aortic area in patients with microscopic tumor involvement may salvage up to 50% of patients but has a 12% mortality rate.[6]

(2) Grossly positive pelvic nodes or multiple microscopically positive pelvic nodes.

(3) Grossly positive adnexal metastasis.

(4) Outer third myometrial invasion and grade 2 or 3 tumors.

D. Medical therapy:
  1. Cytotoxic chemotherapy:
     a. Cisplatin and doxorubicin are the most active agents.
     b. Other active chemotherapeutic agents are paclitaxel, doxorubicin, and ifosfamide. Hexamethylmelamine, etoposide, tamoxifen, tenoposide, methotrexate, dactinomycin, piperazinedione, and topotecan are ineffective (see GOG 129G).
  2. Hormones:
     a. Tumors with positive estrogen or progesterone receptors have a better response to these drugs. Adjuvant oral or intramuscular progestins are equally effective. One-third of patients with a recurrence respond to progestin.
     b. Dosages that have been studied are:
        (1) Depo-Provera, 400 mg IM weekly.
        (2) Provera, 200 mg PO qd. This dose has a 25% overall response rate.[7]
        (3) Tamoxifen, 20 mg PO b.i.d. It has modest activity (GOG 81F).
        (4) Megestrol acetate (Megace), 800 mg PO qd. This dose has insufficient activity.[8]

PROGNOSTIC FACTORS

GOG studies[9,10] revealed important prognostic factors (Table 6–2). Many of these factors require laparotomy, thus giving importance to surgical staging for uterine cancer.

TABLE 6–2.

Uterine factors	Extrauterine factors
Histologic type (worse prognosis = serous/clear cells)	Adnexal masses
Grade (worse prognosis = grade 3)	Intraperitoneal spread
Myometrial invasion	Positive peritoneal cytology
Isthmus–cervix extension	Pelvic node metastasis
Vascular space invasion	Aortic node metastasis
Hormonal receptor status	
Size of cancer > 2 cm	

ROUTE OF SPREAD

- Direct extension to adjacent structures.
- Transtubal passage of exfoliated cells into the peritoneal cavity.
- Lymphatic dissemination: para-aortic, pelvic, inguinal/femoral nodes.
- Hematogenous spread: to lungs (most common), liver, brain, and bone.

FOLLOW-UP

- Follow-up examinations should be scheduled every 3 months for the first 2 years; thereafter, every 6 months for the next 3 years. After 5 years, examination should occur once a year.
- Examination should focus on lymph nodes and pelvic examination. Especially watch for pelvic pain or mass, vaginal bleeding, and respiratory symptoms.
- Tumor markers: follow CA-125 if it was initially elevated.
- Obtain additional laboratory studies or CT scan only as warranted by symptoms.

RECURRENT DISEASE

- Only recurrences at the vaginal cuff can be considered curable.
- Other recurrences can be palliated with progestins or chemotherapy (see earlier Treatment section).

CONTROVERSIES/SPECIAL ISSUES

A. Uncertain primary site:
　　1. Cancer of similar histology may be found in both the ovary and endometrium. If the metastatic pattern is not obvious, the primary site is assigned to the site having the most advanced stage and largest mass. The prognosis is usually better, because the ovarian cancer is investigated earlier due to abnormal uterine bleeding.
　　2. When both the cervix and endometrium seem to be involved in the malignant process to an extent that the primary site is not obvious, the tumor is usually assigned

to the endometrium as the primary site. Certain factors such as the presence of cervical intraepithelial neoplasia or endometrial hyperplasia, positive human papillomavirus (HPV) status (common in cervical carcinoma), or positive carcinoembryonic antigen (CEA) immunostain (common in endometrial carcinoma) may also help identify the primary site.

B. Tumor markers for endometrial cancer: CA-125 is useful only when it is initially elevated. About 20% of clinical stage I or II patients may have an elevated CA-125. An elevated level is predictive of advanced stage and extrauterine metastases.[11] Some clinicians use it in follow-up to detect recurrence.

C. Ultrasound or MRI for diagnosis:
   1. Ultrasonography and MRI may be used to diagnose uterine invasion and lymph node involvement, but these studies are not part of the staging procedures.
   2. An endometrial stripe of less than 5 mm in a postmenopausal woman confers no risk of cancer[12]; a stripe of more than 10 mm correlates with 10% to 20% risk of hyperplasia or cancer. In premenopausal women, an endometrial stripe of less than 12 mm confers no risk of cancer.

D. Methods of determining histologic grade: D&C has 30% to 50% inconsistency with the grade obtained from hysterectomy specimen.[13] Fifteen percent to 25% of cases of atypical hyperplasia noted in endometrial biopsy are upgraded to adenocarcinoma, usually well-differentiated stage I, in the hysterectomy specimen.

E. Methods of determining depth of invasion: gross evaluation of the uterus is 80% to 90% reliable (accuracy decreases with worsening grade). Frozen section assessment is 90 to 95% of cases, consistent with final pathology.[14,15]

F. Adjuvant radiation therapy for patients in the intermediate risk (IR) group:
   1. IR patients are those with the following characteristics: stage IB, IC, occult IIA and B, grade 3.

2. In the July 1999 GOG symposium, Dr. James A. Roberts reported that IR patients in a group that received adjuvant radiation had a survival rate of 97% compared with a 94% survival rate for those in a group that did not receive radiation ($P = .27$). Dr. Jeffrey Bloss argued that over 85% of patients in the IR group would receive unnecessary radiation if pelvic radiation were applied universally to patients in the IR group. (That is, out of 34,000 patients with endometrial cancer, 25,000 would be in the IR group.) Universal adjuvant radiation would prevent 2000 recurrences at the expense of 21,250 (85%) patients receiving unnecessary radiation. Out of 21,250 patients, 2750 would suffer grade 3 and 4 toxicities, and 250 might die from treatment-related complications.

3. The confusion continues: of the 767 listed Society of Gynecologic Oncologist members, 325 (42%) returned completed surveys. Less than 20% of respondents recommended adjuvant radiation therapy in stage IA grade 1 or 2 and stage IB grade 1 endometrial cancer. Adjuvant radiation was recommended by 40% to 50% of respondents in women with stage IA grade 3 and IB grade 2 tumors. Most respondents recommended adjuvant radiation for all women with more than 50% myometrial invasion or grade 3 tumors with any myometrial invasion. Lymph node sampling was attempted in all cases by 48% of respondents. For those who were familiar with GOG Study 99, 20% said they were more likely to recommend adjuvant radiation, and 27% said they were less likely to recommend adjuvant radiation based on the preliminary results. Except in stage IA grade 1 tumors, the likelihood of recommending further therapy in women with all stages and grades was significantly less if a complete staging procedure, including lymph node dissection, had been performed.[16]

4. Recently reported randomized trial of postoperative pelvic radiation (46 Gy) for clinical stage I uterine cancer (PORTEC) demonstrated no survival advantage (85%

no RT, 81% RT), but local regional recurrence was significantly lower in RT group (4% vs. 14%, P <.001).[17] Treatment-related complications occurred in 25% of RT patients versus 6% in control group (P <.0001). However, two-thirds of these were grade 1.

G. Peritoneal cytology positive without other extrauterine spread:

1. Four percent to 6% of patients with positive washings have no other evidence of extrauterine spread. Several small published series show no difference in outcome. Two large series suggest that it is a poor prognostic factor on its own.

2. Some clinicians advocate the use of intraperitoneal p32 versus radiation versus chemotherapy.

H. Tamoxifen and endometrial cancer:[18]

1. Tamoxifen increases the risk of developing endometrial cancer 2.4 times (usually well-differentiated carcinoma), but it reduces the risk of recurrent breast cancer to a much greater degree. Thus, women with breast cancer should continue taking tamoxifen. However, endometrial biopsy should be performed in those with irregular menses.

2. Routine endometrial sampling may diminish the accuracy of biopsy. Screening ultrasound is not reliable because tamoxifen induces submucosal thickening of the endometrium. The addition of progestin to a tamoxifen regimen may reduce its antitumor effectiveness.

I. Hormone replacement therapy (HRT) in endometrial cancer survivors:

1. Advanced endometrial cancers usually are less responsive to hormones because they have fewer estrogen-progesterone receptors. There is a concern that early and well-differentiated cancers may be stimulated by hormonal supplementation. All studies supporting the safety of HRT in endometrial cancer survivors were retrospective and of limited scientific value.

2. A prospective study is underway (GOG 137). Patient needs to be informed about the possible risks and bene-

fits of estrogen replacement. Another option is to not give HRT until the patient is free of disease for 2 years, as 80% of recurrences occur within the first 2 years after diagnosis. In patients who are treated with radiation and still retain their uterus, estrogen replacement occasionally induces residual endometrial proliferation. Thus, 2.5 mg of Provera per day is added in these patients.

REFERENCES

1. ANONYMOUS. Annual report on the results of treatment in gynecological cancer. Int J Gynaecol Obstet 36(Suppl):1, 1991.
2. CHEN SS, SPIEGEL G: Stage I endometrial carcinoma. Role of omental biopsy and omentectomy. J Reprod Med 36:627, 1991.
3. CALAIS G, LE FLOCH O, DESCAMPS P, VITU L, LANSAC J: Radical hysterectomy for stage I and II endometrial carcinoma: A retrospective analysis of 179 cases. Int J Rad Oncol Biol Physics 20:677, 1991.
4. DISAIA PJ, CREASMAN WT: *Clinical Gynecologic Oncology,* 5th ed. St. Louis, Mosby-Year Book, 1997, p 151.
5. ROBERTS JA, ZAINO R, KEYS H: A phase III randomized study of surgery vs. surgery plus adjunctive radiation therapy in intermediate risk endometrial cancer. Proc SGO Gynecol Oncol 68:135, 1998 (Abstract #258).
6. ROSE PG, CHA SD, TAK WK, FITZGERALD T, REALE F, HUNTER RE: Radiation therapy for surgically proven para-aortic node metastasis in endometrial carcinoma. Int J Rad Oncol Biol Physics 24:229, 1992.
7. THIGPEN JT, BRADY MF, ALVAREZ RD, ADELSON MD, HOMESLEY HD, MANETTA A, SOPER JT, GIVEN FT: Oral medroxyprogesterone acetate in the treatment of advanced or recurrent endometrial carcinoma: A dose-response study by the gynecologic oncology group. J Clin Oncol 17:1736, 1999.
8. LENTZ SS, BRADY MF, MAJOR FJ, REID GC, SOPER JT: High-dose megestrol acetate in advanced or recurrent endometrial carcinoma: A gynecologic oncology group study. J Clin Oncol 14:357, 1996.
9. MORROW CP, BUNDY BN, KURMAN RJ, CREASMAN WT, HELLER P, HOMESLEY HD, GRAHAM JE: Relationship between surgical-pathological risk factors and outcome in clinical stage I and II carcinoma of the endometrium: A gynecologic oncology group study. Gynecol Oncol 40:55, 1991.
10. CREASMAN WT, MORROW CP, BUNDY BN, HOMESLEY HD, GRAHAM JE, HELLER PB: Surgical pathologic spread patterns of endometrial cancer. A gynecologic oncology group study. Cancer 60(8 Suppl):2035, 1987.

11. Patsner B, Mann WJ, Cohen H, Loesch M: Predictive value of preoperative serum CA 125 levels in clinically localized and advanced endometrial carcinoma. Am J Obstet Gynecol 158:399, 1988.

12. Granberg S, Wikland M, Karlson B, et al: Endometrial thickness as measured by endovaginal ultrasound for identifying endometrial abnormality. Am J Obstet Gynecol 34:175, 1989.

13. Sant Cassia LJ, Weppelmann B, Shingleton H, Soong SJ, Hatch K, Salter MM: Management of early endometrial carcinoma. Gynecol Oncol 35:362, 1989.

14. Goff BA, Rice LW: Assessment of depth of myometrial invasion in endometrial adenocarcinoma. Gynecol Oncol 38:46, 1990.

15. Noumoff JS, Menzin A, Mikuta J, Lusk EJ, Morgan M, LiVolsi VA: The ability to evaluate prognostic variables on frozen section in hysterectomies performed for endometrial carcinoma. Gynecol Oncol 42:202, 1991.

16. Naumann RW, Higgins RV, Hall JB: The use of adjuvant radiation therapy by members of the Society of Gynecologic Oncologists. Gynecol Oncol 75:4, 1999.

17. Creutzberg CL, van Putten WLJ, Koper PCM, et al: Surgery and postoperative radiotherapy versus surgery alone for patients with stage I endometrial cancer: multicentre randomised trial. Lancet 355:1404, 2000.

18. Cohen CJ, Rahaman J: Endometrial cancer. Management of high risk and recurrence including the tamoxifen controversy. Cancer 76(10 Suppl):2044, 1995.

7 | Uterine Sarcoma
Sara Crowder and Joseph T. Santoso

GENERAL

- Rare (1 to 2 cases per 100,000 women), comprising less than 5% of all uterine cancers.
- The incidence of leiomyosarcoma found in patients operated for presumed leiomyoma is between 0.2% and 0.7%.[1]
- The prognosis is poor (death occurring within 1 to 2 years after diagnosis).

RISK FACTORS

- Unknown except for previous history of radiation.
- In the United States, it is more common among blacks than whites. In Israel, European-American Jews have twice the incidence of Jews of Asian-African origin (Arabic descent).
- Carcinosarcoma occurrence is unusual before age 40. After age 40, occurrence rates increase steadily. Leiomyosarcoma occurs at an earlier age and then plateaus.

SIGNS AND SYMPTOMS

The most common symptoms are uterine bleeding (75% to 95%), pelvic pain (33%), prolapsed necrotic tissue through cervical os, and enlarging uterus (15% to 50%).

DIAGNOSIS

Diagnosis usually is made in a patient with vaginal bleeding by endometrial biopsy or from a malignant polypoid mass protruding through the cervical os. Leiomyosarcoma may also be diagnosed after hysterectomy for presumed leiomyoma.

WORKUP

Same as that for uterine cancer.

STAGING

There is no official FIGO staging. Use uterine surgical or clinical staging.

HISTOLOGY

Note: Ninety percent of uterine sarcomas are carcinosarcoma (most common) and leiomyosarcoma (second most common).

A. Mixed epithelial—mesenchymal (stromal):
   1. Carcinosarcoma (also known as malignant mixed müllerian tumor, or MMMT): consists of epithelial carcinoma (usually endometrioid adenosarcoma) and a mesenchymal sarcoma.
      * *Homologous*—stromal (sarcoma) component is normally found in the uterus; examples: leiomyosarcoma, endometrioid stromal sarcoma, and angiosarcoma.
      * *Heterologous*—stromal (sarcoma) component is from tissue foreign to the uterus: examples: rhabdomyosarcoma, chondrosarcoma, and osteosarcoma.
      The homology status does not have prognostic value.[2]
   2. Adenosarcoma: benign proliferative or inactive endometrium mixed with a sarcoma.
   3. Adenofibroma: both the epithelial (endometrium) and stroma (fibroma) are benign.
B. Smooth muscle:
   1. Leiomyoma: benign smooth muscle, less than 5 mitoses per 10× hpf, and no atypia.
   2. Mitotically active leiomyoma: 5 or more mitoses per 10× hpf but no atypia.
   3. Leiomyosarcoma: malignant smooth muscle, atypia, and 5 or more mitoses per 10× hpf.
   4. Intravenous leiomyomatosis: benign myomas that arise in pelvic veins and can migrate to large vessels; there is a benign but prolonged clinical course.
   5. Disseminated peritoneal leiomyomatosis: small nodules (usually < 1 cm) that seed the peritoneal cavity, typi-

cally in pregnant patients; they should regress postpartum. Biopsy is needed to establish the diagnosis.

C. Stroma:
1. Stromal nodule: benign stroma that forms a well-circumscribed nodule of uniform cells resembling the stromal cells of normal proliferative-phase endometrium.
2. Low-grade endometrial stromal sarcoma (ESS; old name—endolymphatic stromal myosis): malignant tumor with indolent behavior—like a stromal nodule but has infiltrating margin and some mitoses (< 10 mitoses per $10\times$ hpf). Invasion of lymphatic/vascular space is common. Mitotic number has no prognostic significance. Responds to progestin (rich in estrogen and progesterone receptor).
3. High-grade ESS: highly aggressive. Consists of sheets of tumor cells with more atypia and mitoses than in low-grade form. Neither mitoses or cytologic atypia predict recurrence.

TREATMENT

- Early disease is managed surgically with hysterectomy, bilateral salpingo-oophorectomy, peritoneal washing, pelvic and para-aortic node sampling, and omental biopsy. Pelvic radiation offers better local control but has no effect on survival.
- In advanced disease, aggressive staging does not have survival benefit. Adjuvant chemotherapy does not affect the survival of patients with stage I disease.[3]
- For carcinosarcoma, ifosfamide and cisplatin are the most active chemotherapeutic agents with a response rate of less than 20%. The addition of cisplatin to ifosfamide adds more toxicity without affecting survival in comparison with ifosfamide alone.[4]
- In leiomyosarcoma, only doxorubicin (60 mg/m^2) has significant activity with a response rate about 25%. Ifosfamide (1.5 g/day for 5 days) has modest activity as a single agent (17%). Taxol, 175 mg/m^2 every 3 weeks, has some short-term

activity.[5] Etoposide,[6] Trimetrexate (GOG 131D), and topotecan (GOG 87H) have no activity.

- Low-grade ESS is cured by surgery alone. Megace may be beneficial for low-grade ESS (not adjuvant setting). Ifosfamide has a 33% overall response rate for high-grade ESS.[7]

PROGNOSTIC FACTORS

Major factors are the presence of extrauterine metastases and number of mitoses, as well as the degree of atypia (5 mitoses per $10\times$ hpf with atypia or 10 mitoses without atypia).

ROUTE OF SPREAD

There is early hematogenous spread; otherwise, it is similar to uterine cancer.

FOLLOW-UP

Same as that for uterine cancer.

RECURRENT DISEASE

Use chemotherapy or radiation therapy for palliation purposes as noted in the Treatment section, earlier.

CONTROVERSIES/SPECIAL ISSUES

The role of adjuvant cisplatin *plus* ifosfamide versus whole abdominal radiation in optimally debulked carcinosarcoma is being studied in Gynecologic Oncology Group (GOG) study 150. In a similar population, the role of ifosfamide versus ifosfamide and taxol is being studied in GOG 161. The role of postoperative radiotherapy in high-grade sarcoma is being prospectively evaluated in the EORTC-55874 trial.

REFERENCES

1. LEIBSOHN S, D'ABLAING G, MISHELL DR JR, SCHLAERTH JB: Leiomyosarcoma in a series of hysterectomies performed for pre-

sumed uterine leiomyomas. Am J Obstet Gynecol 162:968; discussion 974–976, 1990.

2. PETERS WA 3D, KUMAR NB, FLEMING WP, MORLEY GW: Prognostic features of sarcomas and mixed tumors of the endometrium. Obstet Gynecol 63:550, 1984.

3. OMURA GA, BLESSING JA, MAJOR F, LIFSHITZ S, EHRLICH CE, MANGAN C, BEECHAM J, PARK R, SILVERBERG S: A randomized clinical trial of adjuvant adriamycin in uterine sarcomas: A gynecologic oncology group study. J Clin Oncol 3:1240, 1985.

4. SUTTON GP, WILLIAMS SD, HSIU JG: Ifosfamide and Mesna with or without cisplatin in patients with advanced, persistent, recurrent mixed mesodermal tumors of the uterus. Proc SGO Gynecol Oncol 68:137, 1998 (Abstract #266).

5. SUTTON G, BLESSING JA, BALL H: Phase II trial of paclitaxel in leiomyosarcoma of the uterus: A gynecologic oncology group study. Gynecol Oncol 74:346, 1999.

6. ROSE PG, BLESSING JA, SOPER JT, BARTER JF: Prolonged oral etoposide in recurrent or advanced leiomyosarcoma of the uterus: A gynecologic oncology group study. Gynecol Oncol 70:267, 1998.

7. SUTTON G, BLESSING JA, PARK R, DISAIA PJ, ROSENSHEIN N: Ifosfamide treatment of recurrent or metastatic endometrial stromal sarcomas previously unexposed to chemotherapy: A study of gynecologic oncology group. Obstet Gynecol 87(5 Pt 1):747, 1996.

Ovarian Cancer

Sara Crowder, Christine Lee, and
Joseph T. Santoso

GENERAL

About 24,000 new cases of ovarian epithelial cancer occur annually in the United States, and 13,600 women die annually of ovarian cancer. The lifetime risk is 1.4%. This cancer causes the highest mortality of all gynecologic cancers and is more common in developed countries.

RISK FACTORS

A. Environmental factors: a high incidence of ovarian cancer is noted in industrialized countries. Obesity and alcohol consumption have been weakly linked, and coffee and tobacco are not associated with ovarian cancer. There are conflicting reports on the effects of mumps, talcum powder, and fat intake.

B. Reproductive factors: an increased number of ovulatory cycles correlates with a higher risk of developing ovarian cancer. Cancer is postulated to be generated by aberrant repair of ovarian surface epithelium. Inducing ovulatory cycles using clomiphene increases the risk 2 to 3 times.[1] Conditions that decrease ovulation frequency reduce the risk of cancer, as follows:

1. Birth control pills: decrease risks by 50%, when taken for 5 or more years.
2. Multiparity, multiple births, history of breast feeding.

C. Genetic factors:

1. Five percent to 10% is hereditary (defined as having at least two first-degree relatives with ovarian cancer).
2. With one first-degree relative with ovarian cancer, the risk of developing cancer is 5%.
3. With two first-degree relatives with ovarian cancer, the risk increases to 7%.

D. Three types of hereditary epithelial ovarian cancer:

1. Site-specific: only the trait for ovarian carcinoma is transmitted. This type is very rare.
2. Breast-ovarian cancer syndrome: caused by mutation of the BRCA1 genes (tumor suppressor genes). A patient with a mutant BRCA1 gene has a lifetime risk of up to 85% of developing breast cancer and a lifetime risk of up to 50% of developing ovarian cancer in a selected group. In larger studies, these numbers are lower. Although prophylactic mastectomy probably reduces risk, the exact percentage is not known. Prophylactic oopherectomy reduces risk almost back to 2%.
3. Lynch type-II cancer syndrome: inheritance of nonpolyposis colorectal cancer and endometrial, breast, ovarian, and other gastrointestinal and genitourinary malignancies.

SIGNS AND SYMPTOMS

Most patients are symptomatic (95%), but the symptoms are nonspecific—abdominal discomfort/pressure or dyspareunia, and weight gain from ascites or mass.

DIAGNOSTICS[2]

For the most part, measurements of CA-125 and transvaginal ultrasonography have reduced neither morbidity nor mortality from ovarian cancer in the general population. In patients with hereditary ovarian cancer, measurements of CA-125, pelvic examination, and transvaginal ultrasonography may be done every 6 months (no conclusive study on efficacy). In this high-risk population, prophylactic oophorectomy may be recommended at 35 years of age if childbearing is complete. In this population, there is a 2% risk of developing primary peritoneal carcinoma after prophylactic oophorectomy.

WORKUP

- Complete history and physical examination.
- Tumor marker for epithelial cancer (CA-125), germ cell

tumors (LDH, hCG, AFP), sex cord stromal tumor (inhibin for granulosa cell).
- Chemistry panel, CBC, liver function tests.
- Chest x-ray to evaluate for pleural effusion, lung metastases.
- CT scan of abdomen and pelvis.
- If symptomatic, IVP and/or barium enema to evaluate for bladder and bowel involvement.

STAGING

Surgical staging (FIGO 1986) is as follows:

I: growth limited to the ovaries.
>   **IA:** one ovary, no ascites, no tumor on the external surface, capsule intact.
>   **IB:** both ovaries, no ascites, no tumor on external surface, capsule intact.
>   **IC:** either stage IA or IB with tumors on the surface of one or both ovaries, with capsule ruptured, with ascites containing malignant cells, or with positive peritoneal washings.

II: growth involving one or both ovaries with pelvic extension.
>   **IIA:** extension or metastases to the uterus or tubes.
>   **IIB:** extension to other pelvic tissues.
>   **IIC:** tumor of either stage IIA or IIB on the surface of one or both ovaries, with capsule(s) ruptured, with ascites containing malignant cells, or with positive peritoneal washings.

III: tumor involves one or both ovaries with peritoneal implants outside the pelvis or positive retroperitoneal or inguinal nodes; superficial liver metastasis is stage III. Tumor is limited to the true pelvis but has histologically verified malignant extension to small bowel or omentum.
>   **IIIA:** tumor is grossly limited to the true pelvis with negative nodes but has histologically confirmed microscopic seeding of abdominal peritoneal surfaces.

IIIB: tumor of one or both ovaries with histologically confirmed visible implants of abdominal peritoneal surfaces, none exceeding 2 cm in diameter; nodes are negative.

IIIC: abdominal implants greater than 2 cm or positive retroperitoneal or inguinal lymph nodes.

IV: growth involving one or both ovaries with distant metastases. If pleural effusion is present, cytologic test must show cancer cells. Parenchymal liver metastases.

HISTOLOGY

A. Epithelial (65% of all ovarian cancer): most common epithelial types are serous (20% to 50%, most commonly malignant), mucinous (15% to 25%, may grow large in size, variable histology), endometrioid (5%, about 10% are associated with endometriosis), clear cell (5%, poor prognosis), and Brenner (2% to 3%, mostly benign). About 15% of all epithelial cancers present as low malignant potential.

B. Germ cell (25% of all ovarian cancer): most common are dysgerminoma, followed by mixed germ cell tumors. Other types are immature teratoma, choriocarcinoma, endodermal sinus tumor, and embryonal carcinoma.

C. Sex cord stromal (5% of all ovarian cancer): most common type is granulosa cell tumor. Another type is Sertoli–Leydig.

D. Others: sarcoma, metastatic.

TREATMENT

A. Surgery has two purposes: treatment and staging. The surgery includes hysterectomy and salpingo-oophorectomy (TAH-BSO), omentectomy, obtaining ascites fluid or peritoneal washings, and attempting optimal debulking (< 1-cm residual tumor), lymph node sampling (in early stages).

1. Stage IA to IB, grade 1 and 2, or any stage of low malignant potential tumors of the ovary (see Chap. 9):

   a. Observe and follow with CA-125. Patients with stage IA grades 1 and 2 epithelial carcinomas have a

5-year survival rate of 95% with or without melphalan.[3]

b. Some clinicians will treat grade 2.

2. Stage IA to IB, grade 3, stage II to IV:

a. Chemotherapy: paclitaxel (Taxol) *plus* carboplatin or cisplatin.[4,5]

b. Upon finishing chemotherapy, the patient has three options:

(1) Observation.

(2) Continuation of therapy if disease is regressing but has not disappeared completely.

(3) Consolidation chemotherapy—giving different chemotherapy (commonly, hexamethylamine) to continuously suppress possible recurrence.

B. Survival rates (5-year survival rates for patients with epithelial ovarian cancer) are as shown in Table 8–1.

TABLE 8–1.

Stage	Survival (%)
I	74
II	58
III	30
IV	19

C. Recurrent epithelial cancers:

1. Suspect in patients with GI symptoms, partial or intermittent small bowel obstruction, or new masses on CT.

2. Evaluate common sites of recurrence in the abdominal cavity, new pleural effusions.

3. Treatment options:

a. Secondary debulking is controversial. Generally, it is not effective if the tumor is already resistant to chemotherapy.

b. Salvage chemotherapy.

(1) If recurrence occurs more than 6 months after platinum-based therapy, consider reinduction with platinum-based therapy. With a cisplatin-

free interval (CFI) of 5 to 12 months, there is a 27% response rate; with a CFI of 13 to 24 months, a 33% response rate.[6]

(2) If recurrence occurs less than 6 months after platinum-based therapy, consider topotecan and doxorubicin (Doxil), or doxorubicin, ifosfamide, cyclophosphamide, or weekly paclitaxel.

D. Treatment for germ cell ovarian cancer:

1. Because most of these cancers occur in young women, preservation of fertility should be considered.

2. Surgical approach in a patient suspected of having germ cell tumors: exploratory laparotomy, pelvic washing, unilateral salpingo-oophorectomy, omentectomy, pelvic and para-aortic node biopsy, and multiple peritoneal biopsy (gutters, diaphragmatic, anterior/posterior cul-de-sac sites).

3. Obtain a frozen biopsy of the ovarian mass specimen. If the biopsy finds dysgerminoma, evaluate and obtain a biopsy of the contralateral ovary, as dysgerminoma is bilateral in 10% of cases. In contrast, other germ cell tumors are rarely bilateral ($<$ 5%). If the frozen biopsy shows nondysgerminoma and the contralateral ovary appears normal, leave the ovary intact without biopsy.

4. Chemotherapy: all patients with malignant germ cell tumors should be given adjuvant chemotherapy except for those with stage IA dysgerminoma and stage I, grade 1 immature teratoma. In stage I, grade 1 immature teratoma, survival is 85%.[7] In Europe, patients with stage IA endodermal sinus tumor do not receive chemotherapy (experimental). However, the standard of care in the United States is surgery *plus* bleomycin, etoposide, and platinum (BEP) for all stages.[8]

5. Endodermal sinus tumor grows rapidly. Patients should receive chemotherapy quickly after surgery (preferably before discharge to home). Adjuvant BEP should continue for two more courses after AFP (tumor marker for endodermal sinus) normalizes. AFP usually normalizes

after the first cycle of chemotherapy. Carboplatin is not as effective as cisplatin in germ cell cancer.[8]

6. Recurrent germ cell tumor after chemotherapy can be induced with BEP, vincristine, dactinomycin, cyclophosphamide (VAC), or paclitaxel, ifosfamide (anecdotal evidence).

E. Treatment for sex cord stromal tumor of the ovary (SCST):

1. After surgical removal of the tumor and staging, stage I SCST can be observed. If only the ovary is removed, obtain an endometrial biopsy as up to 25% of patients with granulosa cell tumor also have endometrial hyperplasia/cancer.

2. Patients with other than stage I tumors will benefit from adjuvant chemotherapy consisting of BEP.

3. Radiotherapy can induce a clinical response with occasional long-term remission in patients with persistent or recurrent granulosa cell tumor of the ovary.[9]

PROGNOSTIC FACTORS

- Favorable factors include lower grade, lower stage, well-differentiated tumor, optimal debulking, good performance status, and younger age.
- Poor prognostic factors include clear cell and serous histology, advanced stage, presence of ascites, suboptimal debulking, higher grade, and older age.

ROUTE OF SPREAD

Contiguous, malignant cells travel through the peritoneal fluid in a clockwise fashion, resulting in implantation of tumor throughout the abdominal cavity.

FOLLOW-UP

- First 2 years: evaluate every 3 months, as most recurrences of ovarian cancer occurs within 2 years.
- Third through fifth years: evaluate every 6 months; after 5 years, examine annually.

- Each examination includes pelvic examination, guaiac test, node survey, additional laboratory studies, and CT scans, as indicated.

CONTROVERSIES/SPECIAL ISSUES

- Second-look laparotomy: defined as surgery performed after optimal debulking and chemotherapy and clinically without evidence of disease. It is controversial today because 30% to 50% of patients with negative second looks experience recurrences.
- Nonsurgical candidate: in a patient with high surgical risks, neoadjuvant chemotherapy with platinum and paclitaxel may be given for three cycles. If the tumor responds and the patient's medical condition improves, she may be taken to surgery or may continue with current chemotherapy.[10]
- Patients who desire to retain fertility: in early-stage disease, unilateral salpingo-oophorectomy is recommended for patients with grade 1 tumors.
- Cumulative doses of chemotherapy: no correlation with increased survival has been found with a longer chemotherapy course or an increase in the dose intensity.[11]
- Hormonal replacement therapy: does not increase recurrence rate of cancer.[12]
- Familial ovarian cancer: prophylactic BSO can be offered. Despite surgery, patients have about a 2% lifetime risk of developing primary peritoneal carcinoma.
- Intraperitoneal chemotherapy (IP): in optimally debulked stage III epithelial ovarian cancer, patients who received IP cisplatin *plus* IV cyclophosphamide had longer survival rates and less ototoxicity and myelosuppresion than patients who received IV cisplatin *plus* IV cyclosphosphamide.

REFERENCES

1. ROSSING MA, DALING JR, WEISS NS, MOORE DE, SELF SG: Ovarian tumors in a cohort of infertile women [see comments]. N Engl J Med 331:771, 1994.

2. ANONYMOUS: Ovarian cancer: Screening, treatment, and followup. NIH Consensus Statement 12:1, 1994.

3. YOUNG RC, WALTON LA, ELLENBERG SS, HOMESLEY HD, WILBANKS GD, DECKER DG, MILLER A, PARK R, MAJOR F JR: Adjuvant therapy in stage I and stage II epithelial ovarian cancer. Results of two prospective randomized trials. N Engl J Med 322:1021, 1990.

4. MCGUIRE WP, HOSKINS WJ, BRADY MF, KUCERA PR, PARTRIDGE EE, LOOK KY, CLARKE-PEARSON DL, DAVIDSON M: Cyclophosphamide and cisplatin compared with paclitaxel and cisplatin in patients with stage III and stage IV ovarian cancer. N Engl J Med 334:1, 1996.

5. OZOLS RF, GREER B, BAERGEN R, REED E: A phase III randomized study of cisplatin and paclitaxel (24-hour infusion) versus carboplatin and paclitaxel (3-hour infusion) in optimal stage III epithelial ovarian carcinoma [abstract]. ASCO 18:356a, 1999 (Abstr. 1373).

6. MARKMAN M, ROTHMAN R, HAKES T, REICHMAN B, HOSKINS W, RUBIN S, JONES W, ALMADRONES L, LEWIS JL JR: Second-line platinum therapy in patients with ovarian cancer previously treated with cisplatin. J Clin Oncol 9:389, 1991.

7. NORRIS HJ, ZIRKIN HJ, BENSON WL: Immature (malignant) teratoma of the ovary: A clinical and pathologic study of 58 cases. Cancer 37:2359, 1976.

8. GERSHENSON DM: Update on malignant ovarian germ cell tumors. Cancer 71(4 Suppl):1581, 1993.

9. WOLF JK, MULLEN J, EIFEL PJ, BURKE TW, LEVENBACK C, GERSHENSON DM: Radiation treatment of advanced or recurrent granulosa cell tumor of the ovary. Gynecol Oncol 73:35, 1999.

10. SCHWARTZ PE, RUTHERFORD TJ, CHAMBERS JT, KOHORN EI, THIEL RP: Neoadjuvant chemotherapy for advanced ovarian cancer: Long-term survival. Gynecol Oncol 72:93, 1999.

11. BERTELSEN K, JAKOBSEN A, STROYER J, NIELSEN K, SANDBERG E, ANDERSEN JE, AHRONS S, NYLAND M, HJORTKJAER PEDERSEN P, LARSEN G, et al: A prospective randomized comparison of 6 and 12 cycles of cyclophosphamide, adriamycin, and cisplatin in advanced epithelial ovarian cancer: A Danish ovarian study group trial (DACOVA). Gynecol Oncol 49:30, 1993.

12. ALBERTS DS, LIU PY, HANNIGAN EV, O'TOOLE R, WILLIAMS SD, YOUNG JA, FRANKLIN EW, CLARKE-PEARSON DL, MALVIYA VK, DUBESHTER B: Intraperitoneal cisplatin plus intravenous cyclophosphamide versus intravenous cisplatin plus intravenous cyclophosphamide for stage III ovarian cancer. N Engl J Med 335:1950, 1996.

Low Malignant Potential of the Ovary

Christine Lee and Joseph T. Santoso

INCIDENCE

- Comprises 15% of epithelial ovarian cancers.
- Eighty percent to 90% of cases are found in stage I.
- In rare cases, undergoes malignant transformation to invasive cancer (0.7%).[1]

WORKUP

- Similar to that for epithelial ovarian cancer.
- At the time of exploratory laparotomy, send for a frozen section. If the tumor is frankly invasive or of low malignant potential (LMP), proceed with complete staging for ovarian cancer. Ninety percent of frozen sections are sensitive for invasion. Intraoperative frozen sections that are read as LMP have a sensitivity of 45%.[2] Approximately 30% are upstaged to frankly invasive cancer after the preliminary LMP reading. If the frozen biopsy shows no LMP or invasive cancer, no staging is needed.
- The value of complete staging is not clearly demonstrated. However, most clinicians do complete staging because frozen biopsy is not accurate in making a diagnosis of LMP. Often LMP on frozen biopsy is upgraded to invasive cancer on final pathology review.
- Consider more conservative therapy for young patients or patients desiring future fertility.
- CA-125 is a valuable tumor marker only if it is initially elevated.

STAGING

FIGO staging for LMP of the ovary is the same as that for epithelial ovarian cancer.

HISTOLOGY

- Epithelial in origin; diagnosis is by absence of ovarian stromal invasion.
- Serous adenoma of LMP.

- Mucinous adenoma of LMP. *Note:* Mucinous adenoma of LMP can cause pseudomyxoma peritonei and is associated with advanced stage and a poor prognosis. Most pseudomyxoma peritonei arise from low-grade mucinous tumors of the appendix. LMP of the ovary is not invasive; therefore, it is not malignant and has low potential to metastasize to distant sites. LMP is not considered a "precursor" lesion to frankly invasive ovarian cancer. LMP is a lesion that has all the characteristics of an invasive cancer but without stromal invasion.
- Endometrioid tumor of LMP.
- Clear cell tumor of LMP.

PROGNOSTIC FACTORS

More favorable factors are younger age, early stage, and serous histology demonstrating psammoma bodies and diploid tumors.

TREATMENT

A. Stages I and II: Limited resection with washing, biopsies of peritoneal cavity, omentectomy, diaphragm biopsies, and lymph nodes or TAH-BSO, depending on the patient's age and desire to retain fertility.
B. Stages III and IV: TAH-BSO, omental biopsies, lymph node biopsies, pelvic washings, and peritoneal biopsies.
C. Adjuvant therapy:
   1. Highly controversial: most clinicians do not give adjuvant chemotherapy. (Exception: invasive implants in metastatic cases.)
   2. Tumor reductive surgery can be considered if disease recurs.
D. Survival rate is as shown in Table 9–1.

TABLE 9–1.

Years posttreatment	Survival (%)
5	97
10	95
15	92
20	89

REFERENCES

1. KURMAN RJ, TRIMBLE CL: The behavior of serous tumors of low malignant potential: Are they ever malignant? Int J Gynecol Pathol 12:120, 1993.
2. ROSE PG, RUBIN RB, NELSON BE, HUNTER RE, REALE FR: Accuracy of frozen-section (intraoperative consultation) diagnosis of ovarian tumors. Am J Obstet Gynecol 171:823, 1994.

Sara Crowder, Robert L. Coleman, and Joseph T. Santoso

GENERAL

- Hydatidiform mole (molar pregnancy) occurs in 0.2 to 2 per 1000 pregnancies.[1]
- About 20% of complete moles may have malignant sequelae, and 2% may progress to choriocarcinoma.
- Partial moles have only a 5% incidence of any sequelae, and rarely progress to choriocarcinoma. For survival, see the Controversies/Special Issues section later in this chapter.

RISK FACTORS

- Patients with a prior history of gestational trophoblastic disease (GTD) have a 2% recurrence rate.
- Risk is increased in the extremes of maternal age ($>$ 45 or $<$ 20 years old).
- In Asian or Hispanic patients, folate or vitamin A deficiencies may also increase risk.

SIGNS AND SYMPTOMS

- Hydatidiform moles usually present with elevated βhCG and the following symptoms: vaginal bleeding (97%), passage of molar vesicles, uterine size greater than dates (50%), preeclampsia at less than 20 weeks (25%). The drastic elevation in the βhCG can cause the following symptoms: nausea/vomiting (25%), theca-lutein cysts (30%), and hyperthyroidism ($<$ 10%).
- Persistent GTD or choriocarcinoma may present with symptoms caused by metastases in lung (80%), vagina (30%), brain (10%), liver (10%), or other sites ($<$ 5%). Pulmonary lesions may cause hemoptysis, chest pain, or respiratory distress. Vaginal lesions may produce vaginal bleeding. Hepatic metastasis may cause pain and intraperitoneal bleeding.

Central nervous system lesions may present as an acute focal neurological deficit.

DIAGNOSIS

- Hydatidiform mole: diagnosis is made based on the previously mentioned signs and symptoms, an ultrasound that shows the classic snowstorm pattern, and a markedly elevated βhCG level. Differentiating between complete and partial moles can only be done histologically.
- Persistent GTD or choriocarcinoma: diagnosis is made during the follow-up of a hydatidiform mole after evacuation and based on persistently elevated or rising βhCG levels. Choriocarcinoma may also occur after a normal pregnancy, spontaneous abortion, or ectopic pregnancy. In these cases, choriocarcinoma is usually suspected after a woman with prolonged heavy bleeding is found to have an elevated βhCG level. Choriocarcinoma can also be found in women with no prior known pregnancy and may present as a lung nodule. Any woman diagnosed with metastatic carcinoma of unknown primary, particularly in the lung, should have a βhCG level drawn to rule out a possible choriocarcinoma.

WORKUP

- Pretreatment βhCG: to provide a baseline.
- Chest x-ray: to rule out metastases and to provide a baseline, owing to high risk of pulmonary edema.
- CBC: to provide a preoperative baseline, owing to the risk of bleeding.
- Type and crossmatch: to determine the need for RhoGAM and to prepare for possible transfusion.
- Liver function tests/chemistry panel: for preoperative and metastatic screening.
- TSH level if the patient presents with symptoms of hyperthyroidism.

STAGING OR CLASSIFICATION SYSTEMS FOR GTD

A. FIGO staging:
   I: disease confined to uterus (IA, B, or C, depending on risk factors).
   II: metastasis to pelvis or vagina (IIA, B, or C, depending on risk factors).
   III: metastasis to lung (IIIA, B, or C, depending on risk factors).
   IV: metastasis to distant sites: brain, liver, etc. (IVA, B, or C, depending on risk factors).
   A = no risk factors.
   B = one risk factor.
   C = two risk factors.
   1. Risk factors are:
      a. βhCG greater than 100,000 IU/mL.
      b. Duration of disease greater than 6 months from termination of antecedent pregnancy.
   2. Note any prior chemotherapy given for GTD. Placental site trophoblastic tumors should be reported separately, and histologic verification of disease is not required.
B. NCI/NIH clinical classification (most useful for clinical practice):
   1. Benign GTD:
      A: Complete hydatidiform mole.
      B: Partial hydatidiform mole.
   2. Malignant GTD:
      A: nonmetastatic GTD.
      B: metastatic GTD.
         1: good prognosis, low risk—absence of any risk factor.
         2: poor prognosis, high risk—presence of any risk factor.
   3. Risk factors are:
      a. Duration of disease greater than 4 months.
      b. Pretherapy βhCG level greater than 40,000 IU/mL (prior to any chemotherapy).
      c. Brain or liver metastases.

      d. GTD after term gestation.
      e. Prior failed chemotherapy.
C. WHO prognostic scoring system: see Table 10–1.

HISTOLOGY

A. Three different cell types make up trophoblastic tissue:
    1. Cytotrophoblasts are germinative trophoblasts that do not secrete hormones.
    2. Syncytiotrophoblasts are highly differentiated; they produce βhCG and human placental lactogen (HPL).

TABLE 10–1. WHO Prognostic Scoring System[a]

	Score[b]			
	0	1	2	4
Age (yr)	≤ 39	> 39	—	—
Antecedent pregnancy	Hydatidiform mole	Abortion	Term	—
Interval between end of antecedent pregnancy and start of chemotherapy (mo)	< 4	4–6	7–12	> 12
hCG (IU/L)	$< 10^3$	10^3–10^4	10^4–10^5	$> 10^5$
A, B, and O groups	—	O or A	B or AB	—
Largest tumor, including uterine (cm)	< 3	3–5	> 5	—
Site of metastasis	—	Spleen, kidney	GI tract, liver	Brain
Number of metastases	0	1–4	4–8	> 8
Prior chemotherapy	—	—	1 drug	≥ 2 drugs

[a]Most accurate for determining prognosis, especially for stage II and III disease.

[b]Total score is obtained by adding individual scores. Total score ≤ 4 is low risk; 5–7 is medium risk; ≥ 8 is high risk.

3. Intermediate trophoblasts invade vascular channels and produce HPL more than βhCG.
B. Four different histologic entities with important clinical differences make up GTD:
   1. *Hydatidiform mole* ("molar pregnancy"): shows hyperplasia of cytotrophoblast or syncytiotrophoblast, and edematous chorionic villi. It can be complete (90%) or partial (10%). (For histologic differences between complete and partial moles, see the Controversies/Special Issues section later in the chapter).
   2. *Invasive mole:* occurs when molar tissue has invaded into the myometrium; it is usually only diagnosed following a hysterectomy or by MRI.
   3. *Choriocarcinoma:* anaplastic, malignant cells. Consists of a mixture of cytotrophoblast, intermediate trophoblast, and syncytiotrophoblast in a biphasic or bilaminar pattern. Vascular invasion may be prominent, with extensive hemorrhage and necrosis. Immunohistochemistry shows cells positive for βhCG. Villous structures should not be present. If villi are seen, the diagnosis is likely invasive mole.
   4. *Placental site trophoblastic tumor (PSTT):* develops from intermediate trophoblasts; thus it secretes predominantly HPL and usually demonstrates low levels of βhCG.

TREATMENT

The goal of the treatment and follow-up of hydatidiform moles is to avoid transformation into choriocarcinoma, which is frankly malignant and can be deadly if left untreated. Although the risk of progression to choriocarcinoma is different for complete moles (2% risk) and partial moles (much lower), the treatment and follow-up are the same.

A. Hydatidiform moles:
   1. Evacuation by D&C if the patient desires future fertility. If not, total abdominal hysterectomy is the treatment of choice. In one study, hysterectomy lowered the risk of persistent GTD in all patients with molar pregnancy to 3.5% versus 20% after D&C.[2] Another study looked at

a higher-risk subgroup of women over 35 years old and showed a risk of persistent GTD of 33% after D&C that was reduced to 10% after hysterectomy.[3]

2. Bilateral salpingo-oophorectomy is not necessary as ovarian metastasis is rare and manipulation of theca-lutein cysts should be avoided due to their propensity to bleed. They should resolve on their own in 2 to 4 months.

3. Administer RhoGAM within 72 hours after D&C if the patient is Rh negative and there is an absence of anti-body.

4. Metastatic workup and chemotherapy are needed in any patients with:
   a. Rising βhCG for 2 weeks or more (three weekly titers) during surveillance.
   b. Plateau (± 10%) of the βhCG level for 3 weeks or more.
   c. Elevated βhCG after a normalizing value.
   d. Metastases (usually discovered based on symptoms or examination).
   e. Pathology from the D&C showing choriocarcinoma, PSTT, or invasive mole.
   f. Postevacuation hemorrhage not due to incomplete evacuation.

B. Metastatic workup consists of:
   1. History and physical examination.
   2. Pretreatment βhCG titer.
   3. Chest x-ray.
   4. Chemistry and liver function tests.
   5. CBC.
   Note: CT of the brain, ultrasound of the pelvis, and liver scan are only needed if any of the preceding investigations suggest abnormalities.

C. Chemotherapy:
   1. Nonmetastatic or good-prognosis metastatic GTD can be treated with single-agent chemotherapy. Single-agent methotrexate or dactinomycin achieves a 95% complete remission. If this fails, salvage with the alternative single agent. If both fail, use EMACO (etoposide, methotrexate,

actinomycin-D, cyclophosphamide, Oncovin) or MAC (methotrexate, actinomycin-D, chlorambucil).
2. Poor-prognosis metastatic GTD requires combination chemotherapy front-line. Treat with EMACO. Salvage treatment can use EMA–etoposide-platinum (EMA–EP).

PROGNOSTIC FACTORS

See the NCI/NIH or WHO classification, earlier.

ROUTE OF SPREAD

Most common metastases in GTD are to the lung. Liver and brain metastases also occur and put the patient into the metastatic high-risk category. Metastases to the liver are prognostically worse than those to the brain as they are more likely to exist with widespread disease, and these patients have a worse record of survival.

FOLLOW-UP

- Obtain quantitative βhCG levels every 1 to 2 weeks until the level normalizes, then every 1 to 2 months for 1 year.
- If the level rises or plateaus, a metastatic workup is done and the patient is treated with chemotherapy. Treatment is usually initiated based on the βhCG level, and a histologic confirmation of choriocarcinoma is not needed. Some patients will have choriocarcinoma and others will have only an invasive mole. The distinction is not important in guiding therapy.
- Therapy will be guided based on whether the patient has nonmetastatic, metastatic low-risk, or metastatic high-risk disease according to the NCI clinical classification (see the discussion of staging, earlier).
- Ensure that patients use reliable contraception (so that βhCG can be used as a reliable marker). Oral contraceptives can be used safely in GTD patients. A Gynecologic Oncology Group (GOG) study showed no difference in the risk of postmolar disease or the time to a normal βhCG level between patients who used oral contraceptives and those using barrier contraception.

- If the patient is being treated with chemotherapy for persistent GTD, she can be considered to be in remission after three consecutive weekly negative βhCG titers. After remission, close follow-up is required to watch for recurrence.

RECURRENT DISEASE

- The overall risk of recurrence after 1 year of remission is less than 1%.[4]
- Cranial metastases can be palliated with radiation.
- Lung metastases may be resected. All surgical treatment is then followed with combination chemotherapy. EMACO-resistant diseases may be salvaged with EMA–EP.

CONTROVERSIES/SPECIAL CASES

A. Differences between complete and partial moles:
  1. *Complete moles* occur by two mechanisms:
    a. A haploid sperm fertilizes an "empty egg" (anucleate, contains no maternal genetic material), and the sperm reduplicates itself to make a diploid egg that contains all paternal genes.
    b. Less commonly (5%), dispermy may occur when two haploid sperms manage to fertilize the same empty egg. This again results in a diploid genetic component that is completely paternally derived. (See Table 10–2.)
  2. *Partial moles* occur when an egg with a haploid maternal genetic component is fertilized by two haploid sperms (dispermy). (See Table 10–2.)

TABLE 10–2.

	Complete mole	Partial mole
Histology	No fetal parts	Villi and fetal parts/amnion/RBCs
Villi	Hydropic	Hydropic and normal
Origin	Paternal	Paternal and maternal
Genome	46, XX or 46, XY	69, XXY; 69, XXX; or 69, XYY

B. Survival: See Table 10–3.

TABLE 10–3.

Clinical classification	WHO equivalent	Usual treatment	Survival	Caveat
Nonmetastatic, metastatic low risk	WHO score ≤ 7	Metho- trexate	100%	Requires strict adher- ence to follow-up guidelines
Metastatic high risk	WHO score ≥ 8	EMA–CO	90%	Includes only those treated in recent years

C. PSTT: This is an uncommon variant of GTD. Histology shows predominantly intermediate trophoblast cells. There- fore, because intermediate trophoblasts secrete HPL more than βhCG, HPL is a more useful tumor marker. PSTT can occur after any type of gestational event. The most common symptom is abnormal bleeding with increased uterine size. PSTTs are highly malignant and can be deadly. Response to chemotherapy is poor, and hysterectomy is considered the treatment of choice.

D. βhCG regression: βhCG is cleared renally at a constant rate. The half-life is around 40 hours, so one can estimate the approximate regression time depending on the initial level. In one study of 120 patients followed with molar pregnancies the average time for βhCG to return to normal was found to be 73 days.[5]

E. Prophylactic chemotherapy: This is a controversial treat- ment method. In a study of 71 patients with complete moles who were randomized to receive no therapy versus prophy- lactic chemotherapy, the rate of persistant trophoblastic dis- ease was decreased after prophylactic chemotherapy, but at a cost. The group that received prophylaxis had a delay in the diagnosis of persistant disease and required more chemotherapy to undergo remission.[6]

F. Cerebrospinal fluid (CSF) βhCG levels: βhCG level from spinal tap may be useful in patients with disease that is resistant to therapy. Compare the ratio of the serum βhCG and levels in CSF. A ratio of plasma:CSF less than 60 indicates cerebral metastasis. The treatment protocol is as shown in Table 10–4.

TABLE 10–4.

	Initial	Resistant
Stage I	Methotrexate; if resistant, switch to dactinomycin or vice versa or hysterectomy with adjuvant chemotherapy	Combination chemotherapy or hysterectomy with adjuvant chemotherapy; local uterine resection—pelvic intra-arterial infusion
Stages II and III—low risk	Methotrexate; if resistant, switch to dactinomycin	Combination chemotherapy
Stages II and III—high risk	Combination chemotherapy	Second-line combination chemotherapy
Stage IV—brain metastases	Combination chemotherapy; whole head irradiation (3000 cGy); craniotomy to manage complications	Second-line combination chemotherapy
Stage IV—liver metastases	Combination chemotherapy; resection to manage complications	Hepatic arterial infusion

REFERENCES

1. PALMER JR: Advances in the epidemiology of gestational trophoblastic disease. J Reprod Med 39:155, 1994.
2. CURRY SL, HAMMOND CB, TYREY L, CREASMAN WT, PARKER RT: Hydatidiform mole: Diagnosis, management, and long-term followup of 347 patients. Obstet Gynecol 45:1, 1975.

3. BAHAR AM, EL-ASHNEHI MS, SENTHILSELVAN A: Hydatidiform mole in the elderly: Hysterectomy or evacuation? Int J Gynaecol Obstet 29:233, 1989.
4. MUTCH DG, SOPER JT, BABCOCK CJ, CLARKE-PEARSON DL, HAMMOND CB: Recurrent gestational trophoblastic disease. Cancer 66:978, 1990.
5. YUEN BH, CANNON W: Molar pregnancy in British Columbia: Estimated incidence and postevacuation regression patterns of the beta subunit of human chorionic gonadotropin. Am J Obstet Gynecol 139:316, 1981.
6. KIM DS, MOON H, KIM KT, MOON YJ, HWANG YY: Effects of prophylactic chemotherapy for persistent trophoblastic disease in patients with complete hydatidiform mole. Obstet Gynecol 67:690, 1986.

II | **PATIENT MANAGEMENT/
COMPLICATIONS**

PERIPHERAL NEUROPATHY

Etiology

This condition is associated with administration of cisplatin, paclitaxel, vincristine, and hexamethylmelamine.

Signs and Symptoms

- Paresthesia in a stocking-glove distribution.
- Starts as a tingling sensation, which progresses to numbness and motor weakness.

Workup

- Reduce or stop chemotherapy to determine if related.
- The incidence may be reduced if chemotherapy is given concurrently with amifostine, which functions as a free radical scavenger.

Treatment

Effective treatment is unknown. Possible approaches include a trial of medication with multivitamins, vitamin B_{12}, NSAIDs, narcotics, or amytriptyline, 25 mg PO qd to tid. Some promising results for neuropathic pain relief have been found with gabapentin (300 mg/day, then 300 mg PO bid.

COMPRESSION NEUROPATHY

Etiology

May be a result of compression by surgical retractor or occur following surgery, iatrogenically.

Signs and Symptoms

- Burning or electric shocklike (nociceptive) pain.

- Injury to the obturator nerve (L2-4) impairs adduction of thigh. Injury to the genitofemoral nerve (L1-2) causes numbness in the medial thigh and lateral labia. Lateral cutaneous femoral nerve (L2-3) injury causes numbness on the lateral thigh. Compression of the sciatic nerve (L4, L5, S1,2,3) causes weakness in the hamstring (inability to flex the knee). Ilioinguinal nerve palsy causes severe burning in the groin and vulva.
- In general, the femoral nerve innervates the anterior thigh compartment, the obturator nerve innervates the medial compartment, and the sciatic nerve innervates the posterior compartment.

Workup

Perform a careful neurologic examination. Consider an MRI to rule out spinal compression.

Treatment

Provide palliative treatment with physical therapy if the patient is improving symptomatically. If motor weakness or worsening symptoms are noted, consider obtaining a neurology consultation.

SEIZURE

Etiology

Possible causes include metastatic lesion, drug/alcohol use, electrolyte abnormalities, stroke, or infection.

Signs and Symptoms

- Synchronous tonic-clonic movement of all muscles (generalized seizure).
- Brief loss of consciousness, staring, unresponsiveness (absence seizure).
- Loss of postural control, unconsciousness (akinetic seizure).
- Postictal confusion.

Workup

- ABCs: evaluate airway, breathing, circulation. If no vital signs are noted, call a code.
- If the patient is stable, consider ordering the following laboratory studies: serum electrolytes, glucose, CBC, drug/alcohol screen, ABGs, urinalysis, and/or antiepileptic drug levels, as indicated.
- Obtain a head CT scan and spinal tap to rule out infection (after CT rules out CNS lesion).
- Empty the stomach contents via an NG tube.

Treatment

- Thiamine, 100 mg by IV push, followed by 50 mL $D_{50}W$ by IV push.
- Diazepam, 5 mg IV over 2 minutes (up to 10 mg) or lorazepam, 1 to 4 mg over 2 to 10 minutes IV. Watch for respiratory depression. Because of its short duration of action, benzodiazepine administration is followed by phenytoin.
- Phenytoin, in a loading dose of 16 mg/kg, or 1000 mg IV, followed by 100 mg every 8 hours (not to exceed 50 mg/min). Watch for hypotension and heart block (ECG).
- If the seizure persists, call a neurologist.

STROKE (CEREBRAL INFARCTION)

Etiology

Hemorrhagic or embolic causes.

Signs and Symptoms

Findings vary from unconsciousness to localized motor/sensory deficit, confusion, seizure, headaches, and speech abnormalities.

Workup

- Assess ABCs: give oxygen via nasal cannula. Perform a neurologic examination.

- If vital signs are stable, order a noncontrast head CT scan to avoid confusing blood and contrast.
- Laboratory studies: CBC, PT, PTT, electrolytes, and glucose; ECG to rule out arrhythmia.
- Call a neurologist or neurosurgeon for possible thrombolytic therapy. The duration of symptoms to giving r-tPA therapy is less than 180 minutes.

Treatment

- In embolic stroke, call a consultant for thrombolytic therapy. High blood pressure usually does not need to be treated acutely.
- In hemorrhagic stroke, call neurosurgery consultants. High blood pressure (systolic > 160 mmHg or diastolic > 105 mmHg) may cause rebleeding. Treat with nitroprusside or labetolol.
- The role of heparin after stroke is uncertain—wait for consultants.

ALTERED MENTAL STATUS/ACUTE CONFUSIONAL STATE

Etiology

May occur in association with stroke, postseizure, drugs, alcohol, infection, sundowning, or hypoxemia.

Signs and Symptoms

- Presentation varies from confusion and agitation to unconsciousness.
- In sundowning patients, confusion worsens in the evening and in an unfamiliar environment.
- Patients with delirium tremens or severe alcohol withdrawal may present with agitation, hallucinations, fever, tachycardia, and diaphoresis, which occurs 1 to 3 days after drinking cessation, with a 15% mortality rate.

Workup

- Check oxygen saturation and vital signs, and give supplemental oxygen as needed.
- Perform a neurologic examination and follow progress with the Glasgow coma scale (see Table 11–1).
- Laboratory studies: CBC, electrolytes, creatinine, liver function tests, blood alcohol, drug screens, TSH, ABGs.
- Obtain a CT scan to rule out mass effect or cranial hemorrhage. Perform a lumbar puncture to rule out meningitis if the CT scan shows no herniation.

Treatment

- See Workup for stroke and seizure, earlier.
- For hypoglycemia, give thiamine, 100 mg IV, followed by 50 mL of $D_{50}W$.
- For narcotic overdose, give naloxone, 0.01 mg/kg by IV push (maximum: 2 mg).

TABLE 11–1. Glasgow Coma Scale (GCS)

Eye opening	Response	Score[a]
	Spontaneous	4
	To verbal command	3
	To pain	2
	None	1
Verbal response		
	Oriented and converses	5
	Disoriented and converses	4
	Inappropriate words	3
	Incomprehensible sounds	2
	None	1
Motor response		
	Obeys commands	6
	Localized pain	5
	Normal flexion-withdrawal	4
	Decortication/abnormal flexion	3
	Decerebrate/abnormal extension	2
	None	1

[a]Score: 15 is normal, 11 is normal in intubated patients. Coma is defined as GCS of 8 or lower.

- For benzodiazepine overdose, give flumazenil, 0.2 mg IV; repeat every minute (maximum: 1 mg).
- For sundowning patients, increase lighting and provide familiar belongings. If these actions are not effective, give haloperidol PO or IM; begin at 25 mg and titrate to effect.
- For alcohol withdrawal, give thiamine, 100 mg IV, then PO qd for 3 days; multivitamins; and diazepam, 5 to 20 mg PO every 6 hours.
- If there is no suspicion of herniation on CT scan and meningitis is suspected, a lumbar puncture should be done to obtain a sample for testing (cell count, protein, glucose, Gram's stain, acid-fast stain, India ink stain, fungal/bacterial culture, cryptococcal and bacterial antigen if antibiotics have been given). Save an extra tube in the refrigerator in case the laboratory loses the specimen.
- Order an EEG to rule out psychogenic etiology.

BRAIN/SPINAL CORD METASTASES

Etiology

Many primary cancers produce metastatic lesions to the brain or spinal cord.

Signs and Symptoms

Findings include focal neurologic deficit, weakness, or confusion.

Workup

Obtain a CT or MRI scan. For spinal compression syndrome, order a spinal screen MRI.

Treatment

- In symptomatic patients, start dexamethasone, 10 mg IV, then 6 mg every 6 hours to reduce edema.

- Consult a radiation oncologist for palliative radiation (if the tumor mass is relatively small) or an orthospine consultant (if the tumor mass is larger than can be controlled with radiation). Patients with acute neurologic changes may need emergent radiotherapy.
- Place a Foley catheter to rule out urinary retention. In spinal shock, give fluid bolus and ephedrine (10 to 25 mg IV, slowly) or phenylephrine (50 μg as IV bolus) or epinephrine (1 to 4 μg/kg/min) and titrate to acceptable blood pressure.

Cardiovascular

Joseph T. Santoso

CHEST PAIN

Etiology

- Cardiovascular (angina pectoris, MI, pericarditis, dissection of aneurysm).
- Pulmonary (pneumonia, pneumonitis, pneumothorax, pulmonary embolism).
- Musculoskeletal (Tietze's syndrome, rib injury, herpes zoster).
- GI (peptic ulcer, hiatal hernia, reflux, esophagitis).
- Renal colic.
- Other (stress, psychogenic, tumor mass effect).

Signs and Symptoms

Presentation may vary from vague anginal pain to severe, sharp, or colicky pain.

Workup

- Complete history of onset, duration, location, modifying activities, drugs, medical/surgical history.
- Laboratory studies: CBC, urinalysis, liver function tests, amylase, creatinine.
- ECG to rule out referred pain from ischemic heart disease.
- Chest and upright abdominal x-rays to rule out air below the diaphragm, air fluid level, mass, or renal stone. Consider obtaining a CT scan or an abdominal ultrasound.

Treatment

Treat the underlying disease.

TACHYCARDIA

Etiology

- Anxiety, pain, fever.

- Hypovolemia, bleeding, hypoxemia.
- Arrhythmias.

Signs and Symptoms

Presentation may vary from asymptomatic to hypotension.

Workup

- If the patient is hypotensive, refer to the ACLS algorithm for cardioversion (Appendix F).
- If stable, obtain an ECG.
- Laboratory studies: ABGs, electrolytes, serum creatinine, weight, history of surgery, stool occult blood.

Treatment

Treat the underlying disease.

HYPOTENSION/SHOCK

Etiology

- Pump problems (congestive heart failure, MI, cardiac tamponade, tension pneumothorax, arrhythmias).
- Fluid problems (dehydration, hemorrhage, third spacing from sepsis, ascites or mass compressing vena cava).
- Vessel problems (vasodilation in spinal shock, sepsis, or anaphylaxis).

Signs and Symptoms

Hypotension, low urine output, altered mental status.

Workup

Rule out previously mentioned problems.

Treatment

A. Treat the underlying problem. Watch ABCs (airway, breathing, circulation).

B. Almost always start with fluid replacement before using vasopressor or contractility drugs.

C. Hypovolemia: give crystalloid, colloid, and/or blood. Maintain hemoglobin at 10 to 11 g/dL to improve oxygen delivery. To monitor response, use a Foley catheter, physical examination, central line, or pulmonary artery catheter (when using vasopressor or contractility drugs).

D. General guideline for fluid/blood resuscitation:
   1. Give blood if 2 L lactated Ringer's solution does not stabilize blood pressure.
   2. Give 1 unit of packed red blood cells for each liter of crystalloid infused.
   3. Give 2 units of fresh frozen plasma for each 6 units of red blood cells.
   4. Give 10 units of platelets for every 10 units of red blood cells.
   5. Give 8 units of cryoprecipitate if there is no clot or if fibrinogen is less than 100,000 mg/dL.

E. Low cardiac contractility: start with dopamine, 3 to 5 µg/kg/min IV, and titrate to blood pressure (maximum: 20 µg/kg/min). If patient is not responsive, use norepinephrine, 0.05 µg/kg/min, or epinephrine, 0.05 µg/kg/min, and titrate to effect (maximum for both drugs is 0.4 µg/kg/min).

F. Arrhythmias: see the ACLS algorithms in Appendix F.

G. Excessive vasoconstriction: begin nitroprusside, 0.5 µg/kg/min, and titrate to effect (maximum: 7 µg/kg/min).

H. Excessive vasodilation: see the instructions for epinephrine, earlier.

I. Anaphylactic shock: give fluids; epinephrine, 0.1 to 0.2 mg IV; diphenhydramine, 50 mg IV; ranitidine, 50 mg IV; methylprednisolone, 100 to 250 mg IV.

SUPERIOR VENA CAVA SYNDROME

Etiology

Any compression or infiltration of the superior vena cava from tumor or blood clot.

Signs and Symptoms

Edema/cyanosis of face, neck, shoulder, and arms. It is life threatening when edema compromises the airway or CNS.

Workup

Order a chest x-ray and CT scan of the chest or an angiogram to rule out tumor versus thrombosis.

Treatment

- Elevate the patient's head; give dexamethasone and diuretics.
- Intubate if the airway is compromised.
- For thrombosis, the clinician may use urokinase infusion or order stent placement by an interventional radiologist.
- For tumor, give radiation or chemotherapy (tumor requires tissue biopsy).

CONGESTIVE HEART FAILURE

Etiology

Hypertension, MI, valvular disease, doxorubicin myocardiopathy, pulmonary hypertension (right-sided heart failure), arrhythmias, valvular diseases. Subtypes are left, right, or biventricular failures.

Signs and Symptoms

- Symptoms are caused by inability of the heart to pump blood sufficiently to meet the body's oxygen needs.
- Tachycardia, hypoxemia, bilateral respiratory rales, wheezes, hypotension, low urine output, altered mental status, orthopnea, peripheral edema, jugular venous distention.

Workup

- Examination and laboratory studies: CBC, electrolytes, creatinine.
- ECG: ischemia, ventricular hypertrophy, arrhythmias.

- Chest x-ray: cardiomegaly, pulmonary edema.
- Cardiac echogram or MUGA scan: abnormal ejection fraction ($< 40\%$), pericardial effusion, valvular diseases, abnormal cardiac wall motion.

Treatment

- Supportive treatment: oxygen; bed rest; treat underlying diseases.
- Reduce symptoms.
- Sodium restriction: less than 2 g/day; fluid restriction: less than 2 L/day.
- Diuretic: begin furosemide at 20 mg IV and double every 4 to 6 hours until adequate diuresis is obtained.
- Vasodilator: nitroprusside (begin at 0.5 μg/kg/min IV and titrate to effect; maximum: 7 μg/kg/min), nitroglycerin (10 to 20 μg/min IV), ACE inhibitor (captopril, 6.25 to 12.5 mg PO every 8 hours), calcium channel blockers (nifedipine, 10 mg PO every 6 hours; maximum: 120 mg/day), or morphine, 1 to 3 mg IV (venodilates).

MYOCARDIAL INFARCTION

Etiology

Mainly due to thromboembolic effects obstructing cardiac perfusion; exacerbated by exertion, surgery, shock, and hypoxemia.

Signs and Symptoms

- Left chest pain radiating to left shoulder, arm.
- Tachycardia/tachypnea, hypotension, hypoxemia.
- May be accompanied by heart failure, pulmonary and peripheral edema.

Workup

A. Laboratory studies:
    1. CBC, electrolytes, creatinine.

2. Cardiac enzymes at 0, 6, and 12 hours after admission. CKMB peaks 12 to 24 hours after infarction.
3. LDH (LDH1/LDH2 > 1) peaks within 24 to 48 hours, lasts up to 14 days.
4. Troponin T (last up to 2 weeks).

B. ECG: ischemia (ST elevation → T-wave inversion → Q wave).

C. Chest x-ray: pulmonary edema, cardiomegaly.

Treatment

A. Bed rest with MONA (*m*orphine, *o*xygen, *n*itroglycerin, *a*spirin).
   1. Morphine: 1 to 3 mg IV, titrate to relieve pain.
   2. Oxygen: start with 4 L/min via nasal cannula.
   3. Nitroglycerin: 0.3 to 0.4 mg sublingual, repeat every 5 minutes as needed for chest pain; paste, 1 to 2 inches; or IV infusion, 10 to 20 μg/min increase by 5 to 10 μg every 5 minutes as needed for chest pain. Watch for hypotension.
   4. Aspirin: 160 to 325 mg PO (contraindicated in asthma or active ulcer disease).
   5. Beta blockers: discuss with a cardiologist first because of side effects.

B. Consult a cardiologist for possible thrombolytic therapy or cardiac catheterization as soon as possible.

HYPERTENSION

Etiology

Mostly unknown. Secondary hypertension may be due to renal or endocrine etiologies and mostly occurs in younger patients.

Signs and Symptoms

- Mostly asymptomatic.
- Diagnosis requires two readings with BP higher than 140/90. (see Table 12–1).

TABLE 12–1. Stages of Hypertension and Recommended Follow-Up

Stages	Systolic BP	Diastolic BP	Follow-up
Mild	140–159	90–99	Confirm within 2 mo
Moderate	160–179	100–109	Evaluate within 1 mo
Severe	180–209	110–119	Evaluate within 1 wk
Very severe	> 210	> 120	Treat immediately

Workup

- Examination to identify end-organ damage (eye, renal, CNS).
- CBC, electrolytes, serum creatinine, funduscopic examination, ECG to check for ischemia or ventricular hypertrophy.

Treatment

A. Life-style changes: advise patient to quit smoking, lose weight, exercise, decrease sodium intake, follow a low-fat diet, and reduce alcohol intake.

B. Initiate diuretic or beta-blocker therapy. Alternative drug regimen: ACE inhibitors, calcium-channel blockers. (Oral antihypertensive drugs such as diuretics are not as effective in African Americans and may cause hyperglycemia in diabetics. Remember to check and replace potassium.)
   1. Hydrochlorothiazide, 12.5 to 50 mg q.d.
   2. Furosemide, 40 mg b.i.d. (maximum: 600 mg/day).
   3. Triamterene (potassium sparing): 50 to 100 mg b.i.d.

C. Beta-blockers (cardioselective) are not as effective in African Americans and may mask symptoms of hypoglycemia. *Do not use* in patients with asthma or COPD.
   1. Atenolol, 50 to 200 mg q.d. (start with 50 mg q.d. and increase after 1 to 2 weeks).
   2. Metoprolol, 50 to 100 mg b.i.d. (maximum: 450 mg/day).

D. Calcium-channel blockers:

    1. Nifedipine SR, 30 to 60 mg q.d. (maximum: 120 mg/day, adjust after 1 to 2 weeks).

    2. Verapamil SR, 180 mg q.d. (maximum: 480 mg, increase dose after 24 hours).

    3. Diltiazem SR, 60 mg b.i.d. (maximum: 180 mg b.i.d.).

E. ACE inhibitors (especially useful for renal protection in diabetics: captopril, 25 to 50 mg PO b.i.d.

F. If hypertension is persistent, increase dosage or add a second agent.

G. In acute hypertension (diastolic BP > 120), the goal is to lower blood pressure, but not too quickly. The clinician may use parenteral drugs such as:

    1. Nitroprusside, 1 to 10 μg/kg/min IV. Nitroprusside is usually used for less than 1 week of duration, since drug tolerance develops. Consider switching to PO enalapril.

    2. Labetolol, 20 mg IV; repeat 40 to 80 mg every 10 minutes for a maximum total dose of 300 mg. Maintenance: 0.5 to 2 mg/min; duration: 3 to 6 hours; onset: 5 minutes.

    3. Hydralazines, 5 to 20 mg IV/IM; duration: 2 to 6 hours; onset: 10 to 30 minutes.

    4. Esmolol, loading dose of 500 μg/kg IV; maintenance dose of 50 to 200 μg/kg/min; avoid in patients with congestive heart failure, asthma, or chronic obstructive pulmonary disease.

    5. Furosemide, 10 to 80 mg IV; onset: 15 minutes; duration: 4 hours.

ARRHYTHMIAS

- See the ACLS algorithms in Appendix F.
- Also see Chap. 28.

ASTHMA

Etiology

This is a chronic illness caused by reversible airway inflammation and constriction from various stimuli.

Signs and Symptoms

- Obtain a history of intubation, steroid use, past attacks, previous treatment, precipitating factors (infection, exercise), and bronchospasmic agents (aspirin, beta-blockers, cholinergic eye drops).
- Tachypnea, inability to speak, use of accessory respiratory muscles.
- May be accompanied by respiratory infection.

Workup

- Laboratory studies: CBC, electrolytes, creatinine to diagnose infection and dehydration.
- Spirometry: hospitalize if FEV_1 is less than 30% of predicted value or does not improve to 40% or more after 1 hour of vigorous therapy. If spirometry is not available, use peak flowmeter.
- ABGs: hypoxemia with widened A–a gradient due to increasing dead space. Increasing P_{CO_2} indicates impending respiratory failure.
- Chest x-ray to rule out pneumonia, pneumothorax, atelectasis.

Treatment

- Supplemental oxygen; consider intubation in patients with elevated P_{CO_2} or tiredness.
- For acute asthma: albuterol, 1 to 2 puffs via inhalation every 1 to 2 hours (maximum: 12 puffs) or 0.25 to 0.5 mL 5%

solution via nebulizer every 1 to 2 hours. Beclomethasone dipropionate, 2 puffs q.i.d.
- Prednisone, 40 to 60 mg PO q.i.d. if the patient is not responsive to albuterol, then taper. In severe cases, use methylprednisolone, 0.5 mg/kg IV every 6 hours (35 mg IV for 70 kg every 6 hours). If refractory, consider $MgSO_4$, 1 to 2 g IV over 20 minutes, once.
- Aminophylline (not a first-line agent): load 6 mg/kg ideal body weight via IV. May be reduced if the patient takes PO theophylline. Maintenance dose is 0.5 mg/kg/hour IV. Check drug level (normal is 10 to 20 mg/L).
- Other drugs that may be administered are an anticholinergic agent (ipratropium bromide MDI, 2 puffs q.i.d.) or cromolyn sodium MDI, 2 puffs b.i.d.

CHRONIC OBSTRUCTIVE PULMONARY DISEASE

Etiology

A condition of chronic dyspnea that results in most cases from smoking. In contrast to asthma, its symptoms do not markedly fluctuate.

Signs and Symptoms

Similar to those for Asthma, earlier.

Workup

Similar to that for Asthma, earlier. Spirometry: Patients with an FEV_1 of less than 1 L have a 50% 5-year survival; an FEV_1 of 1.2 to 1.5 represents dyspnea on exertion; FEV_1/FVC of less than 75 indicates chronic obstructive pulmonary disease (COPD).

Treatment

- Supplemental oxygen to keep O_2 saturation around 90%. Excessive O_2 administration may cause apnea.

- An anticholinergic agent is the first-line therapy for most patients with stable COPD: ipratropium bromide, 2 puffs every
  4 to 6 hours.
- Additional agents include bronchodilators (albuterol) and
  steroids (see Asthma, earlier).
- In chronic bronchitis: give Bactrim (double strength), 1 tablet
  b.i.d., or amoxicillin, 250 to 500 mg PO every 8 hours.
- Perform chest percussion *plus* postural drainage.
- Avoid bronchospasmic agents (aspirin, beta-blockers).
- Once the patient is clinically stable, consider administering
  influenza and pneumococcal vaccines.

PNEUMONIA

Etiology

The most common cause is infection. Opportunistic infections
occur most commonly in immunosuppressed patients. Other
causes include tumor, drugs, radiation, and trauma.

Signs and Symptoms

Fever, tachypnea, productive cough.

Workup

- Laboratory studies: CBC, electrolytes, and creatinine to aid
  in diagnosing infection and dehydration.
- Spirometry and ABGs, as for Asthma, earlier.
- Chest x-ray.
- Sputum culture is low yield, as it is usually contaminated.

Treatment

- Give supplemental oxygen.
- Bronchospasms may be treated as for Asthma, earlier.
- Provide antibiotic therapy, as indicated (see Table 13–1).

TABLE 13–1. Recommended Antibiotics for Some Common Pneumonias

Bacteria	Patient characteristics	Treatment
Streptococcus pneumoniae	Outpatient, community	Cefuroxime, 250–500 mg PO b.i.d.
Polymicrobial	Inpatient, Community acquired	*Mildly ill*—cefuroxime, 0.75–1.5 g IV q 8 h *Moderately ill*—ceftriaxone, 1–2 g IV q 12–24 h
Pseudomonas	Inpatient, ICU, aspiration pneumonia	Ceftazidime, 1 g IV q 8–12 h *plus* gentamicin, 5–7 mg/kg IV qd
Mycoplasma	Mostly adult patients	Azithromycin, 500 mg PO on day 1, then 250 mg PO qd on days 2–5

PLEURAL EFFUSION

Etiology

Most commonly tumor related (increased lymph production and decreased lymph evacuation). Other causes are infection (exudate effusion) and trauma (blood).

Signs and Symptoms

Tachypnea with decreased breath sounds, pleuritic pain.

Workup

- Chest x-ray: upright and/or lateral decubitus film to layer the fluid.
- CBC, PT/PTT if the patient has an abnormal bleeding history.
- CT scan if pleural fluid is loculated before doing thoracentesis.

- Send pleural fluid for cytology. If infection is suspected, send for culture. If etiology is unclear, send for LDH, protein, pH, glucose (infection, TB, cancer), amylase (pancreatitis, renal failure), and triglycerides (thoracic duct injury). For comparison, also send for serum LDH, albumin, and glucose.

Treatment

- Treat the cancer with chemotherapy, if possible.
- If the patient is symptomatic, thoracentesis is usually sufficient. If pleurodesis is planned, consider putting in a chest tube (see Chap. 24).

ADULT RESPIRATORY DISTRESS SYNDROME

Etiology

A. Unknown but probably due to severe systemic inflammatory response instead of direct lung injury. Mortality is about 50%.
B. Definition (must meet all criteria):
  1. Pao_2/Fio_2 is less than 250 to 300, regardless of PEEP level.
  2. Bilateral pulmonary infiltrates on chest x-ray.
  3. Not fluid overloaded, pulmonary artery occlusion pressure (PaOP) $\leq$ 18 mmHg.

Signs and Symptoms

Severe hypoxemia; may be accompanied by infection, edema, or trauma.

Workup

- Rule out cardiogenic pulmonary edema by inserting a Swan–Ganz catheter.
- Chest x-ray to rule out other etiology for hypoxemia.
- Laboratory studies: CBC and blood or sputum cultures, as indicated.

- ABGs show an increased shunt as lungs are perfused but not ventilated.

Treatment

- Treat the underlying disorders (ischemia, sepsis, trauma, aspiration, etc.).
- Provide supportive treatment: the goal is to maximize perfusion without incurring further injury to the lungs. Use inotropes to improve cardiac contractility, if possible.
- Keep peak inspiratory pressure below 40 cm H_2O and keep Fio_2 less than 50% (see Chap. 29).

ASPIRATION PNEUMONITIS

Etiology

Anything that reduces mental status (general anesthesia, drugs, alcohol, seizure, etc.). Aspiration of gastric contents has a mortality rate of 50%.

Signs and Symptoms

Aspiration of gastric contents induces lung inflammation, intense bronchospasms, and destruction of alveoli (including the surfactant, producing type 2 pneumocytes). Secondary bacterial infection occurs only in a third of the cases. Finally, food particles obstruct terminal bronchi and cause absorptive atelectasis.

Workup

Obtain a CBC and chest x-ray.

Treatment

- The goal is to maintain airway patency and minimize the extent of damage.

- If possible, place the patient in the left lateral decubitus with head down so that the aspirate may flow only to one lobe and to the mouth.
- Bronchoscopy can be helpful in retrieving small food particles and opening up small bronchioles. However, bronchoscopic lavage may exacerbate the injury by spreading the acidic solution to uninjured lung tissues.
- Prophylactic antibiotics or steroid therapy are not indicated. Instillation of sodium bicarbonate into the trachea is not helpful as pulmonary injury is almost instantaneous following acid aspiration.

PULMONARY EMBOLUS (See Chap. 22)

VENTILATOR AND PULMONARY FUNCTION TESTS (See Appendix E)

ABDOMINAL PAIN

Etiology

- Intestinal obstruction, infarction, or perforation.
- Inflammatory (appendicitis, cholecystitis, diverticulitis, pancreatitis, salpingitis, abscess).
- Retroperitoneal or abdominal bleeding.
- Gastroenteritis (bacterial or viral).
- Renal or biliary colic.
- Other causes (constipation, diarrhea, indigestion).

Signs and Symptoms

Presentation may vary from pain to nausea, vomiting, hypotension, or rebound tenderness.

Workup

- Complete history of onset, duration, location, modifying activities, drugs, and medical/surgical history.
- Laboratory studies: CBC, urinalysis, liver function tests, amylase, creatinine. Pregnancy test as indicated.
- ECG to rule out referred pain from ischemic heart disease.
- Chest and upright abdominal films to rule out air below the diaphragm (perforated viscus), air fluid level (bowel obstruction), mass, or renal stone. Pneumoperitoneum (air in abdominal x-ray) after abdominal surgery may last up to 2 weeks; however, most pneumoperitoneum should have resolved in 1 week or less. Consider obtaining a CT scan or an abdominal ultrasound.[1,2]

Treatment

- Keep the patient NPO and initiate IV access.
- Perform exploratory laparotomy in patients with acute surgical

abdomen (rebound tenderness, worsening pain, severe leuko-cytosis, hypotension, "sick-looking patient").
- More stable patients may be observed while diagnostic tests are completed.

ASCITES

Etiology

- Transudative fluids: tumors, liver cirrhosis, right heart fail-ure, pericarditis, supradiaphragmatic occlusion of the inferior vena cava, anasarca.
- Exudative fluids: ruptured bowel, tuberculosis, pancreatitis, bile peritonitis, tumors.

Signs and Symptoms

Presentation may vary from pain to nausea, vomiting, hy-potension, and shortness of breath.

Workup

- Complete history of onset, duration, location, modifying ac-tivities, drugs, and medical/surgical history.
- Laboratory studies: liver function tests, amylase, serum cre-atinine, electrolytes.
- Diagnostic paracentesis if diagnosis is not tumor. In ovarian cancer, paracentesis may spread tumor.
- ECG if symptoms are accompanied by chest pain.
- Chest and upright abdominal films to rule out air below the diaphragm, air fluid level, or mass. Consider obtaining a CT scan or an abdominal ultrasound.

Treatment

- For shortness of breath, elevate the head of the bed and pro-vide supplemental oxygen. Diuretics are not helpful—and may cause intravascular depletion.

- Watch urine output because ascites may compress the vena cava significantly and reduce preload.
- Perform therapeutic paracentesis if the patient is symptomatic from ascites (even if a tumor is suspected, when benefits outweigh the risks).
- Definitive treatment of ascites from ovarian or peritoneal cancer is tumor debulking followed by chemotherapy.
- Perform percutaneous liver biopsy if cirrhosis is the suspected etiology.

STOMATITIS (ORAL OR ESOPHAGEAL)

Etiology

Chemotherapy such as doxorubicin, methotrexate, 5-FU.

Signs and Symptoms

Painful ulcer (at worst grades 3, 4, patient is unable to swallow).

Workup

Rule out cancer or infection (herpes, candidiasis, *Monilia*).

Treatment

- For mucositis: treat with a soft toothbrush every 4 hours. Rinse with baking soda (1 teaspoon/500 mL water), or xylocaine, 2% viscous 10 mL swish-and-spit as needed (20 minutes). Or: give MXB, 1 to 2 tablespoons 15 minutes before meals and at bed time. MXB is a mixture of Mylanta, 345 mL; xylocaine viscous, 79 mL; and Benadryl, 47 mL—yielding 1 pint. Some patients prefer Hurricane spray or swab.
- For oral candidiasis: begin with 200 mg of fluconazole (Diflucan) PO/IV on day 1, then 100 mg q.d. Continue for 2 weeks after symptoms resolve.
- For oral moniliasis: give clotrimazole troche, 1 lozenge PO 5 times per day for 14 days.

NAUSEA/VOMITING

Etiology

Drug side effects (chemotherapy, morphine), radiation, GI (bowel obstruction, ileus, anastomotic leak), aspiration.

Signs and Symptoms

Presentation may vary from mild nausea to vomiting. Bilious vomiting indicates the source is from the small bowel. Vomiting of bright red blood may indicate a stomach or esophageal source.

Workup

See Bowel Obstruction, Pancreatitis, Acute Cholecystitis, and Jaundice, later in this chapter; see also Chap. 26 (chemotherapy).

Treatment

- Chemotherapy-induced: see Chap. 26.
- Narcotic-induced: usually resolves spontaneously in a few days. May use standard antiemetic drugs for palliation.
- Ileus: minimize narcotic usage; consider using NSAIDs (i.e., Toradol); replace abnormally low potassium, magnesium, and calcium serum levels and wait.
- Bowel obstruction: insert an NG tube for patients with excessive vomiting; order fluid and electrolyte replacement; and consider surgical therapy or palliative gastrostomy.
- Examples of antiemetics are provided in Table 14–1.

ILEUS

Etiology

- Drug effects (narcotics, antipsychotics, anticholinergics, ganglionic blockers, antiparkinsonian drugs).
- Electrolyte imbalance (low potassium, sodium, magnesium, calcium).

TABLE 14–1. Commonly Administered Antiemetic Drugs

Drug	Adult dose	Availability
Prochlorperazine (Compazine)	5–10 mg PO/IM t.i.d.–q.i.d. (max: 40 mg/day); 25 mg PR b.i.d.; 5–10 mg IV	5, 10, 25 PO; 2.5, 5, 25 PR; 5/5 mL; IM; IV
Promethazine (Phenergan)	12.5–25 mg PO/IM/PR q 4–6 h	12.5, 25, 50 PO; supp; IM; IV
Metochlopramide (Reglan)	1–2 mg/kg IV/IM/PO q 2–4 h; may add diphenhydramine (dystonic)	5, 10 PO; 5, 10/5 mL, IM; IV
Dronabinol (Marinol)	5 mg/m^2 PO q 1–3 h (max: 15 mg/m^2 PO per day)	2.5, 5, 10 PO
Trimetho-benzamide (Tigan)	250 mg PO t.i.d.–q.i.d.; 200 mg PR/IM t.i.d.–q.i.d.	100, 250 PO; supp; IM
Dolasetron (Anzemet)	100 mg PO q.d.; 12.5 mg IV	50, 100 PO; IV
Ondansetron (Zofran)	0.15 mg/kg IV or 8 mg PO b.i.d.–t.i.d. q 4 h	4, 8 PO; IV
Granisetron (Kytril)	10 μg/kg IV or 1 mg PO q.d.	1 PO; IV

- Infection or abscess.
- Postoperative period (small bowel function returns first, then stomach, then colon).
- Other (tumor, diabetic neuropathy, uremia, spinal fracture, scleroderma, lupus).

Signs and Symptoms

Patients may be asymptomatic or experience bloating without flatus, nausea, and vomiting.

Workup

- Examination to rule out rebound, point tenderness, and peritoneal sign.

- Abdominal x-ray to rule out bowel obstruction, Ogilvie's syndrome (see Ogilvie's Syndrome, ahead), or constipation.
- Electrolyte levels (including calcium and magnesium).

Treatment

- Keep the patient NPO and provide fluid and electrolyte replacement.
- Treat the underlying problem.
- Avoid administration of predisposing drugs.

CONSTIPATION

Etiology

Drug side effects (narcotics) or mass effect.

Signs and Symptoms

Abdominal or rectal discomfort.

Workup

Rule out tumor obstruction by rectal examination, barium enema, CT scan, or sigmoidoscopy.

Treatment

Differentiate between constipation as a result of obstruction due to tumor or to excessive use of narcotics. Laxative cathartics can be divided into three groups according to outcomes and amount of time needed (see Tables 14–2, 14–3, and 14–4).

DIARRHEA

Etiology

Drug side effects (chemotherapy, especially CPT-11, 5-FU), radiation, or infection.

TABLE 14–2. Stool Softeners That Take Effect in 1 to 3 Days

Drug	Adult dose	Availability
Docusate (Colace)	100 mg PO q.d.–b.i.d.	50 mg, 100 mg PO; 4/mL syrup; 10 mg/mL liquid
Glycerin	1 supp PR prn	4 mL/applicator enema
Lactulose	15–30 mL PO q.d. (max: 60 mL/d)	10 g/15 mL liquid; enema
Psyllium (Metamucil)	1–2 teaspoon PO q.d.–t.i.d.	Powder, dissolve in juice/water

TABLE 14–3. Stool Softeners That Produce Semifluid Stool in 6 to 12 Hours

Drug	Adult dose	Availability
Bisacodyl (Dulcolax)	10–15 mg PO q.d.	5 mg PO; 5 mg, 10 mg PR
Magnesium citrate	120–240 mL PO (max: 300 mL)	Liquid

TABLE 14–4. Stool Softeners That Produce Watery Stool in Less Than 6 Hours

Drug	Adult dose	Availability
Castor oil	15–60 mL PO, once only	Liquid
Polyethylene glycol (Colyte, Golytely)	4 L PO/NG, once	Solution

Signs and Symptoms

Patients may show signs of dehydration and nausea. Diarrhea with colicky abdominal cramping begins in the second and third week of abdominal and pelvic radiation.

Workup

- Order *Clostridium difficile* toxin, ova and parasite in stools, CBC, electrolytes, and creatinine.
- Monitor changes in weight.

TABLE 14–5. Examples of Antidiarrheal Agents Used After an Infectious Cause Is Ruled Out

Drug	Adult dose	Availability
Loperamide	2 mg PO; start 4 mg PO × 1 then 2 mg PO after each loose stool (max: 16 mg/day)	2 PO; 1/5 mL liquid
Atropine/ diphenoxylate (Lomotil)	1–2 tabs PO t.i.d.– q.i.d. prn; start 2 tabs PO or 5–10 mL PO t.i.d.– q.i.d. prn	0.025/2.5 PO; liquid
Atropine/ difenoxin (Motofen)	1 tab PO q 3–4 h; start 2 tabs PO (max: 8 tabs/day)	0.025/1 PO
Bismuth (Pepto Bismol)	2 tabs PO q 1 h prn (max: 8 doses/d); 30 mL PO q 1 h prn	262 PO; 262, 525 mg/15 mL susp
Attapulgite (Kaopectate)	15–30 mL PO prn (max: 8 doses/day); 1–2 tabs PO prn	750 PO; 600 mg/15 mL liquid
Codeine	30–60 g PO t.i.d. prn	15, 30, 60 PO; IM
Tincture of opium	1–4 tablespoons q 4–6 prn	

Treatment

- Replace fluid and electrolytes.
- Administer antidiarrheal agents, as indicated in Table 14–5.
- Pseudomembranous (*C. difficile*) colitis: administer metronidazole, 500 mg PO every 6 to 8 hours; or vancomycin, 125 to 500 mg PO every 6 hours for 7 to 10 days.

BOWEL OBSTRUCTION

Etiology

Adhesions from surgery; fibrosis from radiation or tumor mass.

Signs and Symptoms

Nausea, vomiting, colicky abdominal pain, no flatus or stool.

Workup

- Electrolytes.
- Upright abdominal x-ray to look for air fluid level.
- Gastrografin or barium swallow, which should reach the colon within 1 hour.
- Contrast enema.

Treatment

- Insert an NG tube, administer antiemetics, and initiate fluid and electrolyte replacement.
- Consider surgical resection, especially if pain worsens, to rule out strangulation.
- If the patient is stable, consider palliative gastrostomy or bowel stent (by GI or interventional radiology consultants).

OGILVIE'S SYNDROME (COLONIC PSEUDO-OBSTRUCTION, COLONIC ILEUS)

Etiology

Imbalance in autonomic innervation of the colon (too much sympathetic innervation), surgery, abnormal electrolyte levels.

Signs and Symptoms

Nausea, vomiting, colicky abdominal pain; patients may have flatus.

Workup

Same as that for Bowel Obstruction, earlier.

Treatment

- Insert an NG tube, administer antiemetics, and begin fluid and electrolyte replacement.
- Colonoscopy is sometimes helpful.

- Consider laparotomy if pain worsens or if there is no resolution in a few days as demonstrated by serial abdominal films.

HEMORRHOIDS

Etiology

Venous stasis. Rule out anal fissure, rectal abscess, or tumor.

Signs and Symptoms

Blood in stool. Thrombosed hemorrhoids may cause acute pain.

Workup

Rule out rectal, colon, or metastatic cancer.

Treatment

- Administer bulk-forming agents (fiber) to decrease straining; sitz bath b.i.d.
- Steroids (Anusol HC suppository b.i.d. for 7 to 10 days).
- Surgery, if medical management fails.

GI BLEEDING

Etiology

Ulcerogenic agents (steroids, aspirin, NSAIDs, alcohol, tobacco), severe stress, or trauma (from NG tube insertion).

Signs and Symptoms

- Hematemesis (bright red or black-colored emesis) indicates an upper GI source.
- Hematochezia (bloody stool) suggests a lower GI source.
- Occult blood in stool may indicate an upper or a lower GI source.
- Examination may reveal jaundice, caput medusae, ascites, hepatosplenomegaly, hemorrhoids, or rectal mass.

Workup

- Laboratory studies: CBC, type and cross-match, electrolytes.
- Rule out bleeding from airway, lung, or cancer.

Treatment

- Intubate the patient if the airway is unstable.
- Ensure IV access and insert a Foley catheter. Replace fluid and electrolytes. Consider blood transfusion if bleeding is severe.
- Insert an NG tube to aid in diagnosis (upper versus lower GI bleeding) and to facilitate lavage.
- Call in a GI consultant for endoscopic evaluation and possible vasopressin, electocautery, or sclerotherapy treatment.

ACUTE MESENTERIC ISCHEMIA

Etiology

Atherosclerosis, emboli.

Signs and Symptoms

Nausea, vomiting, or severe abdominal pain exceeding physical findings.

Workup

Maintain a high index of suspicion. If the patient is stable, obtain an arteriogram.

Treatment

Prompt surgery is needed to avoid bowel infarction; mortality is high.

RADIATION PROCTITIS/ENTERITIS

Etiology

Inflammation or fibrosis resulting from radiation therapy.

Signs and Symptoms

Rectal bleeding, frequent small-volume stool.

Workup

Rule out cancer, partial bowel obstruction, or colitis with proctoscopy/sigmoidoscopy, barium enema, or colonoscopy.

Treatment

Administer a retention enema containing hydrocortisone (Cortenema), 100 mg b.i.d. The enema is inserted into the rectum and the patient remains in the left Sim's position for at least 30 minutes. Alternatively, a foam aerosol spray (Cortifoam) is applied to the distal sigmoid junction twice daily. Therapeutic results should be seen within 48 hours. An alternative is Rowasa (rectal suppository or enema), 500 mg (60 to 90 mL) q.d. for 6 weeks.

BOWEL ANASTOMOSIS LEAK

Etiology

May be caused by inaccurate suture or stapler placement, ischemia (especially in the ilocecal area), or inflamed/irradiated bowel, and tension on the suture line. It occurs in 10% to 15% of patients postoperatively after an anastomosis.

Signs and Symptoms

Nausea, abdominal pain, fever, and sepsis. Occasionally, less acute symptoms such as tenesmus, diarrhea, and low back pain result from an abscess on the presacral space.

Workup

- Maintain a high index of suspicion.
- Perform a physical examination and obtain a contrast study with Gastrografin (barium irritates the peritoneal cavity and

is contraindicated) or a CT scan (stool in abdominal cavity and outside the colon).

Treatment

• Perform an exploratory laparotomy to drain the abscess and create a proximal diversion (colostomy). The area of anastomosis, if not grossly disrupted, should be left to heal by itself. The diversional colostomy can be closed at least 2 months after the original surgery, and if a Gastrografin study demonstrates no evidence of anastomotic leak.

COLOSTOMY COMPLICATIONS

Etiology

May be caused by inaccurate suture or stapler placement, ischemia (especially in the ilocecal area), or inflamed/irradiated bowel and tension on the suture line. It occurs in 10% to 15% of patients postoperatively after an anastomosis.

Signs and Symptoms

• Early complications include peristomal abscess, ischemia (stoma dusky color), and retraction.
• Late complications include stomal prolapse, hernia, retraction, and peristomal skin irritation.

Workup

To evaluate the extent of stomal ischemia, put a glass tube into the stoma to inspect the deeper stomal tissue.

Treatment

• If the problem persists, the patient may require further surgery for stoma reconstruction.
• With prolapse, the protruding segment may need to be resected and the stoma reconstructed. (Prolapse occurs more frequently with loop colostomy than with end colostomy.)

- With hernia, stoma reconstruction with a mesh may be needed. If this fails, the stoma may need to be relocated.

HIGH STROMA OUTPUT

Etiology

Decreased absorption because of short gut (when a large segment of bowel is resected or not functioning).

Signs and Symptoms

Dehydration, weight loss, and electrolyte abnormalities.

Workup

Daily weight, I/O recording, electrolytes.

Treatment

Order a low-fat diet and give octreotide (50 to 200 μg SQ, IV, q.d. to t.i.d. to reduce GI fluid secretion), cholestyramine (4 g PO q.d. to b.i.d. to absorb lipid), tincture of opium (1 mL prn PO; 1 mL has approximately 10 mg morphine sulfate). Because the high-output condition may last for weeks, consider starting TPN. Check daily weight to assess fluid loss. If the patient bruises easily, check INR/PT, as vitamin K absorption may also be abnormal.

PANCREATITIS

Etiology

Gallstones, alcohol, hyperlipidemia, infection, drugs, trauma, idiopathic causes.

Signs and Symptoms

- Midepigastric pain, which is worsened after a meal or alcohol. Pain may radiate to the back, is alleviated by sitting up, and is worsened by motion.

- Nausea, vomiting, fever, and tachycardia are common. Jaundice is rare.

Workup

- Laboratory studies: CBC, electrolytes, amylase, lipase, AST, ALT, LDH, GGT, alkaline phosphatase, and bilirubin. Utilize a Foley catheter as necessary. Insert an NG tube if the patient is vomiting.
- ECG to rule out MI.
- Chest x-ray to rule out pulmonary or other abdominal etiology for pain.

Treatment

- Keep the patient NPO; administer fluids, electrolyte replacement, and meperidine for pain.
- Administer TPN if the patient is expected to be NPO for more than 7 days.
- Alcohol withdrawal prophylaxis: diazepam, 10 mg PO/IV t.i.d. to q.i.d.; thiamine, 100 mg q.d. for 3 days; folate, 1 mg for 3 days; multivitamins.

ACUTE CHOLECYSTITIS

Etiology

In 95% of cases, calculous cholecystitis is related to an obstructing gallstone. Bile stasis or fasting is a more common etiology in acalculous cholecystitis.

Signs and Symptoms

Right upper quadrant pain, nausea, vomiting, fever, and tachycardia.

Workup

- Laboratory studies: CBC, liver function tests, electrolytes, amylase.
- Diagnostic tests: ultrasound, HIDA scan.

Treatment

A. Provide supportive treatment; administer IV fluids and an antibiotic.
B. Perform drainage or surgical removal, as necessary.
C. Prophylactic cholecystectomy should only be done in the following cases:
    1. Diabetic patients with increased risks for complications.
    2. Patients with a nonfunctioning gallbladder as seen on oral cholecystogram.
    3. "Porcelain" gallbladder (15% of these are associated with carcinoma).
    4. Any patient with a history of biliary pancreatitis.
    5. Gallstones found at time of laparotomy (15 to 20% associated with acute postoperative cholecystitis).

JAUNDICE

Etiology

- Increased bilirubin production resulting from massive transfusion, hematoma, crush injury, sickle cell anemia, or hemolysis from blood transfusion.
- Decreased bilirubin clearance resulting from cholestatic jaundice, hepatitis, hepatotoxic drug (alcohol is the most common), TPN, shock, sepsis, or biliary obstruction.

Signs and Symptoms

Presentation varies from pain to asymptomatic.

Workup

- Laboratory studies: bilirubin, CBC, liver function tests, hepatitis panel, albumin, PT, urobilinogen.
- Abdominal x-ray to visualize radiopaque gallstone, gas in the biliary tree, or gallbladder.
- Ultrasound to locate gallstone or obstruction.
- Nuclear biliary scan (HIDA): diagnoses acute cholecystitis but is unreliable when bilirubin is greater than 20 mg/dL.
- CT scan to identify mass lesion.

• Percutaneous transhepatic cholangiography, endoscopic retrograde cholangiopancreatography (diagnose with specimen).

Treatment

Provide supportive treatment and manage the underlying disease.

REFERENCES

1. EARLS JP, DACHMAN AH, COLON E, GARRETT MG, MOLLOY M: Prevalence and duration of postoperative pneumoperitoneum: sensitivity of CT and lateral decubitus radiography. Am J Roentgenol 161:781, 1993.
2. LEE DH, LIM JH, KO YT, YOON Y: Sonographic detection of pneumoperitoneum in patients with acute abdomen. Am J Roentgenol 154:107, 1990.

ACUTE RENAL FAILURE/INSUFFICIENCY

Etiology

- Prerenal causes: low renal perfusion from hypovolemia, sepsis, or congestive heart failure.
- Intrarenal causes: renal damage from acute tubular necrosis (hypotension or perfusion leading to tubular ischemia or necrosis), drugs (nephrotoxic, NSAIDs), myo- or hemoglobinuria, contrast agent, nephritis (allergic, autoimmune), hyperuricemia (tumor lysis syndrome), or glomerulonephropathies.
- Postrenal causes: obstructed Foley catheter, obstructed urethra or ureter (from tumor, stone, clot), or neurogenic bladder.

Signs and Symptoms

- Low urine output, weight gain due to water retention, and elevated serum creatinine.
- Secondary symptoms such as congestive heart failure, pulmonary edema, and uremia.

Workup

A. In general, obtain a careful history of drug exposures, dehydration, and blood loss, and perform a physical examination. The fractional excretion of sodium ($F_{E_{Na}}$) test helps differentiate the etiology of renal failure: $F_{E_{Na}}$ of less than 1% indicates a prerenal cause; $F_{E_{Na}}$ of greater than 2% indicates a renal or postrenal cause. $F_{E_{Na}}$ is unreliable in the elderly or in patients with forced diuresis (diuretics, mannitol, or glucose).
B. Prerenal causes:
1. Place a Foley catheter to carefully quantify urine output.
2. Perform a fluid challenge with 500 mL lactated Ringer's or NS in 10 minutes. Improvement in urine output confirms the diagnosis of prerenal etiology.

C. Intrarenal causes: history, physical exam, and renal nuclear scan.
D. Postrenal causes:
1. Place a Foley catheter to rule out neurogenic bladder. If the Foley catheter is already inserted, flush it to rule out obstruction.
2. Perform a cystoscopy or retrograde ureteral contrast study.
3. Order renal sonography to evaluate for obstruction.

Treatment

- In general, avoid nephrotoxic agents (NSAIDs, aminoglycosides, IV contrast agents) and excessive electrolytes such as potassium; ensure adequate but not excessive hydration; monitor I/O closely, and monitor daily weight.
- Prerenal causes: give fluid and/or blood.
- Intrarenal causes: provide supportive care, consider renal dose dopamine (< 6 µg/kg/min) to increase perfusion.
- Postrenal causes: relieve obstruction. If necessary, consult an interventional radiologist to place a percutaneous nephrostomy (PCN). Watch for postobstructive diuresis (replace fluids and electrolytes to maintain a stable daily weight).
- Indications for renal dialysis (hemodialysis or peritoneal dialysis): BUN greater than 100, volume overload, hyperkalemia, pericarditis, severe toxin ingestion, acidosis (pH $<$ 7.15), changes in mental status, seizures, persistent metabolic abnormalities after conservative management.

URETERAL OBSTRUCTION

Etiology

From mass effect or radiation fibrosis.

Signs and Symptoms

Flank pain with fever and elevated serum creatinine.

Workup

- Obtain a renal radionuclide scan to assess the viability of the kidneys.
- Although uremia is viewed by some clinicians as an acceptable way to die in terminal cases, patients should be informed of the option to place a ureteral catheter versus observation.

Treatment

Consult an interventional radiologist to place a PCN. A few weeks after PCN placement, ureteral edema will subside. Then a urologist can place a retrograde ureteral stent to keep the ureter open and discontinue PCN. After placement of the stent, the patient occasionally has postobstructive fluid and electrolytes diuresis for a few days. The treatment consists of aggressive fluid hydration (replacing fluid to maintain weight) and electrolyte replacement.

URETERAL TRANSECTION DURING SURGERY

Etiology

Difficult dissection, adhesion.

Signs and Symptoms

Asymptomatic if found intraoperatively. Postoperative findings may include peritoneal irritation, bowel obstruction, confusion (from reabsorbed toxic urinary wastes), or electrolyte abnormality.

Workup

- Intraoperative: use IVP or indigo carmine to identify the location of the transected ureter. Another option is to place a ureteral stent.
- Postoperative: use IVP or ultrasound or CT scan.

Treatment

A. Transection found intraoperatively:
   1. If transected distal from the cardinal ligament, reim-
      plantation to the bladder (ureteroneocystostomy) is bet-
      ter than uretero-ureteroanastomosis, because the ureteral
      diameter in this area is narrow and repair may result in
      ureteral constriction. If ureteral length is insufficient, a
      psoas hitch or boari flap can be performed. If the ureter
      is still not reaching the bladder, consider using a piece
      of ileum as a conduit (uretero-ileo-neocystostomy—
      make sure the ileum is isoperistalsis with the ureter). A
      more drastic option is to dissect the kidney from Gerota's
      fascia and lower it; the kidney can be lowered approxi-
      mately 5 cm with this approach.
   2. If transected proximal from the cardinal ligament, uretero-
      ureterostomy (preferably on the same side, in a worst-
      case situation, one could perform trans-uretero-ureteros-
      tomy) can be done.
B. Transection found postoperatively:
   1. If the patient is clinically stable, return her to the oper-
      ating room to undergo primary reanastomoses.
   2. If the patient is not clinically stable, place a PCN.
C. See Chap. 24, which provides step-by-step instructions for
   the procedures described in A and B.

HEMORRHAGIC CYSTITIS

Etiology

Associated with alkylating agents (cyclophosphamide and ifosfamide), tumor invasion, and radiation cystitis.

Signs and Symptoms

Presentation varies from hematuria to distended bladder full of
blood clots.

Workup

Perform a cystoscopy to rule out tumor versus radiation/chemotherapy-induced cystitis.

Treatment

- Evacuate all clots: may require Ellick evacuator or TURP catheter, or may require operative cystoscopy.
- Insert a three-way ureteral catheter (22 to 26 French). Use sterile water to irrigate and flush out the blood clot. Removing the clot will permit bladder contraction and, therefore, hemostasis. Continuous irrigation with 50 to 200 mL/h of water can be used. Monitor I/O carefully.
- If bleeding continues, consider continuous intravesical irrigation with: (1) acetic acid 0.25%; (2) 1% aluminum potassium sulfate; (3) 1% silver nitrate; (4) rarely, 1% formalin; (5) aminocaproic acid 5 g PO/IV over 1h and then 1 to 1.25 g/h prn. Formalin is very painful—the patient will need anesthesia—and is contraindicated if the patient has vesicoureteral reflux (obtain a voiding cytourethrogram first). Aminocaproic acid is an antifibrinolytic agent and is contraindicated in thrombus-prone patients or patients with DIC.
- If persistent bleeding seen, consider operative vesicle coagulation.

RADIATION CYSTITIS

Etiology

- Usually occurs 3 to 4 years after radiation.
- With doses greater than 60 Gy, chronic cystitis and hematuria may occur. Acute radiation nephritis occurs within 6 months after irradiation of 20 Gy with symptoms of headaches, leg edema, hypertension, albuminuria, and elevated BUN.
- Chronic nephritis appears about 18 months or later after radiation exposure with symptoms of progressive anemia, hypertension, and renal function impairment.

Signs and Symptoms

Chronic cystitis and/or urinary tract infection.

Workup

- Acute and transient cystitis can be observed with radiation doses greater than 25 Gy and usually requires no treatment.
- With more severe symptoms, rule out urinary tract infection versus inflammation. Urine needs to be cultured to confirm an infection, as urinalysis can be abnormal from either inflammation or infection.
- In intractable cases, consider cystoscopy.

Treatment

- Treat urinary tract infection with antibiotic.
- If the patient has a significant bladder spasm, pyridium (200 mg PO t.i.d.) may help.
- Administration of 10 to 25 mg of urecholine PO t.i.d. may further help with detrusor muscles spasm.
- If patient has hematuria, prescribe as in hemorrhagic cystitis after cystoscopy.

BLADDER ATONY

Etiology

- Between 60% and 70% of patients experience bladder atony after radical hysterectomy.
- Spinal block (from epidural anesthesia or spinal trauma).

Signs and Symptoms

Painless or painful bladder distention.

Workup

Check residual urine volume as noted below.

Treatment

- Leave the Foley or suprapubic catheter in place for a few days postoperatively. In most patients, the bladder regains its function about the same time as the bowel starts to work. When the patient starts eating a regular diet, clamp the catheter for a few hours. Ask the patient to void. Next, measure the residual volume.
- Some limited success with α-adrenergic agents (terazosin) has been seen.
- An alternative is to instill 300 to 400 mL of sterile water into the bladder and reclamp the suprapubic catheter or discontinue the Foley catheter. Ask the patient to urinate (record this volume). Unclamp the suprapubic catheter or insert another Foley catheter to check the residual volume. If the voiding volume is greater than the residual volume and the residual volume is less than 100 mL, remove the catheter. If not, leave the catheter in place for another week, send the patient home, and repeat the procedure the next week.
- In spinal trauma or metastases, administer corticosteroid as discussed in Chap. 11.

OBSTRUCTED URETHRA

Etiology

Vulvar lesion or trauma to the urethra.

Signs and Symptoms

Painful distention of the bladder.

Workup

Attempt to place a urethral catheter.

Treatment

- Try to insert a urethral catheter.

- If this fails, consider inserting a suprapubic catheter at the bedside using the Seldinger wire method and an 8.5 French pig-tail catheter with local anesthesia. If this equipment is not available, a central line kit may do as well.
- An alternative is placement of a PCN.

VAGINAL/CERVICAL BLEEDING

Etiology

- Cancer versus radiation necrosis.
- Trauma.

Signs and Symptoms

Bleeding, pain.

Workup

- Assess vital signs and ABC—see Chap. 12. Stabilize the patient (using two large IV lines, type and cross blood, and IV fluid) as necessary.
- Rule out hypocoagulation. Check International Normalized Ratio (INR), especially in patients with alcohol or hepatitis history—decreased vitamin K–dependent clotting factors.
- Rule out the endometrium as a source of bleeding.
- If the patient is clinically stable, obtain a tumor biopsy for histologic documentation of cancer.
- Visualize the source of bleeding: call for help; prepare a suction canula and irrigation kit (diluted hydrogen peroxide may be needed to dissolve the blood clot).

Treatment

- Initially, apply Monsel (ferric subsulfate) or acetone solution with pressure.
- If bleeding continues, sutures may be needed. If visualization is poor, consider inserting vaginal packing; then take the patient to the operating room to place the suture(s).

- Persistent bleeding from an exophytic cervical tumor may require radiation (which takes a few days) or, alternatively, an interventional radiology procedure to thrombose the arterial blood supply.

VESICOVAGINAL FISTULA

Etiology

- May occur after radiation therapy or hysterectomy.
- Tumor invasion.

Signs and Symptoms

Excessive vaginal discharge, frequent urinary tract infection.

Workup

A. Inject diluted methylene blue in sterile water to the bladder using a Foley catheter. The presence of blue fluid in the vagina increases the suspicion of vesicovaginal fistula.
B. Obtain an IVP to rule out ureterovaginal fistula.
C. Perform cystoscopy to assess number and size of fistula.
D. Rule out other fistulae:
   1. Enterovaginal fistula: use a barium enema study.
   2. Ureterovaginal fistula: use an IVP or indigo carmine.

Treatment

- If fistula size is small, as seen with cystoscopy, and the bladder has not been radiated, conservative management with Foley catheter for a few weeks may allow spontaneous healing. If fistula continues to progress, surgery will be required.
- Most fistulae can be repaired transvaginally; exceptions are those in the trigone, cases in which surrounding tissues have been radiated, or poor exposure.
- The ideal repair time is 3 to 6 months after the initial injury to decrease inflammation.

ANEMIA

Etiology

A. Microcytic (blood loss, iron deficiency).
B. Macrocytic:
1. Folic acid deficiency from alcoholism, malabsorption, hemolytic anemia, pregnancy, some drugs that interfere with folic acid metabolism (anticonvulsants, methotrexate, ethanol, trimethoprim).
2. Vitamin B_{12} deficiency from pernicious anemia, gastrectomy, ileal resection, pancreatic insufficiency, intestinal parasites, intestinal bacterial overgrowth.
C. Normocytic (chemotherapy-induced, chronic disease, chronic renal insufficiency).

Signs and Symptoms

- Microcytic: history of GI or GU bleeding, weakness.
- Macrocytic: glossitis, jaundice, splenomegaly may be present. Vitamin B_{12} deficiency may result in paresthesia, confusion, and decreased vibratory sense.
- Normocytic: history of malignancy, renal failure, autoimmune disease, or chronic infection.

Workup

A. Microcytic:
1. MCV (normal 90 ± 5) is normal in early iron deficiency anemia.
2. Serum ferritin less than 10 g/mL in women indicates low iron stores.
3. Low serum iron (< 50 µg/dL, TIBC > 420 mg/dL). Some of the values may fluctuate. Most diagnostic is absence of iron staining in bone marrow biopsy.

4. Intravascular hemolysis shows elevated haptoglobin. In severe cases, free hemoglobin is seen in urine and may cause renal failure.
5. Extravascular hemolysis shows normal haptoglobin because RBC destruction occurs primarily in the spleen.
6. Reticulocyte count (normal: 30,000 to 80,000) indicates rate of red cell formation. A low count with anemia suggests marrow failure. A high count suggests excessive red cell loss.
7. If there is blood loss, find the source (GI, GU, hematoma, vaginal bleeding, etc.).

B. Macrocytic:
1. High MCV, peripheral smear, serum vitamin B_{12} (normal > 180 pg/mL), RBC folate levels (normal > 6.5 ng/mL).
2. If vitamin B_{12} or folate level is equivocal, obtain serum methylmalonic acid and homocysteine levels.

C. Normocytic: normocytic normochromic smear. Ferritin is usually normal but may be elevated as it is an acute phase reactant. Serum creatinine may confirm renal failure.

D. Obtain a bone marrow biopsy in unclear cases.

Treatment

- Microcytic: ferrous sulfate, 325 mg PO t.i.d., will replace iron in 6 months (normalized serum ferritin). Patients with acute bleeding may require blood transfusion. In cases of severe hemolysis, urine output should be greater than 1 mL/kg/hour with saline infusion. Sodium bicarbonate is infused to keep urinary pH above 6, which improves excretion of hemoglobin.
- Macrocytic: folic acid, 1 mg PO q.d. A higher dose of 5 mg PO q.d. may be given to patients with malabsorption. Vitamin B_{12} deficiency is corrected with cyanocobalamin, 1 mg IM q.d. for 7 days, then weekly for 1 to 2 months until hemoglobin is normalized. Long-term treatment is 1 mg IM once a month.

- Normocytic: the patient may need a blood transfusion or erythropoietin, 10,000 U or 100 units/kg SC or IV 3 times a week. Flu-like symptoms usually appear within 1½ to 2 hours after starting the infusion of erythropoietin and can last for 2 to 12 hours. These side effects are generally self-limiting and do not require dose reduction. Aspirin or ibuprofen before infusion of the drug and a slower infusion rate can help minimize side effects. Check ferritin levels (should be > 100 mg/mL). Administer iron and folate supplements. A contraindication is uncontrolled hypertension. Check hematocrit, reticulocyte count, and blood pressure weekly until the hemoglobin stabilizes (goal is 10 g/dL), then monthly. Increase erythropoietin to 20,000 U 3 times a week if the increase in hemoglobin is less than 1 g/dL. This therapy should be discontinued if after an additional 4 weeks of therapy at the higher dose level the hemoglobin increase is still less than 1 g/dL. About a third of gynecologic oncology patients are resistant to erythropoietin.[1] Once the target hemoglobin is reached, the maintenance dose must be individualized (usually 25 to 50 U/kg, 3 times a week).

SICKLE CELL ANEMIA

Etiology

- Aplastic crisis: infections result in decreased RBC production and survival.
- Sequestration: accumulation of large volumes of blood, resulting in shock and death.
- Painful crisis: microvascular occlusion, which is often precipitated by dehydration or infection.

Signs and Symptoms

Shock, abdominal fullness and tenderness, painful joints.

Workup

Red cell sickling is visible on smear. Hemoglobin electrophoresis is used to differentiate sickle cell trait from disease.

Treatment

- Treat the precipitating events.
- Provide fluids, pain control, oxygen, and blood transfusion, as needed.

THROMBOCYTOPENIA

Etiology

- Decreased platelet production: from chemotherapy or radiation therapy, drugs (ethanol, anticonvulsants), infections, vitamin B_{12} deficiency, HIV infection, marrow infiltration by tumor (myelophthisis).
- Increased platelet destruction: from drugs (heparin, quinidine, valproic acid, penicillin, rifampin, digoxin), immune disorders, consumptive processes (DIC, thrombocytopenia purpura, HELLP).

Signs and Symptoms

Bleeding from gums, IV sites, petechiae, purpura, epistaxis, GI bleeding, ecchymosis.

Workup

- Obtain the history; perform physical examination, and possible bone marrow biopsy.
- Rule out other coagulation disorders.

Treatment

- Stop any drug administration that may be contributing to the condition. Heparin flush occasionally causes thrombocytopenia and thrombocytosis; it should be avoided. Low-molecular-weight heparin causes less thrombocytopenia than regular heparin. Reduce or stop chemotherapy.
- Transfuse 6 to 8 packs of platelets and check the platelet count after 1 hour. It should increase by 60,000 to 80,000. If

there is no increase in platelet count 1 hour after transfusion, suspect platelet antibody (alloimmunization). The threshold for prophylactic platelet transfusion ($<$ 20,000) has been questioned. In one study, limited prophylactic platelet transfusion for platelets ($<$ 5,000) resulted in minor bleeding in 14% of patients and no major bleeding, which is not different from the group who received platelets.[2]

- For patients with alloimmunization, HLA-matched or partially matched products can be obtained from the blood bank. HLA-matched platelets are effective in highly alloimmune patients about 50% of the time. Consider platelet cross-matching, a technique that may improve the efficacy of transfusion, if available at your hospital.

- IL-11 (Neumega) can be effective in some patients when given for 1 to 2 weeks immediately after chemotherapy to prevent severe thrombocytopenia. Consider trying it as prophylaxis in patients with a history of severe chemotherapy-induced thrombocytopenia. IL-11 has not been very effective in studies when given during severe thrombocytopenia. It is also more toxic than GM-CSF and causes fever, fluid retention, pleural effusion, and injection site reactions by releasing IL-6 and other acute phase mediators. Thrombopoietin is still not approved, but trials have shown similar efficacy as IL-11, without much benefit to those who are already severely thrombocytopenic. Most chemotherapy is held until platelet count $>$ 100,000.

NEUTROPENIA

Etiology

Myelosuppressive chemotherapy and radiation therapy may be required. Neutropenia is defined by the patient's absolute neutrophil count (ANC) of less than 500 polymorphonuclear leukocytes/mm^3. The ANC equals WBC $\times$ (% PMN). Most chemotherapy should not be given when ANC is less than 1500 cells/mm^3.

Signs and Symptoms

Asymptomatic, except if accompanied by infection.

Workup

Obtain a history, perform a physical examination, and order a CBC with differential.

Treatment

Granulocyte colony stimulating factor (GCSF) is not indicated for neutropenia alone. See Chap. 26.

DISSEMINATED INTRAVASCULAR COAGULATION

Etiology

Generalized bleeding and thrombosis due to consumptive coagulopathy. It may be caused by shock, hypothermia, sepsis, severe blood loss, or retained fetal products.

Signs and Symptoms

Generalized bleeding from gums, IV sites, or incision sites.

Workup

- Laboratory studies show increased PT, PTT, and FDP; decreased platelets, fibrinogen, and hemoglobin.
- The least expensive diagnostic test is to obtain a venous blood sample in a red-top tube. DIC is present if the blood does not clot after 5 to 10 minutes.

Treatment

A. Treat the underlying process.
B. Provide supportive treatment with fresh frozen plasma, cryoprecipitate, red cell and platelet transfusion, and reverse hypothermia.

C. Transfusion guidelines are as follows (adapt to specific situations):
   1. Give blood if 2 L of lactated Ringer's solution does not stabilize blood pressure.
   2. Give 1 unit of packed red blood cells per 1 L crystalloid.
   3. Give 2 units of fresh frozen plasma after 6 packs of red blood cells.
   4. Give 10 packs of platelets for every 10 packs of red blood cells.
   5. Give 8 packs of cryoprecipitate if there is no clot or if fibrinogen is less than 100,000 mg/dL.

BLOOD TRANSFUSION/COMPONENT THERAPY

See Appendix A.

REFERENCES

1. DEMETRI GD, KRIS M, WADE J, DEGOS L, CELLA D: Quality-of-life benefit in chemotherapy patients treated with epoetin alfa is independent of disease response or tumor type: Results from a prospective community oncology study. J Clin Oncol 16:3412, 1998.
2. FANNING J, HILGERS RD, MURRAY KP, BOLT K, AUGHENBAUGH DM: Conservative management of chemotherapeutic-induced thrombocytopenia in women with gynecologic cancers. Gynecol Oncol 59:191, 1995.

DIABETIC KETOACIDOSIS

Etiology

Severe insulin deficiency is combined with elevated anti-insulin hormones (i.e., epinephrine, growth hormone, glucagon, cortisol), resulting in hyperglycemia, osmotic diuresis (severe dehydration, loss electrolytes), and lipolysis.

Signs and Symptoms

Dehydration, decreased mental status, tachycardia, tachypnea.

Workup

- Rule out underlying disorders: infection, stress, missed insulin dose.
- Obtain a finger stick for blood glucose every hour, check electrolytes every 1 to 2 hours (potassium, anion gap), and arterial blood gas for pH. Evaluation of serum ketones is not useful.

Treatment

Hydrate the patient with IV fluid promptly using normal saline (NS). Switch to D_5 1/2 NS once blood glucose level drops to 250 mg/dL, as continued rapid decrease in blood glucose may cause cerebral edema. Give potassium replacement once the potassium level is less than 4 (pseudohyperkalemia initially). Give insulin, 10 U regular, then infuse 10 U/h. If glucose does not decrease, increase IV insulin and fluid hydration by 50%. Goal: blood glucose of 100 to 200 mg/dL with a normal potassium level.

HYPOTHYROIDISM

Etiology

- Primary (90% cases): chronic lymphocytic thyroiditis/ Hashimoto's thyroiditis.
- Secondary: abnormalities of the pituitary or hypothalamus.

Signs and Symptoms

Cold intolerance, weakness, and slow deep tendon reflexes.

Workup

- Screen with TSH (usually > 20 mU/mL).
- Free T_3, T_4 (if unavailable, obtain the T_4 index, which is an estimate of free T_3).
- Rule out underlying disorders such as infection.

Treatment

- Levothyroxine, 50 to 200 μg/day PO. If the patient is elderly or has heart disease, 12.5 to 50 μg. Check the TSH level in 3 months, adjust ± 25 μg, then check every 6 weeks ± 12.5 to 25 μg. Once the TSH level has normalized, check it yearly.
- Rarely, a patient becomes hypotensive and hypoventilates during the postoperative course. Confirm the TSH level, then treat with thyroxine, 50 to 100 μg IV every 6 hours for 4 days followed with 75 to 100 μg IV q.d. until the patient is able to take it orally.

HYPERTHYROIDISM (GRAVES' DISEASE)

Etiology

- Graves' disease is the most common cause of hyperthyroidism, especially in younger patients.
- Toxic multinodular goiter is a more common cause in older patients.

- Rare cases: iodine induced, thyroid adenoma, subacute thyroiditis, pregnancy related, and patients who take an excessive amount of thyroid hormone replacement.

Signs and Symptoms

- Cold intolerance, weakness, and slow deep tendon reflexes.
- Thyroid storm (hyperautonomous), heat intolerance, brisk deep tendon reflexes, arrhythmias.

Workup

Screen with TSH (exclude hyperthyroidism if TSH > 0.1 mU/mL), free T_3, T_4.

Treatment

- For thyroid storm: Follow symptoms and treat with propranolol, 20 to 60 mg PO or 1 to 2 mg IV every 6 hours. Do not use beta-blockers in patients with asthma as they cause bronchospasm. Instead, use verapamil, 40 to 80 mg PO t.i.d., or reserpine, 1 mg PO or IM or IV every 6 to 12 hours.
- In addition, give propylthiouracil (PTU): load 1000 mg PO, then give 200 to 300 mg PO every 6 hours. Watch for symptoms of hepatitis or agranulocytosis (fever, sore throat, bleeding gums).
- To inhibit thyroid hormone, use a saturated solution of potassium iodide, 1 to 10 drops t.i.d. PO, then wean, or give sodium iodide, 0.5 g IV every 12 hours.
- To block T_4 to T_3 conversion, use dexamethasone, 2 mg PO or IV every 6 hours.

ADRENAL FAILURE

Etiology

- Primary/Addison's disease: deficiency of both cortisol and aldosterone with elevated ACTH.
- Secondary: primary or hypothalamus abnormalities with deficiency of cortisol alone.

Signs and Symptoms

- Nonspecific: anorexia, nausea, vomiting, weight loss, fatigue.
- Orthostatic hypotension, hyponatremia.
- Hyperpigmentation, hyperkalemia, dehydration only in primary adrenal failure.

Workup

- Short cosyntropin stimulation test: administer 250 μg cosyntropin via IV and measure plasma cortisol 30 minutes later. The normal response is a stimulated plasma cortisol level of more than 20 μg/dL. This test detects both primary and secondary adrenal failures.
- Obtain a history of pituitary mass (headaches, visual field loss); known pituitary or hypothalamic disease indicates a secondary etiology. Primary etiology is as described earlier.

Treatment

- Adrenal crisis: if a diagnosis of adrenal failure has been confirmed, give 100 mg of hydrocortisone IV every 8 hours. Also give 0.9% saline with 5% dextrose to correct hypotension. The hydrocortisone dose is then tapered over a few days and changed to oral form. If the diagnosis of adrenal failure has not been confirmed, give a single dose of dexamethasone, 10 mg IV with saline and dextrose. Follow with the cosyntropin stimulation test. Dexamethasone is used because it does not interfere with the test.
- Maintenance therapy: start with prednisone, 5 mg PO every morning and 2.5 mg PO at bedtime. Adjust the dose to minimize symptoms.

Fluid and Electrolytes

Joseph T. Santoso

DEHYDRATION

Etiology

Nausea/vomiting, decreased oral intake, third spacing from surgery or infection, diabetic ketoacidosis, sickle cell crisis, bleeding, congestive heart failure.

Signs and Symptoms

- Presentation varies from subjective sensation of thirst to decreased mental status to coma.
- Examination reveals tachycardia, hypotension, decreased skin turgor, and decreased urine output.

Workup

- History, physical examination with vital signs, urine output, O_2 saturation.
- Laboratory studies: CBC, urinalysis, electrolytes.
- Diagnostic tests: X-ray, CT scan, or exploratory laparotomy, as indicated.
- Daily weight is the best means of monitoring fluid status.

Treatment

A. IV fluid bolus; consider blood transfusion as indicated; increase urine output to more than 1 mL/kg/hour, if possible.
B. IV fluid requirement based on weight in an adult is about 30 to 35 mL/kg/day.
C. In congestive heart failure, the patient may not respond to fluid replacement.
D. Treat the underlying disorder.
E. Suggested fluid types:
    1. Lactated Ringer's (LR): to expand plasma volume. Used during the first 24 hours postoperatively or for replacement

of fluid loss. This solution is preferred for complicated surgical patients. Cannot be mixed with blood transfusion as the excess calcium in the LR may increase clot formation in the blood units.[1] Lactate is converted into bicarbonate and may cause alkalosis. In some patients, potassium supplement may not be needed in the first 24 hours due to potassium release from damaged red cells during the surgery. In the setting of hypovolemia/metabolic alkalosis, LR may worsen alkalosis when lactate is metabolized.

2. 0.9% NaCl: to expand plasma volume. Can cause hyperchloremic metabolic acidosis. The only IV fluid that can be mixed with blood.

3. D_5 0.45% NaCl or 0.45% LR: used after the first 24 hours postoperatively as maintenance fluids in uncomplicated postoperative patients. Addition of D_5 makes it an isotonic solution.

4. Albumin: comes as 5% and 25%. Start with 5%. Roughly, 3 mL of NaCl produces an oncotic pressure equal to 1 mL 5% albumin. May cause hypernatremia.

5. D_5W: 50 g of glucose in 1 L of water. Usually not used for resuscitation.

F. Types of fluid and their composition (see Table 18–1).

TABLE 18–1.*

Solution	Na	K	Ca	Cl	HCO$_3$	HPO$_4$	Osm	Glucose
Extra-cellular fluid	**142**	**4**	**5**	**103**	**27**	3	**290**	—
0.9% NaCl	**154**	—	—	**154**	—	—	**308**	—
Lactated Ringer's	**130**	**4**	2.7	**109**	**28**	—	**272**	—
3% NaCl	**513**	—	—	**513**	—	—	**1026**	—
D_5W	—	—	—	—	—	—	**252**	50 g

*Bold amounts in μ/L; other unspecified amounts in mg/dL.

HYPONATREMIA (Na < 136 mEq/L)

Etiology

See later Workup discussion.

Signs and Symptoms

Presentation varies from asymptomatic to confusion and seizure (when Na < 120 mEq/L).

Workup

A. Obtain accurate sodium level.
   1. Check serum osmolarity (mOsm/kg) = [Na(mEq/L) × 2] + [glu (mg/dL)/18] + [BUN (mg/dL)/2.8].
   2. Correct sodium for hyperglycemia (if present)
      a. Na (corrected) = Na = (Glucose − 5) / 3.5
      b. Na, Glucose (mmol)
B. Based on the calculated osmolarity, differential diagnoses are made:
   1. Hypertonic (P Osm > 280)—usually due to hyperglycemia, mannitol.
   2. Isotonic—hyperlipidemia, hyperproteinemia, glucose, mannitol
   3. Hypotonic—three types, based on ECF volume status. Hypotonic hyponatremia can be divided based on the patient's volume status:
      (1) Hypovolemic: GI loss, third spacing, adrenal insufficiency, renal loss (diuretics/renal damage). Treatment is isotonic NaCl infusion.
      (2) Hypervolemic: CHF, liver disease, nephrosis. Treatments are furosemide, restricting free water to 500 mL/day, 0.9% NaCl infusion.
      (3) Isovolemic: SIADH, renal failure, H_2O intoxication, potassium loss. Treatment is mainly water restriction of less than 500 mL/day.

Treatment

A. In symptomatic hyponatremia (lethargy, seizure, headache), the amount Na required is as follows: [125 − plasma Na] × total body water = mEq Na needed/day. *Note:* 125 is the level of Na at which a seizure is less likely to happen. Total body water is 60% (for male) or 50% (for female) of body weight.
B. *Example:* a patient has acute hyponatremia with a recent serum Na level of 100 mEq/L. Her weight is 50 kg. Na

needed to be replaced is $(125 - 100) \times 0.5 \times 50$ kg $= 625$ mEq. Because 3% hypertonic saline contains 0.5 mEq Na/mL, the volume needed is 625 mEq: 0.5 mEq/mL $=$ 1250 mL. Give this amount of 3% NaCl over 6 hours. Do not allow serum Na to increase more than 12 mEq/mL during the first 24 hours. A too-rapid correction causes central pontine myelinolysis and pulmonary edema.

C. The main principle is: acute hyponatremia, treat acutely (i.e., increase serum sodium 2 mEq/hour). Chronic hyponatremia, treat chronically (i.e., increase serum sodium < 10 mEq/day).

D. SIADH is characterized by:
1. Hypotonic hyponatremic euvolemia.
2. Less than maximally dilute urine (urine osmolality $>$ 100 mOsm/kg).
3. Elevated urine sodium (> 20 mEq/L).
4. Normal renal, adrenal, and thyroid function.

E. Treatment of acute SIADH is acute sodium replacement, as described previously. Chronic SIADH can be treated with water restriction and increased salt intake. Demeclocycline (300 to 600 mg/day) antagonizes the effect of ADH. Demeclocycline is nephrotoxic in patients with liver disease.

HYPERNATREMIA (Na > 144 mEq/mL)

Etiology

See later Workup discussion.

Signs and Symptoms

Presentation varies from asymptomatic to altered mental status and seizure.

Workup and Treatment

A. Always associated with hypertonicity. Check the patient's volume status:
1. Hypernatremia—hypervolemic (Na gain $> H_2O$): TPN, aldosteronism, Cushing's disease, congenital adrenal hy-

perplasia. Treatment: starts with 20 mg furosemide IV and D_5W infusion.

2. Hypernatremia—isovolemic: due to central/renal diabetes insipidus (DI), iatrogenic (TPN), skin loss. In DI, serum osmolarity is much more concentrated than urine osmolarity (dilute urine). Treatment: in DI, use vasopressin 5 U SC or 1 U/hour IV titrated to UO 100 to 200 mL/hr. In iatrogenic causes, treat the underlying disorder, then use D_5W IV or water PO.

3. Hypernatremia—hypovolemic: due to diuretic, glycosuria, renal failure, GI/respiratory loss. Treatment: use 0.9% NaCl until euvolemia. Then use D_5W or ½ NS. In renal failure, use dialysis.

B. Water deficit calculation is as follows:

$$\text{Body water deficit} = \text{Normal body water} - \text{Current body water}$$

$$= [0.6 \times \text{body wt in kg}]$$

$$- \frac{[\text{Normal serum Na in mEq/L} \times (0.6 \times \text{wt})]}{\text{Measured serum Na in Eq/L}}$$

Give only half the amount body water deficit in the first 24 hours. The remaining water can be given in the next 1 to 2 days. Cerebral edema may result from overly rapid correction.

HYPOKALEMIA (K < 3.5 mmol/L)

Etiology

- Due to redistribution: 0.1 U change in pH is equal to 0.6 mEq/L change in serum potassium.
- GI losses: NG tube suctioning, vomiting, diarrhea.
- Renal losses: renal tubular acidosis, diuretics, Cushing's disease, postobstructive diuresis.
- Low potassium intake.

Signs and Symptoms

- Presentation varies from asymptomatic to weakness, paralysis, arrhythmia.

- Progressive ECG changes: frequent PVC → flat or inverted T waves → U wave → depressed S-T segment → prolonged PR → tall P waves → widened QRS.

Workup

Check other electrolytes; rule out underlying disorder; obtain an ECG.

Treatment

- Maximal potassium infusion in unmonitored unit is 10 mEq/hour. In severe hypokalemia (with concerning ECG changes) a central line may be used to increase infusion up to 40 mEq/hour under direct physician supervision and continuous ECG monitoring.
- When serum potassium level is 3 or higher, oral supplementation or slower infusion rate may be substituted.
- Concurrent hypomagnesemia must be corrected simultaneously if hypokalemia is to be effectively corrected.

HYPERKALEMIA (K > 5 mmol/L)

Etiology

- Excessive potassium intake.
- Renal failure.

Signs and Symptoms

- Weakness, hypoventilation.
- Progressive ECG changes: tall peaked T waves → widened QRS → depressed S-T → decreased R-wave amplitude → prolonged PR interval → diminished P waves → widened QRS with prolongation of QT interval → sine wave → cardiac arrest.

Workup

Check electrolytes; rule out underlying disorder; obtain an ECG.

Treatment

A. K < 6.5 with no ECG changes: stop all IV K. Repeat serum K immediately.

B. K < 6.5 with ECG changes (only peaked T wave): give Kayexalate, 100 mg, mixed in sorbitol as a retention enema for 45 minutes every hour or 40 g Kayexalate in sorbitol PO every 2 hours.

C. K > 6.5 or any K level with ECG changes more than T waves:
1. In a patient with intact renal function, who is not taking digitalis, start calcium gluconate (90 mg of elemental calcium in a 10-ml ampule) IV over 2 minutes. Onset of action is minutes, with a duration of about 1 hour.
2. If ECG changes persist or if the patient takes digitalis, give sodium bicarbonate (45 mEq) IV over 5 minutes. Bicarbonate shifts potassium into the cell within 15 to 30 minutes with a 1- to 2-hour duration.
3. If ECG changes persist, give glucose (one ampule D_{50}) and insulin (10 U regular) IV. Another option is saline hydration with furosemide.
4. In patients with renal failure who do not respond to the preceding treatment, consider dialysis.

HYPOMAGNESEMIA (Mg < 1.3 mEq/L)

Etiology

- Chemotherapy: occurs in up to 50% of patients receiving cisplatin.
- GI losses (diarrhea, NG suction, prolonged bowel rest, fistula).
- Alcoholism, diabetic ketoacidosis.

Signs and Symptoms

Arrhythmias, seizures, neuromuscular excitability.

Workup

- Serum magnesium level.
- Obtain history of nephrotoxic drugs (i.e., cisplatin).

Treatment

- Treat the underlying disorder (except for cisplatin toxicity).
- Give magnesium sulfate, 2 g IV and/or 500 mg Mg gluconate tablets PO, 2 to 8 tablets/day.
- Mg gluconate is less effective than $MgSO_4$ but causes less abdominal cramping and diarrhea.

HYPERMAGNESEMIA (Mg > 2.1 mEq/L)

Etiology

Overdose, renal failure.

Signs and Symptoms

Respiratory depression, fatigue, muscle weakness.

Workup

Rule out any underlying disorder.

Treatment

Give calcium gluconate, 90 to 180 mg (10 to 20 mL of a 10% solution) IV over 5 to 10 minutes. In severe or refractory cases, consider dialysis.

HYPOPHOSPHATEMIA (phosphates < 2.5 mg/dL)

Etiology

Poor GI absorption, increased renal excretion or reentrance of phosphate into the cells.

Signs and Symptoms

In severe cases, symptoms include weakness, respiratory or heart failure, paresthesias, and confusion.

Workup

Rule out any underlying disorder; check electrolyte levels.

Treatment

Patients with moderate hypophosphastemia (1 to 2.5 mg/dL) who are without symptoms do not require treatment. Supplementation may be given with 0.5 to 1 g of elemental phosphorous PO b.i.d. to t.i.d. In severe cases ($<$ 1 mg/dL), the patient may receive 0.08 to 0.16 mmol/kg phosphate (or 2.5 to 5 mg/kg elemental phosphate) in 500 mL of 0.45% NaCl IV over 6 hours. IV infusion should be stopped when the serum phosphorous is 1.5 g/dL. Also check and correct concurrent hypokalemia and hypomagnesemia.

HYPERPHOSPHATEMIA (phosphates $>$ 4.3 mg/dL)

Etiology

Tumor lysis syndrome, hypoparathyroidism, pseudohypoparathyroidism, rhabdomyolysis, respiratory or metabolic acidosis.

Signs and Symptoms

Similar to those for hypocalcemia and ectopic calcifications.

Workup

Rule out any underlying disorder. Serum calcium and phosphate vary inversely.

Treatment

- Acute cases without renal failure can be improved using saline hydration.
- In patients with renal failure, give calcium carbonate to bind with phosphate. Initial dosage is 0.5 to 1 g elemental calcium

PO t.i.d. with meals. The dosage can be increased at intervals of 2 to 4 weeks to a maximum of 3 g t.i.d.
- The goal of therapy is to maintain serum phosphorous levels between 4.5 and 6 mg/dL and serum calcium below 11 mg/dL.
- To minimize ectopic calcification, keep the calcium-phosphorous product below 60. If hyperphosphatemia persists, consider giving aluminium hydroxide or carbonate.

HYPOCALCEMIA (Ca < 8 mg/dL; IONIZED Ca < 1.12 mmol/L)

Etiology

- Hypoalbuminemia (pseudohypocalcemia is the most common, no treatment needed).
- Excess hydration.
- Massive blood transfusion (excess blood preservative-citrate).
- Hyponatremia.
- Chemotherapy (cisplatin, cytosine), antimicrobials (pentamidine, ketoconazole, foscarnet).

Signs and Symptoms

- Carpal spasm when blood cuff measurement is inflated above systolic pressure for 3 minutes (Trousseau's sign).
- Twitching of facial muscles when the facial nerve is tapped anterior to the ear (Chvostek's sign).
- Severe hypocalcemia may cause lethargy, confusion, laryngospasm, seizures, or heart failure (prolonged QT interval).

Workup

Rule out any underlying disorder, electrolytes.

Treatment

- Acutely, 2 g calcium gluconate (180 mg elemental calcium or 20 mL of 10% calcium gluconate) IV over 10 minutes, followed by infusion of 6 g calcium gluconate in 500 mL of

D_5W over 4 to 6 hours. The infusion goal is to reach a calcium level between 8 and 9 mg/dL.

- Hypomagnesemia must also be corrected. Patients taking digitalis require continuous cardiac monitoring as hypocalcemia potentiates digitalis toxicity.
- Chronic treatment: calcium carbonate (Tums extra strength, 250 to 500 mg elemental calcium).

HYPERCALCEMIA (Ca > 11 mg/dL; IONIZED Ca > 1.23 mmol/L)

Etiology

- May result from bone metastasis, primary hyperparathyroidism, or increased local osteoclastic activity (as in multiple myeloma and some lymphomas).
- The most common etiology is tumor secretion of a parathyroid hormone–related protein (PTHrP). PTHrP is almost structurally homologous as compared to the parathyroid hormone (PTH). Between 50% and 80% of patients with humoral hypercalcemia have elevated serum PTHrP and suppressed PTH levels.[2] PTHrP induces calcium release into the blood, resulting in polyuria, abdominal pain, and constipation with progressive dehydration, and decreasing renal perfusion. This increases renal reabsorption of calcium and therefore worsens serum hypercalcemia.
- Serum PTH is high in primary parathyroidism and low in malignancy.
- Albumin-corrected serum calcium (mg/dL) = serum calcium (mg/dL) + [0.8 (4 − serum albumin in g/dL)].

Signs and Symptoms and Workup

- Symptoms related to paraneoplastic hypercalcemia usually surface rapidly in contrast to the gradual presentation of primary hyperparathyroidism.
- Neurologically, the patient may complain of nausea, vomiting, and abdominal pain. Additional symptoms include weakness, confusion, coma, arrhythmias, and hypertension. Furthermore, hypercalcemia causes reversible renal tubular deficiency

in concentrating urine. Subsequently, the patient has a large volume of urine which causes further dehydration.
- Acute hypercalcemia causes bradycardia. In moderate hypercalcemia, the QT interval is shortened. In severe hypercalcemia, the QT interval is prolonged. Be careful when using digitalis in patients with hypercalcemia.

Treatment

- Initial treatment consists of vigorous IV hydration. Once the patient is no longer dehydrated, furosemide may be added. Urine output goal is more than 2 L of urine/day. Ethacrynic acid (a loop diuretic) is an acceptable alternative; however, thiazide diuretics should not be used. For more refractory hypercalcemia, pamidronate, calcitonin, and steroids (especially in patients with breast cancer) have been used.
- The most effective agent is pamidronate (Aredia), a bone resorption (osteoclast) inhibitor. For a corrected serum calcium level of 12 to 13.5 mg/dL, administer a single dose of 60 mg IV over a minimum of 4 hours. For a corrected serum calcium level of more than 13.5 mg/dL, administer a single dose of 90 mg IV over 24 hours. Improvement should be seen in 2 days. Allow a minimum of 7 days to elapse before retreatment with pamidronate to allow for full response to the initial dose. The effect may persist for more than 2 weeks. Alternatives are etidronate (Didronel) 20 mg/kg/d, which can be used as a maintenance agent or plicamycin (25 μg/kg over 6 hours), but plicamycin is more toxic.
- The most rapid-acting agent is calcitonin (onset: 2 hours; duration: about 6 to 8 hours; safe usage in renal failure). The dose is 4 IU/kg SQ or IM every 12 hours. Perform skin testing with 1 U (0.1 mL of a 1:10 dilution of calcitonin) to rule out allergy.
- Steroids take several days to lower the calcium level. The dose is hydrocortisone, 100 mg IV every 6 hours for 24 hours, followed with prednisone, 10 to 30 mg/day PO for

about 1 week. If there is no response after 1 week, taper the dose and discontinue use.

- Gallium nitrate is given via continuous IV infusion (200 mg/m^2/day for 5 days). It is nephrotoxic and experience with the drug is limited.
- Phosphate will bind to calcium and decreases its serum level regardless of the etiology of hypercalcemia. Although effective, phosphate administration has complications, including MI, hypotension, acute renal failure, and ectopic calcifications. Use oral phosphate only in mild or moderate hypercalcemia in patients *with* a low phosphate level or as the last resort before dialysis. The dose is 0.5 to 1 g elemental phosphorous t.i.d. PO.

REFERENCES

1. KING WH, PATTEN ED, BEE DE: An in vitro evaluation of ionized calcium levels and clotting in red blood cells diluted with LR solution. Anesthesiology 68:115, 1988.
2. BUNN PA JR, RIDGEWAY EC: Paraneoplastic syndromes, in *Cancer: Principles and Practice of Oncology,* 4th ed, VT Devita, S Hellman, SA Rosenberg, (eds). Philadelphia, Lippincott, 1993, p 2036.

Joseph T. Santoso

MAIN PRINCIPLES OF BLOOD GASES

- Pa_{O_2}: Represents the partial pressure of O_2 in alveoli, with normal value ranges between 80 and 100 mmHg. This value is directly measured. Pa_{O_2} is age dependent (see calculation that follows).
- Pa_{CO_2}: Represents the partial pressure of CO_2 and correlates directly with alveolar ventilation. Low respiratory rate or abnormal low tidal volume causes elevated Pa_{CO_2}.
- O_2 saturation depends on Pa_{O_2}, Pa_{CO_2}, temperature, and 2,3-DPG. O_2 in an arterial blood gas sample is calculated using Pa_{O_2}, Pa_{CO_2}, temperature, and pH. But the level of 2,3-DPG is not accounted for. Most importantly, in a venous sample, the O_2 dissociation curve is at the steepest slope. Consequently, any minuscule inaccuracy in P_{O_2} would cause a significant error in reading the O_2 saturation. Therefore, a co-oximeter should be used for a more accurate value of venous O_2 saturation (mixed venous O_2 saturation) but is not necessary in the arterial blood sample.
- Measured variables in ABGs (more accurate): P_{O_2}, P_{CO_2}.
- Calculated variables in ABGs (less accurate): O_2 saturation, HCO_3, pH.
- Pressure alveolar-arterial (A-a) O_2 gradient equals PA_{O_2} minus Pa_{O_2}.

  $PA_{O_2} = Pi_{O_2} - Pa_{CO_2}/0.8$ (where Pi_{O_2} is equal to 21% × 760 mmHg).

  Pa_{O_2} = the value you get from your ABGs.

  Normal $P(A-a)_{O_2}$ in a 20-year-old person = 5 to 10 mmHg. In chronic obstructive pulmonary disease, a $P(A-a)_{O_2}$ greater than 40 mmHg and is accompanied by an increase in P_{CO_2} and low Pa_{O_2}.

HOW TO READ ARTERIAL BLOOD GASES (ABGs)

A. Normal Pa_{O_2} is greater than 85 to 90 mmHg. Pa_{O_2} decreases with age. To calculate what is normal Pa_{O_2} based on age:

1. Upright position = $104.2 - [0.27 \times$ age (years)].
2. Supine = $103.5 - [0.42 \times$ age (years)].
3. Causes of hypoxemia are hypoventilation, A-V shunt, V/Q mismatch, and diffusion impairment (in critically ill patients, low mixed venous O_2 saturation).

B. P_{CO_2} is normally around 40 mmHg. Look at P_{CO_2} from the blood gas.
   1. If the blood gas P_{CO_2} is greater than 40 mmHg, respiratory acidosis is present.
   2. If the blood gas P_{CO_2} is less than 40 mmHg, respiratory alkalosis is present.

C. Determine if metabolic acidosis or alkalosis is present by obtaining the expected pH based on P_{CO_2} from blood gas:

P_{CO_2}	64	51	40	32	25
Expected pH*	7.2	7.3	7.4	7.5	7.6

*pH = $6.1 + \log [HCO_3 / (0.03 \times P_{CO_3})]$

D. Next, compare the expected pH against the pH from blood gas.
   1. If the blood gas pH is less than the expected pH, metabolic acidosis is present.
   2. If the blood gas pH is greater than the expected pH, metabolic alkalosis is present.
   3. For example, if the blood gas pH is 7.3 and the expected pH is 7.4, then metabolic acidosis is present.

E. HCO_3 is approximately 24 mEq/L.
   1. If the blood gas HCO_3 is less than 24 mEq/L, the buffer has been used (probably acute acidosis).
   2. If the blood gas HCO_3 is around 24 mEq/L, the buffer has returned to normal (probably chronic acid-base imbalance).

MANAGEMENT OF ABNORMAL ABGs (LIST OF DIFFERENTIAL DIAGNOSIS)

Respiratory Acidosis

- Use $P(A-a)O_2$ to generate the differential diagnoses and workup.
- Normal $P(A-a)O_2$: central nervous system (drug overdose,

hypoventilation), paralysis, airway obstruction, chest-wall failure.
- Elevated $P(A-a)O_2$: chronic obstructive pulmonary disease, cystic fibrosis, scoliosis.
- Duration of disturbance = ratio of change in $H+/PCO_2$. In the absence of ABGs, pH and PCO_2 are assumed to be 7.4 and 40. Changes in HCO_3 reflect nonrenal buffering. Patients with chronic conditions will show normalized pH value but never exactly normal HCO_3.

Respiratory Alkalosis

- Normal $P(A-a)O_2$: central nervous system, aspirin, progesterone, pregnancy, high altitude (hyperventilation).
- Elevated $P(A-a)O_2$: infection, pulmonary edema, interstitial lung disease.

Metabolic Acidosis

- Anion gap (unmeasured ion) = $Na - (Cl + HCO_3)$. Normal value: 8 to 12.
- With increased anion gap (KLIK):
  K—Ketoacidosis: diabetes mellitus, starvation, or alcohol abuse.
  L—Lactic acidosis: shock, aspirin.
  I—Intoxication: aspirin, methanol, ethylene glycol.
  K—Kidney failure: accumulation of organic waste.
- Without increased anion gap:
  Renal—renal tubular acidosis I, II, IV, excessive acetazolamide (carbonic anhydrase inhibitor).
  GI—diarrhea, pancreatic fistula.
  Mineral acids—NH_4Cl, $CaCl_2$.

Metabolic Alkalosis

- Hydrogen losses: vomiting, NG suction, diuretics, hypokalemia.
- HCO_3 gain: massive blood transfusion, renal failure, lactate.
- Contraction (hypovolemic) alkalosis.

Pain Control

Sara Crowder and Joseph T. Santoso

GENERAL CONCEPTS

Delivering adequate pain control is one of the most important jobs of a gynecologic oncologist. In general, we are asked to offer short-term, acute pain control (i.e., postoperatively) and long-term chronic pain control (i.e., for painful, progressive disease). Pain management requires a foundation of basic principles and medication information.

- For acute pain: Use immediate-release medications for a short period of time. *Example:* A postoperative patient is given intravenous morphine sulfate intermittently (or with a patient-controlled analgesia [PCA] pump) until she is able to tolerate oral pain medications.
- For chronic pain: Use controlled-release narcotic medications for a sustained effect with immediate-release medications on a prn basis. *Example:* A patient with progressive cancer pain no longer responsive to prn pain medications is admitted and placed on a PCA device with morphine to quickly titrate her 24-hour narcotic needs. Then, the parenteral needs are converted into long-acting tablets or patches that are supplemented with immediate-release medications for breakthrough pain.

PAIN ASSESSMENT

Assessment should start with a complete history and physical examination. Failure to reassess the patient's pain often leads to undertreatment. It is recommended that pain be assessed at regular intervals after initiation of treatment, at each new report of pain, and after giving pain medication. It is also important to differentiate the etiology of pain. The management of pain may be markedly different for different etiology. For example, pain from progressive cancer may require a narcotic dose increase while surgery may be indicated for pain for acute complication such as bowel ischemia.

PAIN MANAGEMENT[1]

- Use the simplest dosage schedules and least invasive pain management modalities first.
- For mild to moderate pain, use (unless contraindicated) aspirin, acetaminophen, or NSAID (World Health Organization [WHO] ladder, step 1).
- When pain persists or increases, add an opioid (WHO ladder, step 2).
- If pain increases, increase the opioid potency or dose (WHO ladder, step 3).
- Schedule doses regularly (i.e., "by the clock") to maintain the level of drug that will help prevent recurrence of pain. Ask for patient and family cooperation in establishing the effective level.
- Administer additional doses "as needed" for breakthrough pain.

ROUTE OF ADMINISTRATION[1]

- *Oral:* the most convenient and inexpensive route.
- *Rectal:* an effective route for delivery when patients have nausea or vomiting. It should not be used for patients with diarrhea, anal/rectal lesions, mucositis, thrombocytopenia, or neutropenia; those who are physically unable to place the suppository in the rectum; or those who prefer other routes.
- *Transdermal (Fentanyl):* patches provide analgesia lasting up to 72 hours. They are not suitable for rapid dose titration and should be used for relatively stable analgesic requirement when rapid increases or decreases in dosage are not likely to be needed.
- *Intermittent Injection or Continuous Infusion:* IV and SC routes provide effective opioid delivery. Methadone may cause skin irritation when infused subcutaneously or intravenously.
- *Patient-Controlled Analgesia (PCA):* the opioid may be administered orally or via a dedicated portable pump to deliver the drug intravenously, subcutaneously, or intraspinally.

- *Intraspinal:* consider this invasive route for patients who develop intractable pain or intolerable side effects with other routes. It is used for intractable pain in the lower part of the body, particularly bilateral or midline pain. Profound analgesia is possible without motor, sensory, or sympathetic blockade. Local anesthetics may be combined with opioids for intraspinal administration.

OPIOID SIDE EFFECTS (MODIFIED FROM REFERENCE 1)

Constipation

A decreased bowel peristalsis results in increased water reabsorption from the stool, leading to hardened stool. Consequently, all patients using opioid medications should be well hydrated in addition to taking a scheduled regimen of stool-softening agents (e.g., docusate sodium). Claims that transdermal fentanyl causes less constipation than oral morphine are promising but need to be confirmed in prospective studies.

Nausea and Vomiting

This side effect occurs in one-third to two-thirds of patients taking opioids. Opioids stimulate the chemoreceptor trigger zone and reduce GI motility, including delayed gastric emptying. Nausea usually resolves after the first week of treatment. An antiemetic such as metoclopramide is recommended as a first-line agent as it also improves gut motility. The role of $5-HT_3$ receptor antagonists such as ondansetron in ameliorating opioid-induced nausea is not clear. An alternative treatment is to switch different opioids to reduce nausea. Switching the route, specifically from the oral to the parenteral, has also been suggested, but the studies supporting this strategy are few.

Nausea and vomiting may become chronic in nature and probably are due to accumulation of active opioid metabolites. A number of strategies are suggested to manage this, including switching the opioid or decreasing the dose where pain is well controlled.

Opioid-Induced Delirium

Rule out acute complications such as sepsis, hypercalcemia, other drug interaction, sun-downing syndrome, and dehydration as other possible etiologies for delirium. In controlling agitation from delirium, haloperidol is the first choice, with methotrimeprazine and chlorpromazine considered as alternatives. Midazolam, a sedating and short-acting benzodiazepine given by continuous infusion, is sometimes necessary, especially in the case of nonreversible delirium. In opioid-induced delirium, consider a dose reduction or an opioid switch.

Respiratory Depression

Patients receiving chronic opioid therapy are usually not prone to respiratory depression.

Subacute Overdose

This side effect may manifest as slowly progressive (hours to days) somnolence and respiratory depression. Before reducing analgesic doses, advancing disease must be considered, especially in the dying patient. Generally, withholding 1 or 2 doses of an opioid analgesic is adequate to assess whether mental and respiratory depression are opioid related. If symptoms resolve after temporary opioid withdrawal, reduce the scheduled opioid dosage by 25%. If symptoms do not abate but the patient complains of or exhibits signs of increased pain, or if symptoms referable to opioid withdrawal occur, consider alternative causes for CNS depression and reinstitute analgesic treatment. Ongoing assessment is essential to maintain adequate pain relief.

Opioid Effect on Libido

Opioids diminish libido, causing sexual dysfunction, reduced testosterone levels in men, and amenorrhea in women. These effects resolve after the opioid has been discontinued.

Other Opioid Side Effects

Dry mouth, urinary retention, pruritus, myoclonus, dysphoria, euphoria, sleep disturbances, and inappropriate secretion of antidiuretic hormone are less common.

MEDICATIONS

IV Medications

- Morphine sulfate: binds to the opioid mu or morphine receptor. According to the WHO, morphine sulfate is the prototype opioid for severe cancer-related pain.
- Meperidine (Demerol): synthetic opioid. Has a quicker onset of action, but shorter duration of pain relief. Its metabolite is a potent convulsant. Side effects may occur from frequent dosing, which may result in a buildup of metabolites. We avoid using it for cancer-related pain.
- Hydromorphone (Dilaudid): five times more potent than morphine. It has a shorter duration of action. May be useful if high doses of subcutaneous opioids are needed.
- Methadone (Dolophine): synthetic opioid that has a long half-life but a short duration of effect; sedation or overdosing can easily occur.

Patient-Controlled Analgesia (PCA)

- An IV pump that allows for a basal rate of a maintenance medication to be delivered automatically (usually hourly) at a dose determined by the physician. It also has a "demand" button that allows the patient to self-administer a certain amount of medication at a certain interval (any more frequent and the patient is locked out); this allows the patient to titrate her own medication needs without having to rely on the availability of nursing staff.
- Morphine is the preferred pain medication for use with PCA. However, other parenteral opioids can be substituted for morphine.

- Examples of PCA orders:
    Morphine sulfate 30 mg/30 mL (or 100 mg/30 mL for high doses).
    Basal (continuous) rate: 1 mg/hour.
    Demand dose: 1 mg.
    Lockout (dose delay): 6 minutes.
    One-hour limit (maximum dose/hour): 11 mL/hour (not including RN bolus).
    RN can bolus 1 to 2 mL/hour prn pain.
    If respiratory rate <10, give 0.4 mg of Narcan IV push; stop PCA, keep IV TKO with D_5W, and call MD.
    Phenergan 50 mg IV q 8 h prn. Benadryl 25 mg IV/IM q 6 h prn.
    Urinary/constipation prn (Foley catheter if no UO in 6 hours, stool softener of choice).
- On postoperative day 1 or 2, the basal rate can be discontinued, and the patient can continue to use the demand button prn as she is transitioned to ambulating and PO intake. The demand button can be discontinued when the patient takes PO pain medication.

Sustained-Release Medications

These medications are usually used for maintenance of chronic pain in conjunction with immediate-release medications (either combined or opioid only) or breakthrough medications (see later discussion). SR medications are used as scheduled doses and not on a prn basis.

Morphine

- *Brand name:* MS Contin.
- Dosing: comes in 15-, 30-, 60-, 100-, and 200-mg tablets.
- Brand-name tablets are blue, purple, orange, gray, and green; strength is indicated on pill.
- Schedule: Recommended dosing is every 12 hours, but many clinicians find that dosing every 8 hours gives better pain control.

Morphine (continued)

- *Brand name:* Oramorph SR.
- Dosing: comes in 15-, 30-, 60-, and 100-mg tablets.
- Tablets are all white but have strength indicated on them.
- Schedule: same as for MS Contin.

Oxycodone

- *Brand name:* Oxycontin.
- Dosing: comes in 10-, 20-, 40-, and 80-mg tablets.
- Brand-name tablets are white, pink, yellow, and green; strength is indicated on pill.
- Schedule: recommended dosing is every 12 hours.

Fentanyl Patch

- *Brand name:* Duragesic.
- Dosing: comes in 25-, 50-, 75-, and 100-μg/hour transdermal patches.
- See later conversion tables for relative potency.
- Schedule: patches need to be changed every 72 hours (q3d).

Common Breakthrough Medications

- Vicodin, or any of the other combined analgesics in Table 20–1.
- Morphine:
    MSIR tablets/capsules—15 or 30 mg.
    MSIR oral solution—10 or 20 mg/5 mL (bottles of 120 mL).
    MSIR oral solution concentrate—20 mg/1 mL (bottles of 30 or 120 mL with dropper marked with 5-mg increments).
    Roxanol oral solution—20 mg/1 mL (bottles same as MSIR concentrate).
    Roxanol T oral solution—20 mg/1 mL tinted and flavored concentrated solution.
- Oxycodone:
    Roxicodone tablets—5 mg.
    Roxicodone solution—5 mg/mL.

TABLE 20-1. Combined Analgesics (Oral Medication)

Name	Medications	Doses available (mg)	Interval	Schedule	Comments
Darvocet	Propoxyphene/ acetaminophen	N-50 (50/325) N-100 (100/650)	q 4 h	IV	For mild postoperative pain
Fiorocet	Acetaminophen/ butalbital/caffeine/ codeine	325/50/40/30	q 4 h	III	Commonly used for tension headaches
Fioronal	Aspirin/butalbital/ caffeine/codeine	325/50/40/30	q 4 h	III	Commonly used for tension headaches
Lorcet	Hydrocodone/ acetaminophen	5/500 7.5/650 10/650	q 4–6 h	III	Like Vicodin
Lortab	Hydrocodone/ acetaminophen	2.5/500 5/500 7.5/500 10/500	q 4–6 h	III	Higher doses allow more narcotic with less acetaminophen
Lortab elixir	Hydrocodone/ acetaminophen	2.5/167 per 5 mL	q 4–6 h	III	Good for patients who cannot take tablets
Percocet	Oxycodone/ acetaminophen	5/325	q 6 h	II	Stronger than Vicodin
Percodan	Oxycodone/ aspirin	5/325	q 6 h	II	Stronger than Vicodin

156

Name	Generic	Strength	Frequency	Schedule	Notes
Roxicet	Oxycodone/acetaminophen	5/325 5/500	q 6 h	II	Stronger than Vicodin
Tylenol with codeine	Codeine/acetaminophen	#2 = 15/300 #3 = 30/300 #4 = 60/300	q 4 h	III	For mild postoperative pain
Tylenol with codeine pediatric liquid	Codeine/acetaminophen	12/120 per 5 mL	q 4 h	V	Good for patients who cannot take tablets or pills
Tylox	Oxycodone/acetaminophen	5/500	q 6 h	II	Similar to Percocet, Roxicet
Vicodin	Hydrocodone/acetaminophen	5/500 ES 7.5/750 HP 10/660	q 4–6 h	III	For mild to moderate postoperative pain
Vicoprofen	Hydrocodone/ibuprofen	7.5/200	q 4–6 h	III	For moderate pain; avoid alcohol

TABLE 20–2. DEA Schedules

Class	Description	Examples
I[a]	High abuse potential, no accepted use	Marijuana, heroin
II[a]	High abuse potential, dependence liability	Morphine, oxycodone
III	Moderate dependence liability	Hydrocodone (Vicodin)
IV	Limited dependence liability	Propoxyphene, benzodiazepines
V	Limited abuse potential	Lomotil

[a]Requires triplicate prescription in some states.

Intensol solution—20 mg/mL.

OxyFast oral concentrate solution—20 mg/mL (30-mL bottle with dropper).

OxyIR immediate-release capsule—5, 10, 15, 20, 30, 40, 50, 60 mg.

DEA schedules are listed in Table 20-2.

CONVERSION TABLES AND FORMULAS

A. To convert another opioid to morphine:
  1. Total the amount taken in a 24-hour period that effectively controls pain.
  2. Multiply by the conversion factor in the table (Tables 20-3 and 20-4). Divide by 2 to allow for incomplete cross-tolerance between narcotics (may need to titrate liberally and rapidly to analgesic effect in first 24 hours).
  3. Divide by number of doses per day (e.g., 6 doses for regular PO morphine every 4 hours, or 2 doses for controlled-release morphine every 12 hours) to determine the individual dose.
B. To convert to transdermal fentanyl (Duragesic):
  1. Determine 24-hour morphine equivalent requirement using the previous tables.
  2. Select the µg/hour dose according to the ranges listed in Table 20–5. For dosage requirements greater than 100 µg/hour, multiple patches may be used.

TABLE 20–3. Oral and Parenteral Opioid Analgesic Equivalencies and Relative Potency of Drugs as Compared with Morphine

Narcotic agonists	Parenteral (mg)	Oral (mg)	Conversion factor (IV to PO)[a]	Duration
Morphine	10	30	3	3–4 h
Controlled-release morphine (MS Contin, Oramorph SR)	NA	30	NA	12 h
Methadone (Dolophine)[b]	10	20	2	4–8 h
Hydromorphone (Dilaudid)	1.5	7.5	5	2–3 h
Fentanyl[c]	100 µg	NA	NA	1 h
Meperidine (Demerol)[d]	75	300	4	2–3 h
Levorphanol (Levo-Dromoran)[b]	2	4	2	3–6 h
Oxymorphone (Numorphan)	1	6	6 (rectal)	3–6 h
Codeine	130	200	1.5	3–4 h
Oxycodone (Oxycontin,	NA	30	NA	3–5 h
Roxycodone, Percodan, Tylox)[e]				
Hydrocodone (Vicodin, Lortab)	NA	200	NA	3–5 h
Propoxyphene (Darvon, Darvocet)[b,d,e]	NA	200	NA	3–6 h

TABLE 20-3. Oral and Parenteral Opioid Analgesic Equivalencies and Relative Potency of Drugs as Compared with Morphine (Continued)

Narcotic agonists	Parenteral (mg)	Oral (mg)	Conversion factor (IV to PO)[a]	Duration
Partial agonist				
Buprenorphine (Buprenex)[f]	0.3	NA	NA	4–6 h
Mixed Agonist-Antagonists				
Pentazocine (Talwin)	Partial agonists and mixed agonist-antagonists have limited usefulness in cancer pain. They should not be used in combination with narcotic agonist drugs. Converting a patient from an agonist to an agonist-antagonist could precipitate a withdrawal crisis in the narcotic-dependent patient.			
Nalbuphine (Nubain)				
Butorphanol (Stadol)				

NA = not available.

[a]Conversion factor listed is for chronic dosing—single doses can require 6:1 factor.

[b]Long half-life; observe for drug accumulation and side effects.

[c]Available in transdermal system (Duragesic) supplying 25, 50, 75, or 100 μg/hour.

[d]Not recommended for long-term or high-dose use because of CNS toxic metabolites (normeperidine, norpropoxyphene).

[e]With the exception of Roxycodone and Darvon, these drugs are combined with ASA or acetaminophen in 325- to 750-mg doses. Dosage must be monitored for safe limits of ASA or acetaminophen.

[f]Partial agonist can produce withdrawal in opioid-dependent patients.

TABLE 20–4. Conversion Factors (Other Opioids to Morphine)

From oral	To oral morphine	From parenteral	To parenteral morphine
Methadone	1.5	Methadone	1
Hydromorphone	4	Hydromorphone	6.7
Meperidine	0.1	Meperidine	0.13
Levorphanol	7.5	Levorphanol	5
Codeine	0.15	Codeine	0.08
Oxycodone	1	Oxymorphone	10
Hydrocodone	0.15	Buprenorphine	25
Oxymorphone (rectal)	5		

3. Patch duration = 72 hours. To effectively titrate the dose, prescribe a prn dose of morphine or other narcotic, especially during the first 12 hours. Increase the dose based on the average amount of additional narcotic required over the next 72-hour period.

TABLE 20–5. Conversion of Morphine to Fentanyl Patch Per 24 Hours

Parenteral morphine (mg/24 hours)	Fentanyl patch (Duragesic) equivalent (μg/hour)
8–22	25
23–37	50
38–52	75
53–67	100
68–82	125
83–97	150

TABLE 20–6. Amount of Rescue Analgesic at Which a 25-μg/hour Increase in Duragesic Is Recommended

Oral	Mg/24 hours
Codeine	300
Oxycodone	45
Hydrocodone	45
Morphine	90
Hydromorphone	12

TABLE 20–7. Equianalgesic Conversion of Parenteral Opioids to MS Contin

Current parenteral opioid	IM/IV/SC dose and schedule	Approximate equianalgesic regimen of MS Contin tablets
Morphine	5 mg q 4 h	3 MS Contin tab 15 mg q 12 h
	10 mg q 4 h	3 MS Contin tab 30 mg q 12 h
	20 mg q 4 h	3 MS Contin tab 60 mg q 12 h
	33 mg q 4 h	3 MS Contin tab 100 mg q 12 h
Hydromorphone (Dilaudid)	1 mg q 4 h	2 MS Contin tab 30 mg q 12 h
	2 mg q 4 h	2 MS Contin tab 60 mg q 12 h
	4 mg q 3 h	3 MS Contin tab 100 mg q 12 h
Methadone (Dolophine)	5 mg q 6 h	2 MS Contin tab 15 mg q 12 h
	7 mg q 4 h	2 MS Contin tab 30 mg q 12 h
	20 mg q 4 h	3 MS Contin tab 60 mg q 12 h
	50 mg q 6 h	3 MS Contin tab 100 mg q 12 h
Meperidine (Demerol)	75 mg q 4 h	3 MS Contin tab 30 mg q 12 h
	150 mg q 4 h	3 MS Contin tab 60 mg q 12 h
	250 mg q 4 h	3 MS Contin tab 100 mg q 12 h
Levorphanol (Levo-Dromoran)	2 mg q 6 h	2 MS Contin tab 30 mg q 12 h
	4 mg q 6 h	2 MS Contin tab 60 mg q 12 h
	9 mg q 4 h	4 MS Contin tab 100 mg q 12 h

TABLE 20–8. Equianalgesic Conversion of Oral Opioids to MS Contin

Current oral product	PO dose and schedule	Approximate equianalgesic regimen of MS Contin tablets
Morphine—immediate release (MSIR)	10 mg q 4 h	2 MS Contin tab 15 mg q 12 h
	30 mg q 4 h	3 MS Contin tab 30 mg q 12 h
	80 mg q 4 h	4 MS Contin tab 60 mg q 12 h
	100 mg q 4 h	3 MS Contin tab 100 mg q 12 h
Hydromorphone (Dilaudid)	4 mg q 4 h	3 MS Contin tab 15 mg q 12 h
	8 mg q 4 h	3 MS Contin tab 30 mg q 12 h
	10 mg q 4 h	2 MS Contin tab 60 mg q 12 h
	25 mg q 4 h	3 MS Contin tab 100 mg q 12 h
Methadone (Dolophine)	10 mg q 6 h	2 MS Contin tab 15 mg q 12 h
	20 mg q 6 h	2 MS Contin tab 30 mg q 12 h
	30 mg q 4 h	2 MS Contin tab 60 mg q 12 h
	70 mg q 4 h	3 MS Contin tab 100 mg q 12 h
Meperidine (Demerol)	100 mg q 3 h	2 MS Contin tab 15 mg q 12 h
	200 mg q 3 h	2 MS Contin tab 30 mg q 12 h
	600 mg q 3 h	4 MS Contin tab 60 mg q 12 h
	1000 mg q 3 h	4 MS Contin tab 100 mg q 12 h
Levorphanol (Levo-Dromoran)	2 mg q 6 h	2 MS Contin tab 15 mg q 12 h
	4 mg q 6 h	2 MS Contin tab 30 mg q 12 h
	6 mg q 4 h	2 MS Contin tab 60 mg q 12 h
	14 mg q 4 h	3 MS Contin tab 100 mg q 12 h

TABLE 20–8. Equianalgesic Conversion of Oral Opioids to MS Contin (*Continued*)

Current oral product	PO dose and schedule	Approximate equianalgesic regimen of MS Contin tablets
Oxycodone	10 mg q 4 h	2 MS Contin tab 15 mg q 12 h
	20 mg q 4 h	2 MS Contin tab 30 mg q 12 h
	40 mg q 4 h	2 MS Contin tab 60 mg q 12 h
	100 mg q 4 h	3 MS Contin tab 100 mg q 12 h

REFERENCE

1. Pain (PDQ). National Cancer Institute. Available: http://cancer-net.nci.nih.gov/pdq/pdq_supportive_care.shtml.

Joseph T. Santoso

FEVER

Etiology

- Benign: atelectasis, postoperative period, tumor fever (diagnosis of exclusion).
- Serious: infection (UTI, pneumonia, abscess, cellulitis, wound breakdown), thromboembolic (DVT, PE), ureteral obstruction, HIV.
- Rare: tuberculosis, infective endocarditis, drugs, connective tissue diseases, thyroiditis sarcoidosis, Q fever, hemolytic anemia, factitious fever, fever of unknown origin.

Signs and Symptoms

Fever—defined as consecutive temperatures >38°C (100.6°F) more than 6 h apart, after first 24 h of surgery, or single temperature >39°C (102.5°F)—with or without pain.

Workup

- History and physical examination.
- For the first 48 hours after surgery, the clinician need only to examine the patient if clinically well.
- If abnormal physical findings are noted, obtain CBC, urinalysis, urine and blood cultures, and chest x-ray, as indicated to rule out infection. CT scan or ultrasound for abscess.
- Obtain a Doppler sonogram of the lower extremities if DVT is suspected; VQ scan to rule out PE.
- Order an IVP to rule out ureteral obstruction (get creatinine first before injecting contrast agent).

Treatment

Treat accordingly to etiology.

ABSCESS OR PERITONITIS (PELVIC/ABDOMEN)

Etiology

Bacteria from bowel (perforation, anastomotic leak, tumor invasion).

Signs and Symptoms

Localized abdominal/pelvic pain, which is generalized after peritonitis sets in; fever; tachycardia; pain; hypotension (severe case).

Workup

- History and physical examination.
- CBC, blood culture, creatinine, CT scan, or ultrasound.

Treatment

- Start with ampicillin, gentamicin, and metronidazole while awaiting results of culture sensitivity.
- The abscess may be drained percutaneously or the clinician may choose to perform exploratory laparotomy.

CELLULITIS

Etiology

Staphylococcus aureus and streptococci.

Signs and Symptoms

- Erythema, painful skin lesion.
- Fever, mild tachycardia.

Workup

- CBC. Wound culture may not help because cellulitis resolves by the time the culture result comes back.
- Rule out underlying abscess or seroma.

Treatment

- Oxacillin, 1 to 2 g IV every 6 hours, or cefazolin, 1 to 2 g IV every 8 hours. Use vancomycin, 1 g IV every 12 hours if the patient is allergic to penicillin.
- Cellulitis in a diabetic patient with foot ulcer may benefit from the addition of metronidazole, 500 mg IV every 6 hours. Alternatively, use cefoxitin, 1 to 2 g IV every 8 hours.

NECROTIZING FASCIITIS

Etiology

Polymicrobial bacterial invasion of muscle and fascia, which may lead to gangrene.

Signs and Symptoms

- Fever, tachycardia, pain, pus, black ischemic wound.
- Third spacing from sepsis (low urine output).

Workup

- History and physical examination (crepitus).
- Foley catheter, IV access.
- CBC, blood culture, creatinine, CT scan, or ultrasound.

Treatment

Start with ampicillin, gentamicin, and metronidazole while awaiting results of culture sensitivity, and perform immediate surgical debridement to healthy and well-vascularized tissue once diagnosis suspected.

WOUND/INCISIONAL INFECTION

Etiology

Polymicrobial bacteria in high-risk patients (obese, diabetic, smoker, prior radiation) or contaminated wound.

Signs and Symptoms

Pain, fever, wound drainage, tachycardia.

Workup

- CBC, creatinine.
- Examine incision with cotton swab to rule out fascial dehiscence or subcutaneous abscess.

Treatment

- Give cefoxitin, 1 to 2 g IV every 8 hours.
- Drain abscess or seroma and pack wound with dry-wet dressing.

URINARY TRACT INFECTION/CYSTITIS

Etiology

Mostly *Escherichia coli*. Others are *S. aureus,* chlamydia, ureaplasma, and *Neisseria gonorrhea.*

Signs and Symptoms

Dysuria, polyuria, fever.

Workup

- Urinalysis, urine culture.
- In patients with multiple infections, rule out urologic abnormalities (e.g., fistula).

Treatment

- Trimethoprim/sulfamethoxazole (TMP/SMX) 160/800 mg PO b.i.d. for 3 days.
- Ofloxacin, 200 to 400 mg PO/IV every 12 hours.

PYELONEPHRITIS

Etiology

Usually *E. coli.*

Signs and Symptoms

Fever, flank pain, dysuria.

Workup

CBC, urine and blood cultures, creatinine.

Treatment

- If the patient is clinically stable, give trimethoprim/sulfamethoxazole (TMP/SMX) 160/180 mg PO b.i.d. for 10 to 14 days as outpatient.
- If more ill, use ofloxacin, a third-generation cephalosporin, or gentamicin.
- If enterococcal infection is found, give ampicillin, 1 g IV every 6 hours.
- If symptoms do not resolve within 2 days with antibiotics, order an IVP, an ultrasound, or a CT scan to rule out renal abscess, calculi, or foreign body obstruction.

FEBRILE NEUTROPENIA

Etiology

- Related to myelosuppressive antibiotics and mostly gram-negative infection.
- Various definitions: We use the 1998 GOG chemotherapy manual; temperature greater than 38°C documented twice within a day or a single temperature greater than 38.3°C once, both accompanied by absolute neutrophil count of less than 1000/mm^3.

Signs and Symptoms

Fever, tachycardia, weakness, abscess.

Workup

- CBC, chest x-ray, blood and urine cultures.
- Consider removing a central line if erythema and pus are seen at the site.

Treatment

- Hospitalize all patients with febrile neutropenia.
- Follow neutropenic precautions (hand washing by visitors, minimize rectal examination, brush teeth with a soft brush, no raw vegetables).
- Start ceftazidime, 2 g IV every 8 hours, combined with gentamicin 5 to 7 mg/kg IV every 24 hours, while awaiting culture results and continue until the patient has been afebrile for more than 2 days with an improvement of ANC greater than 1000/mm^3.
- If line sepsis is suspected, consider adding nafcillin or vancomycin.
- If fever persists for 1 week or more, consider adding fluconazole or amphotericin while awaiting fungal cultures.
- GCSF 300 μg/day may decrease the duration of neutropenia.[1]
- In hospitalized low-risk patients who have fever and neutropenia during cancer chemotherapy, empirical therapy with oral ciprofloxacin and amoxicillin-clavulanate is as safe and effective as IV antibiotics.[2,3] Low risk is defined as: neutropenia expected to resolve within 10 days after the onset of fever, hemodynamically stable, absence of abdominal pain, nausea, vomiting, diarrhea (passage of six loose stools daily), neurologic/mental status changes, line infection, or new pulmonary infiltrates.

LINE SEPSIS

Etiology

Mostly *S. aureus* and streptococci.

Signs and Symptoms

- Locally, erythema and pus at the catheter insertion site.
- Systematically, tachycardia and fever; hypotension in severe cases.

Workup

- CBC, blood culture.
- Remove the catheter in patients with systemic septic symptoms and inflammation/pus at the insertion site.
- Seventy-five percent of patients with systemic septic signs but no clear source of infection are not infected. The line can be rewired with a new catheter; send the tip of the old catheter in for culture. If the culture of old catheter reveals 15 or more colonies, remove the catheter.

Treatment

Give nafcillin, 1 to 2 g IV every 6 hours. If the patient is allergic to penicillin or the culture is staphylococcus coagulase negative, use vancomycin 1 g IV every 12 hours.

PNEUMONIA (SEE CHAP. 13)

PANCREATITIS AND CHOLECYSTITIS (SEE CHAP. 14)

REFERENCES

1. CRAWFORD J, OZER H, STOLLER R, JOHNSON D, LYMAN G, TABBARA I, KRIS M, GROUS J, PICOZZI V, RAUSCH G, et al: Reduction by granulocyte colony-stimulating factor of fever and neutropenia induced by chemotherapy in patients with small-cell lung cancer. N Engl J Med 325:164, 1991.
2. FREIFELD A, MARCHIGIANI D, WALSH T, CHANOCK S, LEWIS L, HIEMENZ J, HIEMENZ S, HICKS JE, GILL V, STEINBERG SM, PIZZO PA: A double-blind comparison of empirical oral and intravenous antibiotic therapy for low-risk febrile patients with neutropenia during cancer chemotherapy. N Engl J Med 341:305, 1999.
3. KERN WV, COMETTA A, DE BOCK R, LANGENAEKEN J, PAESMANS M, GAYA H: Oral versus intravenous empirical antimicrobial therapy for fever in patients with granulocytopenia who are receiving cancer chemotherapy. International Antimicrobial Therapy Cooperative Group of the European Organization for Research and Treatment of Cancer. N Engl J Med 341:312, 1999.

Joseph T. Santoso

ARTERIAL THROMBOSIS

Etiology

Same as for Deep Venous Thrombosis, later.

Signs and Symptoms

5 Ps (pulselessness, pain, pallor, paresthesias, paralysis).

Workup

Check pulse, Doppler sonogram.

Treatment

- Heparin versus surgical embolectomy/angioplasty versus heparin and thrombolytic therapy. Call a vascular surgery consultant.
- If using heparin, use a high dose (20,000-U bolus). Then titrate the heparin according to the patient's level of pain. Disregard PTT initially: this value may be misleading as the PTT in the serum sample may be high, but in the nonperfused area it would be extremely low. The risk of losing an extremity is higher than the risk of a bleeding complication during the first 2 days of heparin therapy.

DEEP VENOUS THROMBOSIS

Etiology

Virchow's triad (hypercoagulation, stasis, vessel injury), deficiency of protein C or S or antithrombin III, SLE/HIV, atrial fibrillation (5% risk of CVA), and family history.

Signs and Symptoms

Extremity tenderness, edema, erythema, low-grade fever.

Workup

Doppler sonogram of the extremity.

Treatment

- Heparin (fractionated, unfractionated) and warfarin per protocol (see later discussion).
- Prior to surgery, consider placing a vena caval filter.
- If a line is in place and functional, it may be left in situ for antibiotic therapy. If nonfunctional, we prefer to remove and replace as needed for vascular access.

PULMONARY EMBOLISM

Etiology

Similar to that for Deep Venous Thrombosis, earlier.

Signs and Symptoms

Tachypnea, tachycardia, agitation, chest pain.

Workup

- ABGs show hypoxemia with acute respiratory alkalosis, and an increased A-a gradient because emboli create an area of the lung that is ventilated but not perfused (dead space).
- Chest x-ray may show Hampton's hump, Westermark's sign—it is ordered to rule out pneumothorax, pneumonia, or aortic dissection.
- ECG may show T-wave inversion in leads V1-4—it is ordered to rule out angina pectoris or MI.
- VQ scan is diagnostic in most cases.
- Doppler sonogram of the lower extremity is helpful only if it is positive. Almost one-third of patients with proven pulmonary embolism have negative noninvasive leg studies.
- Pulmonary angiogram in equivocal cases or in patients with pneumonia.
- Spiral CT scan of the chest is an alternative noninvasive test.

Treatment

- Heparin and warfarin per protocol (see later discussion) for 6 months[1] or longer.
- Thrombolytic therapy is rarely used. In a UPET-NIH study of randomized urokinase versus heparin alone, the study showed that the clot lysed sooner but did not affect mortality. In smaller studies, thrombolytic therapy seemed to work more effectively in patients with shock. The complication that causes the most concern is intracranial hemorrhage. Relative contraindications to thrombolytic therapy are major surgery (< 10 days), trauma (including CPR), and history of major bleeding.
- Embolectomy in rare cases.

UNFRACTIONATED HEPARIN PROTOCOL[2]

1. Calculate using total body weight: _____ kg to get the dose of heparin.
2. Bolus heparin at 80 U/kg = _____ U IV.
3. IV heparin infusion at 18 U/kg/hour = _____ U/hour.
4. Warfarin, 5 mg PO q.d. to start on first day of heparin administration.
5. Laboratory studies: obtain PTT, INR, CBC (baseline) now; CBC with platelet count q.d.; STAT PTT 6 hours after heparin bolus; INR q.d. (start on third day of heparin administration).
6. Adjust heparin infusion based on the sliding scale that follows:

PTT < 35 sec	80 U/kg bolus = _____ U
(< 1.2 × normal)	Increase drip 4 U/kg/hour = _____ U/hour
PTT 35–45 sec	Give additional 40 U/kg bolus = _____ U
(1.2–1.5 × normal)	Increase drips 2 U/kg/hour = _____ U/hour

7. Order a PTT 6 hours after any dosage change, adjusting heparin infusion by the sliding scale until PTT is therapeutic (46 to 70 seconds). When two consecutive PTT are therapeutic, order PTT (and readjust heparin as needed) every 24 hours. Make changes as promptly as possible.

PTT should reach 1.5 to 2.5 times normal within 24 hours. The recurrence rate for thromboembolism was 10-fold greater in those who did not achieve therapeutic PTT within 24 hours (24.5% versus 1.6%).[2] Check hematocrit and platelets daily to detect bleeding or heparin-induced thrombocytopenia (HIT). If heparin infusion is changed, monitor PTT every 6 hours.

FRACTIONATED HEPARIN PROTOCOL

- Agents: enozaparin, dalteparin, ardeparin.
- With or without evidence of pulmonary embolism, give enoxaparin 1 mg/kg SC each day.
- Overlap with warfarin as with unfractionated heparin.
- Randomized trials have demonstrated equal efficacy to unfractionated heparin but with reduced side effects (bleeding, thrombocytopenia).
- Dalteparin and ardeparin are approved for deep venous thrombosis.

WARFARIN PROTOCOL

- Warfarin can be started on the first day of heparin therapy and is safe and effective.[3] Initiate therapy with 5 mg warfarin q.d. to achieve an INR between 2 and 3 within 4 to 5 days. Using a higher dose only increases complications of excess anticoagulation without shortening the time to achieve full anticoagulation.[4]
- Monitor INR daily until it is therapeutic. Taper monitoring to every 2 to 3 days, then weekly, and then monthly.
- Patients can develop a hypercoagulable state in the first few days of warfarin treatment because warfarin can induce protein C and S deficiency (vitamin K–dependent endogenous anticoagulant).
- Continue IV heparin for at least 2 days after warfarin range is achieved as an INR does not achieve steady state for a while (long half-life of warfarin).[5]
- Continue warfarin therapy for 6 months.[6]

FACTORS THAT POTENTIATE THE EFFECTS OF WARFARIN

- Drugs: amiodarone, cimetidine, clofibrate, corticosteroids, danazol, disulfiram, erythromycin, felbamante, fluconazole,

isoniazid, ketoconazole, lovastatin, metronidazole, miconazole, moricizine, omeprazole, phenylbutazone, phenytoin, piroxicam, propafenone, propranolol, quinidine, sulfinpyrazone, trimethoprim/sulfamethoxazole.
- Others: liver disease, hyperthyroidism, decreased vitamin K intake, ileal resection.

SPECIAL ANTICOAGULATION SITUATIONS

Long-Term Warfarin Treatment (i.e., Atrial Fibrillation) Prior to Surgery

- Admit the patient 3 days prior to surgery to stop warfarin and to begin heparin. Maintain PTT at 1.5 to 2.5 seconds times the baseline. Six hours prior to surgery, stop heparin and check PTT; 24 to 48 hours postoperatively, resume heparin infusion (without bolus). On postoperative days 3 and 4, restart warfarin.
- An alternative to 3-days-prior admission is to give SC adjusted-dose heparin: 10,000 U of heparin SC is given every 12 hours (8 A.M. and 8 P.M.). Check PTT 6 hours after the morning dose, it should be 1.5 times baseline. If not, increase the dose by 2000 U. Recheck PTT 6 hours after the morning dose the next day and adjust as necessary. Decrease by 2000 U if PTT is more than 2.5 times baseline. The maximum total dose is 20,000 U SC every 12 hours. Always check the PTT 6 hours after each dose adjustment.

Acute PE/DVT Prior to Surgery

- Delay surgery for 3 to 6 months if possible.
- If unable to delay, place a vena caval filter preoperatively and add heparin and subsequent warfarin postoperatively. The filter increases the incidence of DVT about 10%[7] and may not fully protect the patient from microemboli.

Bleeding During Anticoagulant Therapy

See Table 22–1. Consider diagnostic procedures according to bleeding sources (hematuria: rule out UTI; IVP to rule out nephrolithiasis; cystoscopy to rule out radiation cystitis; endoscopy to rule out GI bleeding; CT scan to rule out intra-abdominal bleeding or CNS involvement).

Elective Cardioversion

- The risk for embolic complications following cardioversion without anticoagulation is about 5%.
- Patients should be anticoagulated at least 3 weeks before cardioversion, and therapy continued for 4 weeks afterward.

DRUG INTERACTION

- Cimetidine and ranitidine can decrease hepatic metabolism of warfarin.
- If the PT value is excessively elevated in a patient who receives warfarin and these H_2 blockers, substitute famotidine or sucralfate.

MANAGEMENT OF PATIENTS RESISTANT TO ANTICOAGULANT THERAPY

- Resistant to heparin: obtain antithrombin (AT) III level (normal value is 80% to 120% of "normal"). For example, you have given your patient heparin at 7000 U/hour, but her PTT remains 30. This usually indicates that antithrombin III level is less than 80%. Theoretically, a level of less than 70% indicates hypercoagulation. Heparin can be increased or you can add AT III (synthetic AT III, cryoprecipitate, or fresh frozen plasma).
- Resistant to warfarin: evaluate whether the patient takes her medication correctly or is taking supplemental vitamin K. Foods containing high levels of vitamin K include broccoli, brussels sprouts, cabbage (raw), chickpeas, lettuce, and spinach (raw).[8]

MANAGEMENT OF THE OVERLY ANTICOAGULATED PATIENT RECEIVING WARFARIN

See Table 22-1.

TABLE 22–1.

Nonbleeding patient	First, repeat the test. INR < 6: Hold warfarin for 2–3 days; INR 6–10: give 0.5–1 mg vitamin K (phytonadione) PO; INR 10–20: give 3–5 mg vitamin K PO or SC. Can repeat q 12 h if INR remains high; INR > 20: give 5–10 mg vitamin K SC. May repeat q 12 h if INR remains high.
Bleeding patient	Give 10 mg vitamin K SC or IV; give fresh frozen plasma, 2 to 6 U. *Note:* IV is more effective than SC method in giving vitamin K.[9]

MANAGEMENT OF THE OVERLY ANTICOAGULATED PATIENT RECEIVING HEPARIN

- If the patient is not bleeding clinically, stop the heparin and wait (heparin's half-life is 30 to 90 minutes).
- In the bleeding patient, consider adding protamine sulfate, 1 mg/100 U heparin given (maximum: 50 mg) via IV slowly. Watch for hypotension.

HEPARIN-INDUCED THROMBOCYTOPENIA/THROMBOSIS

- If the platelet count is greater than 100,000, continue heparin. Diagnosis is made by the platelet aggregation test. Treatment includes observation and elimination of heparin. Only give platelets to bleeding patients. Platelet level should return to normal in a few days.
- If anticoagulation is needed, consider dextran or ancrod (which depletes fibrin). Initial ancrod dosage is 2 U/kg IV over 6 hours, subsequent dose is based on fibrinogen level.
- Low-molecular-weight heparin (LMWH) has a lower incidence of heparin-induced thrombocytopenia but is less responsive to protamine.

REFERENCES

1. SCHULMAN S, RHEDIN AS, LINDMARKER P, CARLSSON A, LARFARS G, NICOL P, LOOGNA E, SVENSSON E, LJUNGBERG B, WALTER H: A com-

parison of six weeks with six months of oral anticoagulant therapy after a first episode of venous thromboembolism. N Engl J Med 332:1661, 1995.

2. RASCHKE RA, REILLY BM, GUIDRY JR, FONTANA JR, SRINIVAS S: The weight-based heparin dosing nomogram compared with a "standard care" nomogram. A randomized controlled trial. Ann Intern Med 119:874, 1993.

3. HULL RD, RASKOB GE, ROSENBLOOM D, PANJU AA, BRILL-EDWARDS P, GINSBERG JS, HIRSH J, MARTIN GJ, GREEN D: Heparin for 5 days as compared with 10 days in the initial treatment of proximal venous thrombosis. N Engl J Med 322:1260, 1990.

4. HARRISON L, JOHNSTON M, MASSICOTTE MP, ET AL: Comparison of 5 mg and 10 mg loading doses in initiation of warfarin therapy. Ann Intern Med 126:133, 1977.

5. HIRSH J, DALEN JE, DEYKIN D, POLLER L, BUSSEY H: Oral anticoagulants. Mechanism of action, clinical effectiveness, and optimal therapeutic range. Chest 108(4 Suppl):231S, 1995.

6. KEARON C, GENT M, HIRSH J, WEITZ J, KOVACS MJ, ANDERSON DR, TURPIE AG, GREEN D, GINSBERG JS, WELLS P, MACKINNON B, JULIAN JA: A comparison of three months of anticoagulation with extended anticoagulation for a first episode of idiopathic venous thromboembolism. N Engl J Med 340:901, 1999.

7. DECOUSUS H, LEIZOROVICZ A, PARENT F, PAGE Y, TARDY B, GIRARD P, LAPORTE S, FAIVRE R, CHARBONNIER B, BARRAL FG, HUET Y, SIMONNEAU G: A clinical trial of vena caval filters in the prevention of pulmonary embolism in patients with proximal deep-vein thrombosis. N Engl J Med 338:409, 1998.

8. BOOTH SL, ET AL: Vitamin K contents of foods. J Food Comp Anal 6:109, 1993.

9. RAJ G, KUMAR R, MCKINNEY WP: Time course of reversal of anticoagulant effect of warfarin by intravenous and subcutaneous phytonadione. Arch Intern Med 159:2721, 1999.

CANCER CACHEXIA

Etiology

Unknown—probably related to tumor cytokines.

Signs and Symptoms

Progressive weight loss, anorexia.

Workup

Rule out adrenal or thyroid insufficiency.

Treatment

Megestrol acetate (40 mg/mL suspension) may be given to increase appetite. Begin with 10 mL/day PO, then titrate up to 20 mL to avoid nausea.

Dronabinol, 2.5 mg PO b.i.d. before meals, may be given. Caution: this drug may cause hallucinations or agitation.

BONE PAIN

Etiology

Granulocyte colony stimulating factors (GCSF), paclitaxel, or metastatic cancer.

Signs and Symptoms

Bone pain.

Workup

- Rule out joint or bone diseases.
- Obtain a plain x-ray film if the pain is localized, and a bone scan if the pain is generalized.

Treatment

- Local radiation can be administered to bone metastases to palliate pain or to reduce the risk of bone fracture. However, the radiation itself may make the bone more brittle. In some long bone metastases, the femur may need to be internally fixed with a steel rod prior to radiation to prevent fracture.
- In a patient with multiple bone metastases, strontium 89 may be used to palliate pain. Strontium 89, a calcium analog, is a beta emitter that is taken up by osteoblasts in the area of bony metastases to control tumor growth.
- Bone pain from GCSF or paclitaxel may be treated by discontinuing drugs and administering NSAIDs.

WOUND DEHISCENCE

Etiology

Infection, obesity, malnutrition, ischemia, prior radiation site, chronic cough.

Signs and Symptoms

Varies from serosanguineous discharge to exposed bowel.

Workup

Rule out abscess, cellulitis, or evisceration.

Treatment

- For superficial dehiscence with intact fascia, clean the wound and pack with a wet-to-dry dressing. More contemporary management would be to use accuzyme (containing papain enzyme) q.d. at the wound site to digest necrotic tissues. Once the wound is clean, use fibracol (collagen alginate wound dressing/packing) q.d. In a large wound, the growth of granulation tissue can be encouraged with the use of vacuum-assisted closure.

- If fascia is opened and bowel is outside the fascia, cover the bowel with moist clean towels. Emergency exploratory laparotomy and repair should be done. If the fascia is intact and only subcutaneous separation is found, use a wet-to-dry dressing t.i.d. Once granulation tissue proliferates, the wound can be approximated with tape, suture, or skin graft.

INCISIONAL HERNIA

Etiology

Infection, obesity, malnutrition, ischemia, prior radiation site, chronic coughs. Occurs in 2% of patients undergoing gynecologic surgery, 5% of those with gynecologic oncologic surgery, and 25% after emergency laparotomy.

Signs and Symptoms

Presentation is usually asymptomatic; acute abdominal pain may occur with torsed or trapped bowel.

Workup

CT scan in nonemergency cases.

Treatment

Repair is indicated when symptomatic. A small fascial defect (< 4 cm) can be repaired using mass closure technique with permanent monofilament suture. A larger defect will require a Marlex mesh and a drain. Recurrent hernia occurs in up to 25% of cases after the initial repair.

LYMPHEDEMA

Etiology

- Destruction of the lymphatic system from radiation or surgery causes stagnation in the lymphatic channel, which eventually leads to a permanent fibrotic channel.

- Patients with cervical cancer who are treated with radical hysterectomy, lymphadenectomy, and pelvic radiation may experience up to 23% risk of lymphedema.[1] In patients with vulvar cancer undergoing radical vulvectomy with bilateral groin dissection, the incidence of lymphedema ranges from 26% to 69%.[2]

Signs and Symptoms

Presentation varies from asymptomatic to painful, edematous lower extremities.

Workup

Rule out deep venous thrombosis.

Treatment

- Lymphedema may occur painlessly after surgery and can be alleviated with limb elevation and exercise. If inflammation sets in, the patient may complain of calf tenderness, which may be relieved with anti-inflammatory medications and limb elevation. Chronic lymphedema results in stiff, nonpitting lymphedema unresponsive to any treatment and can be severely debilitating.
- Treatment is mainly palliative with limb elevation and moderate exercise. Avoid vigorous exercise because it increases blood flow to the limb (more than the residual lymph channel can remove) and exacerbates the edema. The Casley-Smith[3] and the Lerner massage techniques[4] incorporate compression garments, lymphatic massage, skin/nail care, exercise, and patient education.
- Diuretics, warfarin, and surgery to remove fluid are ineffective methods.[5] Diuretics are mainly effective in high-sodium, low-protein edema, which is the opposite situation to that of lymphedema. Pneumatic compression devices, if fitted appropriately, may help.

REFERENCES

1. MARTIMBEAU PW, KJORSTAD KE, KOLSTAD P: Stage IB carcinoma of the cervix, the Norwegian Radium Hospital, 1968-1970: Results of treatment and major complications. I. Lymphedema. Am J Obstet Gynecol 131:389, 1978.
2. KARAKOUSIS CP, HEISER MA, MOORE RH: Lymphedema after groin dissection. Am J Surg 145:205, 1983.
3. CASLEY-SMITH JR, BORIS M, WEINDORF S, LASINSKI B: Treatment for lymphedema of the arm—the Casley-Smith method: A noninvasive method produces continued reduction. Cancer 83(12 Suppl Am):2843, 1998.
4. LERNER R: Complete decongestive physiotherapy and the Lerner Lymphedema Services Academy of Lymphatic Studies (the Lerner School). Cancer 83(12 Suppl Am):2861, 1998.
5. MCELRATH TJ, RUNOWICZ CD: Preventing and managing lymphedema. Contemp OB Gyn 115, 2000.

III | SYNOPSIS OF PROCEDURES

GENERAL

- Preoperative note: prior to major procedures, all patients require a preoperative evaluation with a note reflecting the pertinent information.
- The preoperative summary should clearly reflect actual surgical procedures performed. We find it useful at times to outline here the findings and procedures to ensure an accurate representation of the case and to help with subsequent operations (e.g., bowel surgery).
- Postoperative note: postoperative evaluation and notation should be done following surgery to report the following: pain control, level of consciousness, vital signs, laboratory studies, output, and clinical evaluation (wounds, drains, etc.).

SAMPLE PERIOPERATIVE NOTES

A. Preoperative note:
1. Date of planned surgery.
2. Diagnosis.
3. Proposed procedure.
4. Laboratory studies: (pertinent laboratory findings and ABGs, pulmonary function tests, etc.).
5. Radiology: ECG (include pertinent cardiovascular workup).
6. Consent: signed/obtained (minors, guardians)/method (phone/person).
7. Components of informed consent are discussion of procedure, risks, benefits, and alternative treatment.

B. Operative note:
1. Date of surgery.
2. Preoperative diagnosis.
3. Postoperative diagnosis.
4. Procedure.
5. Surgeons.
6. Anesthesia (if local, provide the type and amount used).

7. Estimated blood loss.
8. Fluids (provide all components: crystalloid, colloids, blood products).
9. Output (provide all sources: urine, ascites, drains).
10. Complications.
11. Indications (include medical co-morbidities if applicable).
12. Findings (all findings from the procedure, normal and abnormal; include diagram, if pertinent).
13. Procedure in detail.
14. Specimens.

EXAMPLES OF PROCEDURES (ORGAN BASED)

CENTRAL NERVOUS *(Joseph T. Santoso)*

Lumbar Puncture

- *Indications:* to evaluate infection, tumor, cytology.
- *Contraindications:* increased intracranial pressure (clinical, radiographic, etc.).
- *Preoperative prep:* lumbar puncture tray supply.
- *Consent:* risks—headache, bleeding, infection, paralysis (rare).
- *Description:* the patient is placed in the lateral decubitus position with arched back, and the skin is prepared over the site of entry. Apply local anesthesia (1% lidocaine) to skin and subcutaneous tissue. Place a spinal needle (22-gauge) at L4 or L5 (on or below a plane with the iliac crest), enter the lumbar vertebra, and angle cephalad until the interspace is entered. Advance the needle until it punctures the ligamentum flavum, epidural space, and arachnoid dura. Confirmation will occur with leakage of spinal fluid. Measure the entry pressure and collect tubes for cultures, glucose/protein, and cytology. Remove the needle and apply a dressing.

- *Postoperative care:* keep the patient supine and well-hydrated. Give analgesics for headache as needed. For persistent spinal headache, consider a blood patch.

PULMONARY *(Joseph T. Santoso)*

Emergent Cricothyroidotomy

- *Indications:* Immediate airway access after conditions that injure the oropharynx, coma, upper airway obstructions, unsuccessful endotracheal intubation.
- *Preoperative prep:* protect the cervical spine, particularly in the trauma patient.
- *Consent:* risks—bleeding, infection, injury to recurrent laryngeal nerve and tissues (vocal cords), esophageal perforation.
- *Description:* place patient in the supine position, with head extended and midline; perform sterile prep. Identify and palpate the cricothyroid membrane. Incise skin vertically (approximately 1 cm) in the midline and incise the membrane. Insert the knife handle, rotate 90 degrees, and insert a pediatric (endotracheal) ET tube or the largest accommodating tube/catheter. Begin ventilation with a bag valve (Amboo) unit with 100% oxygen. An alternative, temporary solution is to make a cricothyroid puncture with a large-caliber Angiocath and remove the needle. Connect to an oxygen Y-connector to serve as a ventilator. This temporary approach will provide about 20 minutes of time (beyond that, the CO_2 level will rise to toxic levels).

Tube Thoracostomy (Chest Tube)

- *Indications:* pneumothorax ($> 20\%$ of lung volume), symptomatic pleural effusion, pleurodesis.
- *Contraindications:* multiple loculations.
- *Preoperative prep:* thoracostomy tube (28- or 36-French tube for effusion, 8.5-French tube for pneumothorax), and chest x-ray (consider lateral decubitus position to delineate volume

and flow of effusion). Have a suction-collection device (Pleurovac) ready.

- *Consent:* risks—bleeding, infection, injury to adjacent organs (heart, lung, spleen, liver, breast prosthesis), and reexpansion pulmonary edema. Alternatives—observation, thorascopic exploration and placement.

- *Description:* place the patient in the supine position with a wedge under the thoracic spine and elevate the arm to increase the intercostal space. Prepare and drape over the fifth intercostal space (nipple location in nonpendulous breast), at the midaxillary line. Inject 1% lidocaine to skin and subcutaneous tissue, periosteum, and pleura. Incise (3 cm) parallel to the rib, one interspace below the desired position. Use a large, blunt clamp (Péan) to place a 28- to 36-French tube. Tunnel subcutaneous tissue over the cephalad aspect of the rib into the pleural space. Open the clamp and spread the pleura. Palpate the lung to confirm penetration. Grasp the tip of the chest tube with the clamp and insert it into the pleural space, aiming cephalad and posterior beyond the most proximal hole of the tube. Suture the tube to the chest wall with number 1 prolene and apply a pressure dressing with petroleum gauze. Connect to the collection/suction apparatus.

  Many central line placement-related pneumothoracics can be adequately treated with a unidirectional valve catheter (Cook Catheter). Use the Seldinger technique to anatomically place this 8.5 French catheter (see description for Central Venous Access, later). Although this catheter does not necessarily require wall suction, the surgeon should ensure the direction of air flow is ex vivo.

- *Postoperative care:* obtain a chest x-ray after the procedure and daily while the tube is in place. The last hole in the chest tube is marked and should appear inside the chest on x-ray. For pneumothorax, the suction is generally applied at -20 cmH$_2$O pressure for 2 days and water seal for 1 day. If resolution of pneumothorax is achieved, remove the tube. For pleural effusion, apply suction (-20 cmH$_2$O) for 1 day and water seal at -2 cmH$_2$O until output is less than 100 mL/24 hours. The tube may be removed or pleurodesis performed.

- *Tube removal:* obtain a chest x-ray prior to removal to confirm resolution of the problem. Administer analgesia, and remove the dressing and suture. Ask the patient to inhale and perform a Valsalva maneuver. Remove the tube during exhaling. Apply petroleum gauze and a pressure dressing. Obtain a chest x-ray a few hours after tube removal to rule out recurrence of pneumothorax. *Note:* in the patient with a bilateral chest tube, consider removing one tube on one day and the other tube the next day. This approach reduces the risk of recurring pneumothorax bilaterally.

Pleurodesis

- *Indications:* to prevent pleural fluid reaccumulation.
- *Contraindications:* pleural infection.
- *Preoperative prep:* a chest tube should have been placed, as noted earlier, and pleural fluid collection should be less than 100 mL/24 hours.
- *Consent:* risks—infection, pain, inability to prevent fluid reaccumulation, and pneumothorax. Alternatives—same procedure done using thoracoscopy or open lung procedure.
- *Description:* sclerose the pleura with bleomycin, tetracycline, or (most commonly) talc. Recipe: 10 g sterile talc is mixed with normal saline and 20 mL of 2% lidocaine for a total volume of 200 mL. Give additional IV or PO pain medication. Insert the solution into the pleural cavity via a chest tube. Clamp the chest tube for 4 hours and ask the patient to change position to allow the talc solution to evenly bathe the pleural cavity. Adjust it back to -20 cm pressure of H$_2$O suction for one day.
- *Postoperative care:* if the chest x-ray confirms full expansion on the following day, place the chest tube on a water seal for another day. Obtain a chest x-ray daily. If the lung continues to be expanded, pull the chest tube and repeat a chest x-ray. If pneumothorax persists or is loculated, consider placing

more chest tubes or calling a cardiothoracic consultant to decorticate the pleura.

Thoracentesis

- *Indications:* diagnostic evaluation or therapeutic evacuation of symptomatic pleural effusion.
- *Preoperative prep:* thoracentesis kit or 18-gauge Angiocath with supplies (3-way stopcock, syringe, "male-to-male" extension tubing, 18-gauge free needle vacuum bottle), and chest x-ray.
- *Consent:* risks—pneumothorax (1% to 3% risk), bleeding, infection, injury to adjacent organs (heart, lung, spleen, liver), and re-expansion pulmonary edema (especially if a large volume of fluid is removed). Alternatives—thoracostomy tube or thorascopic evaluation.
- *Description:* position patient sitting, leaning forward over pillows or a table. Percuss the chest to determine fluid level. Prepare the site and drape in a sterile fashion. Inject local (1% lidocaine) anesthetic into skin and pleura, and verify position by entering the pleural cavity and aspirating fluid. Insert a thoracocentesis needle one interspace below the percussed fluid level but not lower than the eighth intercostal space. Track the needle in Z-fashion and insert over the cephalad aspect of the rib. Remove pleural fluid, but not more than 1400 mL (may cause hypotension). Remove the needle or device. Apply a dressing (adhesive bandage). Consider sending the fluid for differential cell count, Gram stain, cultures (bacterial, fungal, mycobacterial), cytology, protein, glucose, amylase, LDH, and pH, as indicated.
- *Postoperative care:* chest x-ray.

Endotracheal Intubation

- *Indications:* to ventilate, oxygenate, or protect the airway in patients with respiratory compromise.
- *Contraindications:* obstructive airway (laryngeal edema, tumor, or some spinal cord injury).

- *Preoperative prep:* suction, appropriate laryngoscope, oxygen, and ET tube. Call for respiratory therapist assistance.
- *Consent:* risks—spinal cord injury, dental or tracheal trauma, esophageal intubation, aspiration, bleeding, and recurrent laryngeal nerve injury. Alternatives—nasotracheal tube or cricothyriodotomy.
- *Description:* the patient is placed in supine position with the head in a sniffing position. Preoxygenate with 100% O_2 via mask to achieve a peripheral O_2 saturation of 100%. Anesthetize the oropharynx with topical anesthetic. Perform a direct laryngoscopy. Visualize the true vocal cords and place a #7 to #8 ET tube under direct visualization. Inflate the cuff to seal the airway. Secure the tube at the lip (approximately 22 cm). Auscultate for equal breath sounds bilaterally. Connect the ET tube to a ventilator and obtain a chest x-ray.
- *Postoperative care:* obtain a chest x-ray daily while intubated (see Chap. 29, regarding ventilator management).

CARDIOVASCULAR *(Joseph T. Santoso)*

Central Venous Access

- *Indications:* vascular access for chemotherapy, fluid resuscitation, central venous pressure monitoring, parenteral nutrition, frequent blood draw, and lack of peripheral access.
- *Contraindications:* hypocoagulable state, bleeding diatheses, and superior vena cava syndrome.
- *Preoperative prep:* laboratory studies—CBC and platelets; get PT/PTT if there is a history of bleeding abnormality.
- *Consent:* risks—pneumothorax (1% to 2%), arterial puncture and thrombosis, brachial plexus injury, thoracic duct injury, and infection. Alternatives—peripheral central access (PICC line or long line, Passport) or femoral line.
- *Description:* (1) *Subclavian technique:* place the patient in supine, Trendelenburg position. Prepare the skin around the subclavian area and drape in a sterile manner. Anesthetize the skin with 1% lidocaine. Attach an 18-gauge needle to a 10-

mL syringe with 3 mL normal saline. Insert 1 cm below the clavicle and at the middle third of the clavicle to yield dark venous blood. Place the catheter using the Seldinger wire method (e.g., place a guide wire with an adapter through the needle). Retract the needle. Make a small incision with a scalpel along the guide wire at the skin to accommodate the vein dilator. Advance the vein dilator to the anticipated level of venous entry. Advance the catheter to the 15-cm mark (for left insertion) and to the 12-cm mark (for right insertion). Suture the catheter to the skin. (*Note:* if you persistently hit the clavicle, try moving the arm to a different position.) (2) *Internal jugular technique:* the landmarks are the triangle formed by the sternal and clavicular muscles of the sternocleidomastoid. Insert the search needle (22-gauge) at the level of cricoid, lateral to the carotid, aiming toward the ipsilateral nipple. Then continue as indicated above. (3) *Femoral line technique:* the vein is medial to the artery. Technique of insertion is similar to above.

- *Postoperative care:* obtain a chest x-ray.

Pulmonary Artery/Swan-Ganz Catheter Placement

- *Indications:* unclear volume status/preload status, hypoxemia management assistance, and generally sick patients whose perfusion needs to be monitored.
- *Contraindications:* hypocoagulable state, bleeding diatheses, superior vena cava syndrome, left bundle branch heart block.
- *Preoperative prep:* laboratory studies—CBC and platelets: get PT/PTT if there is a history of bleeding.
- *Consent:* risks—pneumothorax, arterial puncture and thrombosis, brachial plexus injury, thoracic duct injury, and infection. Alternatives—echocardiogram to assess preload status.
- *Description:* the procedure is started as for a central line placement. Once the cordice is placed, prepare the catheter by inserting the plastic protector sleeve, checking all the ports, and ensuring the balloon is intact. Insert the catheter to the 20-cm mark (right atrium) and inflate and float the

balloon. The pressure wave monitor should demonstrate right atrial, right ventricle, right pulmonary artery, and wedge tracing. The balloon is then deflated, and the catheter usually is noted to be at the 50-cm mark.

- *Postoperative care:* obtain a chest x-ray.

Radial Arterial Line

- *Indications:* continuous blood pressure monitoring and frequent blood gas analysis.
- *Contraindications:* lack of ulnar artery perfusion.
- *Preoperative prep:* palpate both ulnar and radial arteries to confirm arterial anastomosis (Allen's test).
- *Consent:* risk—infection, bleeding, ischemic necrosis of hand, and injury to adjacent nerves.
- *Description:* prepare the skin and drape in a sterile fashion. Use 1% lidocaine as a local anesthetic. Insert a 20-gauge Arrow radial arterial catheter into the artery, noting pulsatile blood flow. When connected to a pressure transducer, an arterial waveform will appear. Use a single 3-0 silk to suture the catheter to the skin. (If a pulse is not palpable, consider using Doppler to identify the approximate location or perform an arterial cut-down). Other arterial line sites are femoral, dorsalis pedis, and brachial. For the brachial artery, watch for arterial thrombosis—which may cause the patient to lose the entire arm from necrosis.

Venous (Long Saphenous) Cut-Down

- *Indications:* IV access.
- *Contraindications:* availability of veins elsewhere and bleeding diathesis.
- *Preoperative prep:* sterile preparation and draping.
- *Consent:* risk—infection, bleeding, injury to adjacent tissues, edema, loss of potential vein graft for cardiac bypass in the future.
- *Description:* make a superficial skin incision over and ante-

rior to the medial malleolus. Identify the vein, and pass two #0-polyglycolic sutures under the vein. Nick the vein and insert and tie catheter. Remove this line within 24 hours to reduce infection.

BREAST *(Robert L. Coleman)*

Fine Needle Aspiration (FNA)

- *Indications:* diagnostic and therapeutic evaluation of palpable lesion, cyst, or mass.
- *Preoperative prep:* 25-, 22-, or 20-gauge needle; 10- or 20-mL syringe; antiseptic (iodine or Hibiclens) skin prep; sterile gloves; and 5 mL 1% lidocaine without epinephrine.
- *Consent:* risk—hematoma formation, infection (rare), and pain. Alternative—biopsy or localization.
- *Description:* perform a thorough breast examination. Prepare the area in proximity to the mass with iodine or Hibiclens solution and drape in sterile fashion. A small (if any) skin wheel is raised with the 1% lidocaine solution. Pass the free needle or needle attached to a syringe through the skin to the cyst or mass of interest fixed between the thumb and fingers. A slight "give" will be felt when a cyst wall is entered, and drainage of the fluid can be achieved with negative pressure. Draw the needle in and out of the cyst and rotate to evacuate the lesion. If the fluid is clear but suspicious, or if the fluid is not clear or bloody, make a slide and send it for cytology. Otherwise, no slide is necessary. If no cyst is encountered, make several passes to obtain a tissue plug for a slide or a sample jar for histologic processing. Apply pressure to the area for 5 minutes to reduce hematoma formation. Palpate the area to feel for residual masses. If a mass is palpated, further biopsy is necessary. If not, the area should be examined in 1 to 2 weeks for follow-up. Consider obtaining a mammogram before biopsy, because hematoma from the biopsy may make mammogram interpretation difficult.

Open Breast Mass Biopsy

- *Indications:* bloody nipple discharge, a persistent mass, suspicious mammography, nipple retraction or elevation, or skin changes such as erythema, edema, and induration.
- *Preoperative prep:* lidocaine 1% and minor surgical set (scalpel, scissors, needle driver, clamps, suture, electrocoagulation, skin retractors).
- *Consent:* risks—hematoma formation, change in breast contour (especially with small breasts), and infection. Alternatives—core biopsy, fine needle aspiration (FNA).
- *Description:* prepare the area and drape as in the FNA procedure described earlier. Administer anesthesia. Most incisions can be circumareolar in a curvilinear fashion. Dissect the area to the lesion. Hemostasis is important. Large and adequate specimens are wedged, although a smaller sample may be taken from a larger lesion. Send at least 1 g of tissue for receptor status. Fresh tissue should be sent immediately as receptors are heat liable and require freezing within 30 minutes.

GASTROINTESTINAL *(Robert L. Coleman and Joseph T. Santoso)*

Paracentesis

- *Indications:* diagnostic evaluation or therapeutic evacuation of symptomatic ascites.
- *Contraindications:* severe abdominal adhesions, bowel obstruction.
- *Preoperative prep:* paracentesis kit or 18-gauge Angiocath with supplies (3-way stopcock, syringe, "male-to-male" extension tubing, 18-gauge free needle vacuum bottle).
- *Consent:* risks—bleeding, infection, injury to adjacent organs (bowel, liver, spleen, etc.), persistent ascitic leak, and hypotension (due to large volume removal). Alternative—peritoneal shunt.
- *Description:* through clinical (percussion) and/or radiographic (ultrasonic) guidance desired sites are marked. Pre-

pare the skin and drape in a sterile manner. Administer local anesthetic to infiltrate the skin and subcutaneous tissue. While advancing the needle, confirm an intraperitoneal location. Use Z-track technique to advance the kit apparatus or Angiocath into the peritoneum while attached to a syringe. Remove or retract the needle and attach to a 3-way stopcock via the connector. The tubing connector then is inserted into the vacuum bottles or to dependent drainage. When complete, remove the needle or kit apparatus and apply a bandage. Consider sending the fluid for differential cell count, Gram stain, cultures (bacterial, fungal, mycobacterial), cytology, protein, glucose, amylase, LDH, and pH, as clinically indicated.

Splenectomy

- *Indications:* metastatic or residual ovarian cancer, control of splenic bleeding, ideopathic thrombocytopenia purpura (ITP), and surgical staging for lymphoma.
- *Preoperative prep:* adequate exposure during celiotomy and knowledge of upper abdominal anatomy.
- *Consent:* risks—bleeding, infection, pseudocyst from distal pancreatectomy, and vascular compromise of the stomach fundus. Alternatives—depends on the indication. For carcinomatous involvement, chemotherapy may obviate the need for resection. For hematologic disorders, medical therapy may be attempted. This surgery is performed as an elective procedure laparoscopically in some centers; however, techniques requiring morcellation may be contraindicated from a pathologic standpoint.
- *Description:* divide the ligamentous attachments (phreno-splenic cephalad; phrenocolic and splenocolic caudally; gastrosplenic inferior and medially) through the celiotomy or through a subcostal incision. They are usually avascular but may contain large vessels if the patient has primary hypersplenism or portal hypertension. Ligate the short gastric vessels doubly, taking care not to avascularize the fundus of the

stomach. With division of the omentum along the greater curvature of the stomach, access to the splenic vessels is made. Within the hilum, there are multiple splenic vessels. Visualize and individually ligate the splenic artery and vein, which are adjacent to the pancreas. If the distal pancreas was not disrupted or ligated in the specimen, no drain is necessary. However, if distal pancreatectomy was performed, place a 19-French Blake or similar Jackson-Pratt drain in the splenic bed. Check for accessory organs.

- *Postoperative care:* hematologically, Howell-Jolly bodies are present and siderocytes are common. Leukocytosis and increased platelet counts are generally observed. If thrombocytopenia was noted preoperatively, the platelet count often returns to normal within 2 days. Leukocytosis may be present for months. The most frequent complication is lower left lobe atelectasis. Other complications include subphrenic hematoma and abscess. Patients should receive pneumococcal prophylaxis with PneumoVax 0.5 mL IM.

Omentectomy

- *Indications:* ovarian cancer, uterine cancers, tubal cancer.
- *Preoperative prep:* bowel prep.
- *Consent:* risks—bleeding, infection, and injury to bowel and spleen. Alternatives—omental biopsy.
- *Description:* identify the omentum and the transverse colon. Sharply dissect the omentum off the transverse colon. Dissect the colonic mesentery free from the omentum until the lesser sac is entered. Skeletonize, ligate, and transect the short gastric vessels along the greater curvature of the stomach. The remaining omental vessels should be skeletonized, ligated, and transected, taking care not to injure the splenic vessels. Inspect all vascular pedicles for hemostasis.
- *Postoperative care:* consider leaving the NG tube in place for 24 to 48 hours. Distention of the stomach may result in bleeding from the short gastric pedicles.

Liver Biopsy/Wedge Resection

- *Indications:* liver metastases, chronic liver disease, hepatitis, and liver insufficiency or failure.
- *Contraindications:* bleeding diathesis and poor exposure.
- *Preoperative prep:* none.
- *Consent:* risks—bleeding, infection, and loss of liver function.
- *Description:* place two heavy, absorbable sutures on a large blunt needle in an inverted "V" fashion on the liver edge sufficient to excise a 2-by-1-cm biopsy. Tie the sutures with care not to lacerate the liver. Excise the specimen and achieve hemostasis with electrocautery. For biopsy, use Tru-cut needle to advance near outside margin of tissue of interest. Advance internal stylet into tissue of interest. Then, while holding internal stylet at appropriate locale, advance outer sheath to obtain specimen. Use electrocautery to achieve hemostasis.
- *Postoperative care:* monitor hemoglobin for 48 hours to watch for bleeding.

Intestinal Bypass

- *Indication:* radiation bowel injury and obstruction.
- *Preoperative prep:* bowel prep if possible, prophylaxis antibiotics with spillage.
- *Consent:* risks—bleeding, infection, and anastomotic leaks. Alternatives—ostomy and bowel resection.
- *Description:* examine the small and large bowel for evidence of obstruction. Identify the distal most unobstructed bowel that appears healthy. In the case of small bowel, bring it parallel with the ascending colon. Make a small incision in the antimesenteric margin of the colon and the small bowel. Insert a gastrointestinal anastomosis (GIA) (55- to 60-mm) stapler in the colon and small bowel, and close and fire it to create a side-to-side anastomosis. Close the remaining defect with a thoracoabdominal (TA) stapler or with hand-sewn closure with 3-0 silk. Irrigate the abdomen with a copious amount of normal saline (for spill of GI contents). Check patency and look for leakage.

- *Postoperative care:* An NG tube is commonly used for a few days, but its usefulness is questionable.

Small Bowel Resection

- *Indications:* obstruction, cancer involving bowel, radiation injury, conduit, and bladder augmentation.
- *Preoperative prep:* gastric lavage or standard bowel prep.
- *Consent:* risks—leakage, ischemia, bleeding, trauma, and infection. Alternatives—bypass.
- *Description:* dissect the area of interest free, and transilluminate the mesentery for a vascular pattern. It should also be palpated for arterial branches. Score the mesentery with electrocautery for 4 to 5 cm in a wedge-like fashion. This ensures adequate blood supply to the remaining bowel to be reanastomosed. Ligate and divide the individual vascular pedicles from just underneath the bowel to the mesenteric scoring with 2-0 silk or synthetic absorbable suture. The devascularized bowel segment to be resected is easily appreciated, and transection of the bowel lumen is made just adjacent to this area in a vascularized location. The angle of the transection should bevel away from the mesentery where the base is slightly longer than the antimesenteric side. Staple the bowel lumen across with a GIA (55- or 60-mm) stapler or transect it with bowel clamps. Once the bowel has been removed, approximate the antimesenteric surfaces of the intestine and fix them with a 3-0 silk suture at two locations. The corners of the antimesenteric surface are nicked, and the GIA stapler is passed down the antimesenteric line and is fired. Use a TA-60 or equivalent stapler to close the lumen. Palpate the area for an acceptable lumen. No cautery should be used around the staple line as this will conduct the current and risk subsequent necrosis and leakage. Close the mesenteric defect with a 3-0 synthetic absorbable suture, taking care not to injure the vascular supply to the segments. If a handsewn anastomosis is to be accomplished, two layers of suture are needed for watertight closure. Close the first layer of mucosa-muscularis with

a 3-0 synthetic absorbable suture, with the knots oriented to the intestinal lumen. Place them on the posterior wall first and work around sequentially (interrupted). Place the second seromuscular suture with 3-0 silk or equivalent, also circumferentially. This layer may be done as a continuous suture. Closure of the mesentery is accomplished as described.

- *Postoperative care:* patients are usually fed when they are truly hungry or if they pass flatus. An NG tube is commonly used for a few days, but its usefulness is questionable.

Large Bowel Resection [Low Anterior Resection (LAR), Posterior Exenteration]

- *Indications/consent/preoperative prep:* similar to small bowel resection. Also includes conduits, colostomy, and posterior exenteration.
- *Description:* the technique for segmental resection is similar to that described for small bowel resection, earlier. Care is taken to evaluate mesenteric vascular supply, and knowledge of the vascular anatomy is important. For sigmoid resection with planned reanastomosis (low anterior resection), the superior hemorrhoidal vessels are transected at the pelvic inlet or at a suitable area above the area of disease. Place the patient in the low lithotomy position to allow for primary rectal anastomosis. In the deep pelvis, the vascular supply becomes lateral (below the peritoneal reflection) and ligation of these vessels must be made. Creation of the posterior rectal space greatly facilitates the dissection, but care must be taken in the presacral area as superficial vessels can be injured and may be difficult to coagulate. The lower rectal transection may be accomplished with a GIA stapler or a reticulated TA-60 stapler. The vagina is often transected separately and the rectovaginal space developed. Mobilize the proximal sigmoid or descending colon from its peritoneal attachments at the splenic flexure to eliminate tension on the proposed anastomotic line. This may require transection of the splenocolic and gastrocolic ligaments. Tension may also be released by

carefully incising the mesenteric root to the ligament of Trietz. To accomplish a low rectal anastomosis, open the proximal end of the sigmoid after mobilization. Be sure to place a bowel clamp above this site to reduce spillage potential. Remove the suture line and size the bowel lumen (most often a 29F or 33F). Place a purse-string suture near the luminal end. Use the end-to-end anastomosis (EEA) stapler and place the acorn in the proximal segment. Take care to ensure a clean suture line by having an intact purse-string suture around the acorn stem. Next, place the EEA device through the anus and to the suture line of the rectal stump. Bring the sharp trocar out just above or below the previous staple line. Remove the trocar to reveal a stem receptacle that is lined up with the proximal segment. Take care to align the mesentery so as not to stricture it. Obtain closure of the device by twisting it until the appropriate line is seen in the staple window. Fire the device and open it approximately 2.5 turns. Then gently rotate the EEA stapler out of its location. Once the device is outside the patient, it is opened and should reveal two complete donuts of tissue, ensuring an intact suture line. Insert a proctoscope and visualize the suture line. Fill the pelvis with fluid to look for escaping air. If air is observed, place reinforcement 3-0 sutures to make the anastomosis watertight. If there is concern about the integrity of the anastomosis, a diverting loop colostomy should be performed. If an exenterative procedure is to be accomplished with resection of the anus (proctocolectomy), the perineal phase with transection of the attachments to the levator is done from the low lithotomy position. This area is quite vascular and receives arterial supply from both the superior rectal vessels and the hemorrhoidal branches of the internal pudendal artery. Pararectal tissue is also resected with the specimen.

Incisional Hernia (Primary and Mesh Closure)

- *Indication:* hernia that is symptomatic or has nonreducible contents.

- *Preoperative prep:* bowel prep.
- *Consent:* risks—infection of tissues or mesh, enterotomy, secondary hernia, and wound seroma. Alternatives—abdominal binder and primary tissue approximation ("vest over pants").
- *Description:* with a large ventral hernia resulting from a vertical skin incision, a transverse incision may be chosen to allow for proper visualization of the lateral anterior rectus sheath. A vertical incision may also be chosen but will require more extensive subcutaneous mobilization. The peritoneal sac is encountered and tissue is dissected free of the attachments to the fascia. Once the sac is free it is entered and the sac resected; it is then closed with absorbable suture. The fascial edges are freshened by judicious removal of avascular scar tissue. If adequate mobilization of the fascia can be made to allow for primary closure, this may be accomplished and closed with delayed absorbable or permanent suture. The "vest over pants" closure is performed when the fascia can be mobilized enough to be sutured to the undersurface of the opposing side. An alternative for tissue that cannot be mobilized to approximation is to perform relaxing incisions that are parallel to the incisional defect and allow closure of the primary defect. Because the rectus muscles and posterior rectus sheath are intact under these incisions, herniation does not occur. If mesh is required for closure, it is commonly placed between the parietal peritoneum and under the surface of the fascia to minimize the exposure of the synthetic material to the subcutaneous tissue. Permanent mesh (Prolene or Marlex) is commonly used, although other choices are available (Gore-Tex, nylon, etc.). The mesh is attached with permanent suture (like 0 prolene), starting cephalad or laterally and trimming the mesh to allow for at least a 2-cm margin on the fascial edge. The area is irrigated and closed. Subcutaneous tissue and drains are not commonly used unless there is large mobilization of subcutaneous tissue or if the patient is obese (> 5 cm of subcutaneous fat). Meticulous care is necessary to minimize subsequent infection.

- *Postoperative care:* patients should be instructed to do no heavy lifting for at least 4 weeks and gradually return to normal lifting over 3 months.

Gastrostomy Tube

- *Indications:* prolonged gastric decompression and/or enteral feeding needs.
- *Contraindications:* tumor involvement of the stomach wall. Relative contraindication for percutaneous placement in presence of ascites.
- *Consent:* risks—bleeding, infection, gastric leakage, and skin breakdown. Alternatives—NG tube, feeding jejunostomy, and parenteral nutrition.
- *Preoperative prep:* choice of tube—Mallenkrodt, MIC, feeding tube, Foley. More permanent types are the Stamm and Glassman operations.
- *Description:* the procedure is usually performed as part of a celiotomy but may be done percutaneously by interventional radiology or endoscopically (PEG). At celiotomy, inspect the midportion of the body of the stomach and mobilize it to the lateral abdominal wall to choose a site that will allow for fixation to the anterior abdominal surface without tension. Use the electrocautery device to make a cruciate or stab wound in the stomach to enter the mucosa. Place two concentric circumferential purse-string sutures with 2-0 silk around the stab wound. Then create a stab wound on the abdominal wall and make a track to the stomach. Pass the selected tube through and into the stomach. A large Mallenkrodt tube (33 French) is a common choice. Draw and tie the purse-string sutures. Place three stay sutures (2-0 silk) seromuscularly in the stomach and to the anterior abdominal wall at strategic sites around the stoma. Fix the sutures and secure the tube to the skin with a 2-0 nylon suture. An MIC tube has a section that needs to be fed into the proximal duodenum. Feeding J-tubes may be placed directly into the jejunum or fed through the duodenum by external manipulation.

- *Postoperative care:* the tube may be attached to drainage postoperatively. Immediate care should include occasional irrigation to keep patent, especially if used primarily for drainage or for relief of obstructive symptoms in a patient with advanced disease undergoing palliation only.

Peritoneal Access

- *Indications:* intraperitoneal chemotherapy, immunotherapy, radiotherapy, or gene therapy.
- *Contraindications:* intestinal adhesions, infection, bowel obstruction.
- *Consent:* risks—intestinal perforation, infection, bowel obstruction or erosion, catheter intestinal fistula.
- *Preoperative prep:* choice of catheter—the author prefers to use a vascular access device such as Life port or mediport. Either attachable or preattached devices may be used, although more flexibility is possible with the attachable variety. Fenestrated peritoneal catheters such as groshong or dialysis catheters are associated with higher infection and perforation rates in this setting. Heparin flush solution.
- *Description:* this device may be placed at the time of celiotomy, or percutaneously with fluoroscopy or laparoscopy. Choice of location is dependent on the duration of use. For repeated use, the author prefers to place the port device over the costal margins to provide an adequate backstop for needle placement. Make a separate stab wound and place the catheter into the abdominal pelvic cavity. Then make a subcutaneous tunnel with a Péan clamp or appropriate tissue-tunneling device to the costal region. Make a transverse skin incision at the costal margin, and create a pocket in the subcutaneous tissue to accept the port. Although the catheter is necessary. This incision should not be over the middle of the port. Fix the port into place with a permanent suture such as 3-0 prolene or nylon. Irrigate the line with heparin flush solution and access it through the skin to rule out obstruction.

  If the device is placed percutaneously, draw a marker over

a suitable region for entry as determined by ultrasound. This may be an area of ascites, free of intestine or tumor. If laparoscopy is used, this area may have the same vital characteristics. Make a small incision to place the catheter using the Seldinger technique as described earlier under Central Venous Access. Once the catheter is placed correctly by fluoroscopic confirmation or direct visualization, make the upper incision at the costal margin as previously described. Take care to minimize handling of the distal end as microperforations and lacerations are a frequent cause of adhesion formation and infection. The lines should go down the paracolic gutters and not be placed directly on the bowel surface if possible.

Ostomy: Colon and Ileal

Colostomy

The best location is midway between the umbilicus and anterior iliac crest. Have the stoma health care provider mark the site preoperatively. Select the most distal site of the large intestine. At the stomal site, carry a 3-cm circular skin incision down to the subcutaneous tissue and fascia of the rectus sheath. Bring the end of the colon through the stoma and suture it to the fascia with interrupted 2-0 silk. Evert the stoma to the skin to form a "rosebud" with interrupted 2-0 polyglycolic acid suture. The suture goes from the skin edge, to serosa of colon, to the edge of the stoma.

Small Intestinal Ostomy

Formation of the small bowel stoma in a rosebud fashion is more critical than for the large bowel because of its irritating contents and the need to have a snug-fitting appliance. The mucosa is formed into a rosebud with at least a 1-cm margin above the skin. Rosebud sutures are 3-0 synthetic absorbable materials placed at the skin margin, to the base of the adjacent bowel seromuscular tissue, to the distal mucosa, and tied. This promotes eversion of the stoma.

Vascular Injuries (Tacs, Instruments [Bulldog, Satinsky Clamp], Fibrin Glue, Gelfoam, Type of Suture to Be Used, Needle)

* *Description:* injury to the vascular structures commonly occurs in situations where co-morbidity exists, disease is extensively retroperitoneal or fibrotic, or if previous surgery and/or treatment (such as radiation therapy) has been administered. Knowledge of anatomy and quick and decisive strategies are important to reduce morbidity. Surgeons should be familiar with instruments developed for vascular surgery, such as a Satinsky clamp or bulldog clamps, which allow immediate ligation and isolation of arterial bleeding. Venous bleeding usually can be transiently controlled with external pressure. Certain clamps and instruments may cause more injury because of the arrangement of their "teeth" or the sharpness of their edges. Adequate exposure is critical to effective and swift closure. Familiarity with vascular sutures is also critical for effective arterial and venous closure. The surgeon should know how to manipulate and tie 4-0 to 5-0 prolene and nylon suture material. Vascular needles, often on both edges of the suture material, are very effective in closing venous bleeding because the size of the needle hole in the tissue is small enough to ensure hemostasis by coagulation. Care must be taken to avoid significant angulation of the vessel, which may lead to venous turbulence and subsequent clot formation. Vascular clips are very helpful for bleeding vessels that may be grasped. They are less effective for holes in major veins because of slippage and often create bigger problems trying to manipulate the defect for closure. Adequate exposure is necessary to choose this technique versus suture. In situations of pelvic bleeding from a bony location such as the sacrum, choices are limited except for suture, packing, and external compression from sterile tacs. A tac placer will hold the tac at a right angle so it may be placed directly into the sacrum. Patients with disseminated intravascular coagulation present more difficult cases and may re-

quire a pelvic pack to "catch-up" on coagulation abnormalities before definitive (if any) control is attempted. Generalized oozing may be controlled with a variety of procoagulant mixtures such as Gelfoam, thrombin spray, fibrin glue, or Surgicell. These may be placed over capillary leakage with good results. More extensive bleeding will not be controlled by these devices and should not be attempted.

Appendectomy

- *Indications:* staging for ovarian cancer, inflammatory changes, mass, or alteration of the organ.
- *Preoperative prep:* bowel prep is similar to any celiotomy where bowel resection is contemplated. Elective surgery on the appendix has not proven cost-effective in adults given the low risk of appendicitis in this age group. However, removing an appendix that appears normal is recommended for staging of borderline and invasive ovarian or peritoneal malignancies, given the 20% microscopic involvement and its utility in delineating a primary site of cancer in ambiguous cases.
- *Consent:* risk—bleeding, infection, mucocele (buried stump).
- *Description:* free the appendix of peritoneal attachments, if they are present. Score the mesentery and identify the mesenteric branches of the appendicular artery and vein and separately clamp them. After dividing these vessels, take care to divide the appendicular artery. You may divide the appendicular stump a number of ways, but it may also be simply removed with three consecutive hemostats placed at the base. Division is made between the outer two clamps to remove the organ. Tie 3-0 absorbable suture below the most proximal clamp and secondarily to the remaining clamp. Exposed mucosa does not require burying or cauterization.

RETROPERITONEAL NODES *(Joseph T. Santoso and Robert L. Coleman)*

Pelvic Node Sampling

- *Indications:* evaluation for nodal metastasis, reduction of nodal tumor bulk, or staging of endometrial, cervical, or ovarian cancers.

- *Contraindication:* pulmonary/supraclavicular metastases, poor surgical risk.
- *Consent:* risks—bleeding, injury to adjacent organs, and infection. Alternatives—CT-guided biopsy.
- *Description:* identify the landmarks (the bifurcation of common iliac, external iliac, hypogastric arteries/veins, and the ureter). The borders of resection are:
  (1) Superior: middle of common iliac artery.
  (2) Lateral: genitofemoral nerve.
  (3) Distal: circumflex iliac vein.
  (4) Medial: ureter.

Para-aortic Node Sampling

- *Indications, contraindications, consent:* similar to those for Pelvic Node Sampling, earlier.
- *Description:* identify the landmarks [aortic bifurcation, inferior vena cava (IVC), ovarian vessels, inferior mesenteric artery, ureter, and duodenum]. The borders are:
  (1) Laterally: ureter.
  (2) Distally: middle of common iliac artery.
  (3) Medially: around the IVC and aorta.
  (4) Superiorly: inferior mesenteric artery (IMA) or renal vein (dissection above the IMA for palpably suspicious nodes or staging procedures of the ovary and uterus).

Superficial Inguinal–Femoral Lymphadenectomy

- *Indications:* surgical staging for vulvar cancer or removal of bulky tumors.
- *Contraindications, consent:* similar to those for Pelvic Node Sampling, earlier.
- *Description:* identify the landmarks (inguinal ligament superiorly, the border of the sartorius muscle laterally, and adductor longus medially). The anterior limit is the superficial subcutaneous fascia (Camper's fascia), and the posterior limit is the cribriform fascia overlying the femoral artery, vein, and deep

nodes. Preserve the saphenous vein, if possible. An adequate skin flap thickness will maintain its blood supply and its viability. After the removal of the superficial nodes, approximate the Camper's fascia with 2-0 polyglycolic acid suture in a continuous fashion. Place a Jackson Pratt drain under Camper's fascia. The skin can be closed with stapler or suture.

- *Postoperative care:* remove the drain when the output is less than 10 mL/24 hour or there is any sign of infection.

Deep Inguinal—Femoral Lymphadenectomy

- *Indications, contraindications, consent:* similar to those for Superficial Inguinal–Femoral Lymphadenectomy, earlier.
- *Description:* Continuing with the superficial lymphadenectomy, open the cribriform fascia over the fossa ovalis. Then move this fascia medially as part of the specimen. Identify the femoral artery and vein and dissect free to remove the deep nodes (usually three to five nodes). The most superior deep node is Cloquet's node. The femoral vessels can be protected by transposing the sartorius muscle from its insertion onto the anterior iliac spine and suturing it to the inguinal ligament.

Lymphatic and Sentinel Node Mapping

- *Indications:* identification of the sentinel node.
- *Contraindications:* intolerance to isosulfan blue dye or radionucleotide.
- *Preoperative prep:* lymphazurin 1% (5-mL vial), radionucleotide scan sulfur colloidal technetium-99 (^{99}Tc), and handheld columnated gamma probe.
- *Description:* the procedure is currently being evaluated in vulvar and cervical cancers. Both situations are best served by performing a ^{99}Tc scan prior to the operating room with available images for localization. In the operating room, inspect the tumor site. Administer the equally divided isosulfan blue dye intradermally and subcutaneously. For the vulva, lightly massage the adjacent skin to ensure lymphatic uptake of dye. In the cervix, take care not to penetrate the cul-de-

sac or through the central cavity of the tumor. Some spillage of contrast is expected from the cervix. There is a short window of time for both sites where the lymph nodes are blue; therefore, initial exploration of the appropriate regional basin (groin, pelvis) should be performed to encounter the dye. Prior to dye injection in the vulva, make a web map using the hand-held gamma probe to mark the sites of the most local radioactivity. Sentinel nodes may be blue, hot (by gamma probe), or both; note their location and characteristics for pathology. Sentinel nodes may undergo ultrastaging with serial sectioning and immunostaining with cytokeratin. Until the technique is validated, an accompanying lymphatic dissection should be the standard of care. Wide ranges of nodal drainage basins are encountered in the pelvis, including the para-aortic regions. Carefully inspect all sites. ^{99}Tc scans may be performed up to 24 hours prior to the procedure. More remote scans require second injection of radiocolloid.

- *Postoperative care:* inform patients about significant but transient tissue staining with the dye. False intraoperative oxygen desaturations may also be encountered as a result of the dye interacting with measured hemoglobin species.

UTERUS/CERVIX *(Robert L. Coleman, Joseph T. Santoso, and Joseph A. Lucci, III)*

Hysteroscopy

- *Indications:* to diagnose intrauterine pathology.
- *Contraindications:* uterine infection, uterine cancer, bleeding diathesis.
- *Preoperative prep:* preoperative doxycycline is needed only in patients at risk or those with a history of pelvic inflammatory disease (PID). To prevent cervical laceration or uterine perforation, laminaria may be placed 12 to 24 hours prior to the procedure. NSAIDs given to prevent cramping.
- *Consent:* risks—uterine perforation, bleeding, media-related complications (hyponatremic encephalopathy, air embolism), infection. Alternatives—ultrasound, CT scan.

- *Description:* under anesthesia or sedation, identify the cervical os and prepare it with Betadine. One percent lidocaine may be injected into the cervix. Dilate the cervical os progressively to accommodate the hysteroscope. The most common media are 3% sorbitol and 1.5% glycine.
- *Postoperative care:* maintain strict I & O and check electrolytes.

Dilation and Evacuation

- *Indications:* molar pregnancy.
- *Contraindications:* normal pregnancy.
- *Preoperative prep:* ultrasound confirming diagnosis. Laboratory studies—quantitative serum βhCG, CBC, thyroid panel (for patients with hyperthyroid symptoms), creatinine, liver function tests, electrolytes. Chest x-ray and type (including Rh) and crossmatch blood.
- *Consent:* risks—bleeding, infection, uterine/cervical perforation, injury to adjacent organs. Alternatives—hysterectomy, chemotherapy.
- *Description:* start 40 U of oxytocin injection in 1 L of lactated Ringer's solution (LR) and start infusing as the cervical os is dilated. Use the largest suction canula (if uterus is 14 weeks gestation, try #12 or #10). Once the uterus is completely evacuated, curette the uterine wall with the largest steel curette (to prevent uterine perforation). Completion is noted by the grittiness of the uterine surface and a decrease in bleeding.
- *Postoperative care:* give another liter of LR with 40 U oxytocin at 125 mL/hour. Give full-dose Rhogam as necessary. Check postoperative hematocrit and administer pain medications. A reliable contraceptive method should be used for 1 year.

Total Abdominal Hysterectomy

- *Indications:* various.
- *Contraindications:* bleeding diathesis, normal pregnancy in most cases, cervical cancer with stage IA2 or higher.
- *Preoperative prep:* laboratory studies—CBC, urine pregnancy test, electrolytes.

- *Consent:* risks—bleeding, infection, injury to adjacent organs, fistulas, infertility, incontinence.
- *Description:* give the patient general anesthesia and place in the supine position. Prepare and drape in the usual sterile fashion. Entry may be made with a Pfannenstiel, Maylard, Cherney, or midline incision. A Pfannenstiel incision is performed by making a transverse incision approximately 2 cm above the symphysis pubis and extend it sharply to the rectus fascia. Then incise the fascia bilaterally with the curved Mayo scissors, and separate the muscles of the anterior abdominal wall in the midline with sharp and blunt dissection. Grasp the peritoneum between two pickups, elevate it, and enter it sharply with the scalpel. Explore the pelvis and abdomen and note findings. Place a retractor in the incision and pack the bowel away with moist laparotomy sponges.

Place two Péan clamps on the cornua and use for retraction. Clamp the round ligaments on both sides, transect, and ligate with #0 polyglycolic acid sutures. Alternatively these may be cauterized and divided. Incise the anterior leaf of the broad ligament along the bladder reflection to the midline from both sides. Then gently dissect the bladder off the lower uterine segment and cervix with a sponge stick or sharply with Metzenbaum or electrocautery. Double clamp the infundibulopelvic ligaments (ovarian vessels) on both sides, transect, and ligate with #0 polyglycolic acid sutures. Be sure hemostasis is achieved. Skeletonize the uterine arteries bilaterally by dividing the medial leaf of the broad ligament parallel to ureter, clamp with Heaney clamps, transect, and ligate with #0 polyglycolic acid sutures. Again, hemostasis was achieved. Clamp the uterosacral ligaments on both sides, transect, and ligate in a similar fashion. Amputate the cervix and uterus with the cautery. Close the vaginal cuff angles with figure-of-eight stitches of #0 polyglycolic acid and transfix to the ipsilateral cardinal and uterosacral ligaments. Close the remainder of the vaginal cuff with a series of interrupted #0 polyglycolic acid sutures, and check for hemostasis. Close the fascia with running #0 polyglycolic acid sutures and ensure hemostasis. Close the skin with staples.

Radical Hysterectomy

- *Indications:* stage IA2, B, and IIA cervical cancers; stage II endometrial cancer.
- *Contraindications:* more advanced cancer, poor surgical risks.
- *Preoperative prep:* enema or magnesium citrate to empty the rectum and sigmoid colon and ease dissection of the recto-vaginal space.
- *Consent:* risks—bleeding; infection; injuries to bowel, bladder, ureter; urinary retention; fistula; failure to remove all cancer; sterility; bowel obstruction. Alternative—chemoradiation.
- *Description:* after induction of anesthesia, insert a Foley catheter. Prepare the patient and drape in the usual sterile manner. Access to the abdominal cavity may be achieved by midline, Cherney's, or Maylard's incision. Explore the upper abdomen and pelvis and document findings. In high-risk cancers evaluate the pura-aortic region for metastatic spread. Place a self-retaining retractor and pack the bowel. Obtain pelvic washing for endometrial cancer. Place a long clamp (Carmalt) over the utero-ovarian ligament bilaterally for traction. Identify the left round ligament, ligate it near pelvic side wall with #0 polyglycolic acid sutures (or electrocautery), and transect it. Open the broad ligament along the infundibulopelvic (IP) ligament. Develop the perirectal space bluntly with the following margins: cardinal ligament anteriorly, sacrum posteriorly, ureter and rectum medially, and hypogastric vessels. Open the anterior broad ligament to create a sharp bladder flap. Develop the paravesical space by identifying the following margins: superior vesicle artery and bladder medially, external iliac vessels and obturator internus laterally, cardinal ligament posteriorly, and pubic symphysis anteriorly. Palpate the parametria for evidence of tumor involvement. Perform the previously described procedures on the right side. Skeletonize the IP ligament and retract the ureter away from the IP ligament. For bilateral salpingo-oophorectomy, identify the IP ligament, clamp, cut, and ligate it bilaterally. For ovarian preservation, clamp the utero-ovarian ligament, cut, and ligate it bilaterally. If

pelvic radiation is contemplated after surgery, consider transposing the ovaries out of the radiation field. Skeletonize the superior vesicle artery, mobilize it laterally, and trace it retrograde to identify the uterine artery. Then skeletonize the uterine artery, double ligate, and cut it at its origin. Mobilize it medially and anteriorly away from the ureter. Next, free the ureter from the medial leaf of the broad ligament and Wertheim's canal (cardinal ligament). Repeat these procedures on the other side. Cut the medial leaf of the broad ligament over the rectovaginal septum. Then develop the rectovaginal space bluntly. Skeletonize the uterosacral ligaments, clamp, cut, and ligate them near the sacrum in a successive manner to free the 2- to 3-cm posterior margin. Clamp the cardinal ligaments, cut, and ligate them along the pelvic side wall until the lateral margin of 2 cm is achieved. Clamp the paravaginal tissues, cut, and ligate them bilaterally. Cross-clamp the vaginal tissue and cut to remove the specimen. Then close the vaginal cuff.

- *Postoperative care:* measure spontaneous voiding and residual volume after the patient tolerates a regular diet. The urinary catheter may be discontinued if residual volume is less than 100 mL and spontaneous voiding volume is more than 100 mL. The use of prophylactic antibiotic is controversial. Bladder muscle tone may increase with 10 to 25 mg bethanechol chloride PO every 6 to 8 hours.

Vaginal Hysterectomy

- *Indications, contraindications, consent, risks:* similar to those for Total Abdominal Hysterectomy, earlier.
- *Description:* place a weighted speculum into the vagina, and grasp the cervix with a toothed tenaculum. Inject 10 mL of 1% xylocaine with 1:200,000 epinephrine into the cervix circumferentially. Then incise the cervix with the scalpel, and dissect the bladder away from the pubovesical cervical fascia anteriorly with a sponge stick and Metzenbaum scissors. Enter the anterior cul-de-sac sharply. Repeat the same procedure posteriorly to enter the posterior cul-de-sac without difficulty.

Next, clamp the uterosacral ligament on either side, cut, and ligate it with #0 polyglycolic acid sutures. Ensure hemostatis. Then clamp the cardinal ligaments on both sides, transect, and ligate them in a similar fashion. Serially clamp the uterine arteries and the broad ligament with Heaney clamps, transect, and ligate them bilaterally. Again ensure hemostasis. Clamp both cornua with Heaney clamps, cut, and then deliver the uterus. Ligate the pedicles and check for hemostasis. Close the peritoneum with a purse-string suture of #2-0 polyglycolic acid. Close the vaginal cuff angles with figure-of-eight stitches of #0 polyglycolic acid on both sides, and transfix to the ipsilateral cardinal and uterosacral ligaments. Close the remainder of the vaginal cuff with figure-of-eight stitches of #0 polyglycolic acid in an interrupted fashion.

Laparoscopic-Assisted Vaginal Hysterectomy (LAVH ± BSO)

- *Indications, contraindications, consent, risks:* similar to those for Total Abdominal Hysterectomy, earlier.
- *Description:* The use of the laparoscope for assistance in vaginal hysterectomy is primary for cases in which the vaginal approach is technically challenging or not accommodating for removal. Dissection from the laparoscopic procedure can include transection of the ovarian vessels (if salpingo-oophorectomy is warranted), transection of the uterine vessels, transection of the cardinal and broad ligaments, or transection of the uterosacral ligaments (in this case, only a colpotomy is required for uterine removal). To avoid injury, it is important not to deviate from the practices and techniques used in an abdominal hysterectomy.

Cervical Cold Knife Conization

- *Indications:* abnormal endocervical curettage (ECC), discrepancy between Pap smear and directed biopsy, unsatisfactory colposcopy (cannot see the entire transformation zone), microinvasive cancer on biopsy.
- *Contraindications:* invasive cancer.

- *Consent:* risks—bleeding, infection, cervical incompetence, injury to adjacent organs. Alternative—loop electrocautery excision procedure (LEEP).
- *Description:* delineate the abnormal area with colposcopy and acetic acid. Insert hemostatic sutures at 3 and 9 o'clock. Define the area to be excised and cone it with a beaver blade. After completing the cone, mark the specimen with a suture at 12 o'clock. Obtain hemostasis with cautery. Curette the endocervix, and then curette the endometrium. Recheck hemostasis (using Monsel solution or more cautery).

LEEP

- *Indications, contraindications:* same as those for Cervical Cold Knife Conization, described earlier.
- *Consent:* risks—bleeding, infection, cervical incompetence, injury to adjacent organs. Alternative—cold knife conization, laser ablation, cryotherapy.
- *Description:* similar to the procedures for Cervical Cold Knife Conization, described earlier. In an office setting, visualize, stain, and anesthetize the cervix in a paracervical fashion with 1% lidocaine, with or without epinephrine. LEEP systems come with individual settings and loops designed for tailored cutting and coagulation. Removal of the transformation zone may require more than one pass; however, orientation of the tissue should be made for accurate pathologic evaluation. Occasionally, a second central pass is required for an endocervical lesion. This is usually accomplished with a 1-by-1-cm loop. Ink the margins to enable the pathologist to correctly orient the upper endocervical margin. A curette of the remaining endocervical tissue is helpful for final clinical triage based on final pathologic assessment.

Vaginectomy

- *Indications:* extensive vaginal dysplasia, massive vault prolapse.
- *Contraindications:* invasive cancer.

- *Consent:* risks—bleeding, infection, trauma to adjacent organs (bladder and rectum). Alternatives—ablative techniques (if focal), radiation therapy (rare).
- *Description:* this procedure is most commonly performed in a limited, directed fashion leaving normal unaffected vagina behind (partial vaginectomy). In this case, prepare the vagina with Lugol's solution (similar to Cervical Cold Knife Conization, earlier). Infiltrate areas of demarcation with 10 mL of 1% lidocaine with 1:200,000 epinephrine and incise sharply with a 5- to 10-mm margin. Make this incision to the subcutaneous tissue, then free the tissue from the underlying septa and carefully resect it. If the uterus has been previously removed, enter the peritoneal cavity at the apex of the vagina. Complete vaginectomy begins with infiltration of 1% lidocaine with 1:200,000 epinephrine in the submucosa and circumferential incision of the vaginal mucosa at the introitus. Vertical incisions are made from the grasped and inverted vaginal apex to the hymenal remnant. Dissection occurs in the rectovaginal and vesicovaginal septa. If the uterus is to remain, create drainage canals by leaving a small lateral strip of mucosa intact which is imbricated around with a polyglycolic acid suture. If no uterus is present, remove the vaginal mucosa in strips and approximate the retained subcutaneous tissue with sequential purse-string sutures of polyglycolic acid.

Trachelectomy

- *Indications:* cervical pathology (dysplasia, polyps, nonmalignant pain and bleeding, dyspareunia) in a patient with prior supracervical hysterectomy.
- *Contraindications:* invasive cancer.
- *Consent:* risks—bleeding, infection, trauma to adjacent organs, particularly the bladder and rectum. Alternative—conization.
- *Description:* prepare the surgical field as for a total vaginal hysterectomy. Grasp the cervical stroma and make a circumferential incision to detach the vagina. Dissect the rectovagi-

nal and vesicovaginal septum in a manner similar to that for vaginal hysterectomy. Entry of the peritoneum anteriorly can be difficult depending on the degree of scarring from prior surgery. Clamp the residual vascular supply from descending branches of the uterine artery and ascending branches of the vaginal artery as well as the uterosacral and lower cardinal ligaments and ligate with absorbable suture. Closure of the vagina is similar to that described for vaginal hysterectomy.

Colposcopy and Cervical Biopsy

- *Indication:* certain abnormal Pap smear.
- *Contraindication* (*relative*): gross cervical tumor.
- *Preoperative prep:* colposcopy, smoke evacuator, LEEP machine, Monsel solution.
- *Consents:* bleeding, infection, cervical stenosis or incompetence, pain.
- *Description:*
    1. Apply 3% to 5% acetic acid to the cervix. (If still not able to see, use Lugol's solution.)
    2. Viewing the cervix through colposcopy, identify transformation zone to determine whether colposcopy is satisfactory or not.
    3. If it is satisfactory, evaluate the cervix and biopsy the lesion if the cervix shows any of these features.
        a. Acetowhite.
        b. Punctation.
        c. Mosaic pattern.
        d. Atypical blood vessel.
    4. Obtain ECC.
    5. Apply Monsel solution to the cervical lesion if bleeding is encountered.

VULVA (*Robert L. Coleman and Joseph T. Santoso*)

Laser/Cavitronic Ultrasound Surgical Aspirator (CUSA)

- *Indications:* dysplasia, hyperkeratotic lesions of the vulva, human papillomavirus (HPV).

- *Contraindications:* known or unknown invasive disease.
- *Consent:* risks—recurrent disease, overlooking invasive cancer (both about 20%). Alternatives—wide local excision.
- *Preoperative prep:* vulvoscopy to target lesions.
- *Description:* (1) *laser*—appropriate knowledge of laser energy and tissue effects are required for this technique. Our practice is to utilize the CO_2 laser at 20-W superpulse mode with hand-held columnator. The spot size should be sufficiently small (1 mm) to generate power densities that vaporize tissue without lateral thermal injury. The depth of ablation for vulva dysplasia in hair-bearing areas should be to the third surgical plane (reticular dermis) demarcated by chamois-colored tissue weeping extracellular fluid (approx. 3 mm). Condyloma requires less vaporization depth. This targeted plane is variable in the vulva and much thinner in the labia minor and clitoral regions (approx. 2 mm). Take care not to ablate too deeply in order to limit postoperative scarring. Make small circular motions to ablate the tissue systematically, removing charred areas frequently. If charred areas are not removed, they will heat to very high temperatures, increasing lateral and deep thermal injury. Once the tissue of interest is vaporized, apply a burn solution (silvadene or zinc oxide). (2) *CUSA*—this tool causes cavitational disruption of water-bearing tissue. Our preference is to set the amplitude at 0.7 with 60% suction. Brush the hand-held device over the tissue of interest. The targeted depth is similar to laser. A retrieved specimen in the aspirate may be sent to pathology for evaluation. Postoperative care is similar to that for laser therapy.
- *Postoperative care:* frequent follow-up and aggressive care of the perineum will maximize recovery from these wounds. Narcotics are usually required for 1 to 2 weeks for pain control. Patients are instructed to irrigate the wound over the toilet after each voiding or bowel movement, and then dry the area with a hair dryer. When the tissue is dry, an ointment is applied (silvadene cream or zinc oxide) to the wound site. Estimated time of healing is about 3 to 6 weeks.

Wide Local Excision (WLE)

- *Indications:* vulvar pathology (dysplasia, mass, pigmentation, cysts).
- *Contraindications:* known invasive cancer.
- *Preoperative prep:* targeted lesion via vulvoscopy or palpation.
- *Consent:* risks—infection, wound breakdown. Alternatives—ablation.
- *Description:* outline the area of interest and appropriate margin with a marking pen. Make an incision of the skin to the subcutaneous tissue, although for superficial lesions the depth may be limited to the deep dermis. Remove the skin carefully and orient for the pathologist. Closure of the defect may require reapproximation if the subcutaneous tissue has been entered. Reapproximation mobilizes the surrounding tissue from the subcutaneous fat to allow for tensionless approximation. Flaps are occasionally needed to close the defect, as described later in this chapter, under the heading "Reconstructive Surgery."
- *Postoperative care:* inspect the vulvar wound weekly until it is determined that the skin is healing and the closure is progressing. If the wound has opened, it should be dressed appropriately by the patient.

Skinning Vulvectomy

- *Indications:* same as for WLE, earlier, except more extensive disease; Paget's disease; hidradenitis suppurativa.
- *Contraindications:* known invasive cancer.
- *Consent:* same as for WLE. Patients also need to be aware of changes in appearance (color, structure, anatomy) depending on the technique used for closure (primary, skin graft, flaps).
- *Description:* outline the vulvar skin with a marking pen. The medial margin is the hymenal ring and urethra. Occasionally, the clitoral hood needs resection because of disease but should be spared if not involved. The lateral incisions should not cross the labiocrural folds. Dissection occurs as in WLE.

Closure without graft (skin) requires extensive mobilization to be tension free. Otherwise a skin graft is prepared and a suture bolstered into place as described toward the end of this chapter under the subheading "Skin Graft."

Radical Local Excision

This name is preferred (also known as wide radical local excision, modified radical vulvectomy, radical wide excision).

- *Indications:* invasive vulvar carcinoma.
- *Preoperative prep:* radiographic evaluation of the pelvic nodes. May be combined with sentinel node mapping, lymphoscintigraphy.
- *Consent:* risks—wound breakdown, infection, bleeding.
- *Description:* in general, the lateral border is the labiocrural fold. The medial border is the introitus with a free margin of at least 1 cm. If the margin is less than 1 cm, the incision should be extended up the vagina or onto the thigh. The deep border is the inferior fascia of the urogenital diaphragm. If the tumor is within 5 mm of the anus, consider using pre- or postoperative radiation.

Radial Vulvectomy

- *Indications, preoperative prep, consent:* similar to those for Radical Local Excision, earlier. Stage IB to stage III squamous vulvar carcinoma, good surgical candidate.
- *Description:* the vulvar incision is carried laterally, as described earlier for Radical Local Excision. The deep border extends to the periosteum over the pubic symphysis, the fascia lata, and the inferior fascia of the urogenital diaphragm. Remove the bulbocavernosus, ischiocavernosus, and superficial transverse perineal muscles. Because of vascularity, use cautery after the initial skin incision. Identify and tie the vessels supplying the vulva (internal pudendal artery). The medial border should have a 1- to 2-cm margin. If the distal urethra has been cut, leave a Foley catheter in place for 2 weeks to allow for granulation and epithelialization of the tract.

Groin Nodes (Superficial/Deep)

- *Indications:* staging or resection of the regional nodal basin for invasive vulvar cancer staging.
- *Preoperative prep:* correct positioning of the patient for the procedures allows for exposure of the vulva and the groin. The vulva and groin are prepared. If the procedures are to be done separately, the groin should be done first to reduce the risk of infection.
- *Consent:* risks—bleeding, infection, lymphangitis, lymphedema, lymphocyst, wound breakdown. Alternatives—groin irradiation.
- *Description:* the common groin incision is transverse, parallel to the inguinal ligament, and approximately 3 cm caudal. Carefully dissect the subcutaneous tissue by electrocautery. Identify the Scarpa's layer and separately incise it. Then raise flaps over the underlying nodal tissue, keeping the Scarpa's layer intact. The limits of dissection are visualized as the following: cephalad— the inguinal ligament; lateral—the sartorius muscle; caudal— Hunter's canal (meeting of the sartorius and adductor longus muscle); medial—adductor longus muscle. Meticulous dissection and attention to vascular and lymphatic drainage isolates the venous tributaries of the femoral vein. Circumferential dissection around the centrally working margins will produce the nodal specimen. Ligation of the saphenous vein and/or its accessory may be necessary; however, this practice may be associated with greater morbidity. The superficial dissection generally removes the nodal tissue medial to the fossa ovalis and the nodes along the medial aspect of the femoral vein. If positive nodes are found in the superficial nodal bundle, the fossa ovalis may be incised to access the deeper nodes along the femoral vein or between the artery and vein. Cloquet's node is the cephalad-most node in this chain below the inguinal ligament. Make the area hemostatic, and insert a 20-French Jackson-Pratt or 19-French Blake drain and bring it through a separate stab wound. Reapproximate the Scarpa's layer with 3-0 polyglycolic acid suture, and staple the skin or close it with a subcuticular stitch. Fix the drain with a 2-0 nylon or permanent suture. If

exploration of the pelvic nodes is necessary, make a separate incision above the inguinal ligament, and perform a retroperitoneal dissection. Alternatively, a vertical skin incision can be made to incorporate the groin and the low pelvic nodes.

GENITOURINARY *(Robert L. Coleman)*

Uretero-Ureterostomy

- *Indications:* fibrosis or stenosis of the ureter, segmental obstruction, damage or nicking of the ureter requiring resection.
- *Consent:* risks—ureteral leak, fibrosis, obstruction. Alternatives—ureteral resection with reimplantation, ureteroureterostomy, or utereoneocystostomy.
- *Description:* dissect the ureter free from its peritoneal attachment, giving particular care to its vascular supply. Remove the area of interest, and freshen the edges of the ureter. If the ureter is narrowed, make a small longitudinal incision with an iris scissors to allow for a larger anastomosis (spatulate). Place a 7- to 9-French ureteral catheter in the renal pelvis to the bladder. Place 4-0 synthetic absorbable sutures full thickness through the ureteral wall. Pass a drain under the anastomosis, and reretroperitonealize the ureter, if possible.
- *Postoperative care:* ureteral stents are left in place for 14 days and removed at cystoscopy. A follow-up voiding cystogram with IVP is done at 6 and 12 weeks postoperatively.

Ureteral Reimplantation with Psoas Hitch

- *Indications, consent:* similar to that for Uretero-Ureterostomy, discussed earlier. This procedure is usually required when the segments of ureters cannot be reapproximated.
- *Description:* close the distal ureteral stump with an absorbable suture. Prepare the proximal end as previously described. Mobilize the bladder through dissection of the Retzius' space. The bladder should reach the proximal ureter. Make a cystostomy with electrocautery, and create a separate stab wound with a Kelly clamp. Identify the tip of the proximal ureter with a 3-0

absorbable suture and grasp it with the Kelly clamp. Create a mucosa-to-mucosa anastomosis with 4-0 absorbable suture. If length is sufficient, tunnel the ureteral stump under the bladder mucosa for 3 to 4 cm to provide an antireflux mechanism. Pass a double J stent to the renal pelvis. Create the "hitch" by passing several interrupted 0 synthetic sutures from the bladder muscularis to the psoas fascia. Closure of the bladder proceeds in the standard two-layer fashion. Place a retroperitoneal drain and reperitonealize the area with 3-0 absorbable suture.

Ureteroneocystostomy

- *Indications:* irreparable ureter injuries close to the bladder are best repaired by direct ureteral reimplantation; fistulas.
- *Preoperative prep:* none, since such an injury is usually unexpected.
- *Consent:* failure of anastomosis, ureteral constriction, renal failure, bleeding, infection.
- *Description:* the damaged distal segment of the ureter is excised to obtain fresh edges. The bladder is mobilized to obtain a tension-free anastomosis. Next the dome of the bladder is opened and a curve clamp is used to tunnel the bladder wall where the distal ureter can pass. This submucosal passage also serves to prevent urinary reflux. The distal ureteral end is then spatulated and sutured into the bladder mucosa, using interrupted absorbable sutures. Most clinicians place a ureteral stent through the implanted ureter.
- *Postoperative care:* intravenous pyelogram 4 to 5 weeks after the procedure, then followed by removal of the ureteral stent.

Boari Flap

- *Indications:* anticipated excess tension on the ureter from a ureteroneocystostomy.
- *Consent:* similar to that for Ureteroneocystostomy.
- *Description:* make a wedge around the distribution of the superior vesical artery. The base of the wedge should be about one-half the length of the flap, which should be about 8 to 9

cm. Make a full-thickness incision, and evert the flap. Create a tube using 4-0 synthetic absorbable suture, starting at the distal end of the flap. Suture the ureter at full thickness to the end of the flap. Insert a ureteral stent in the renal pelvis. Closure of the flap, placement of a drain, reperitonealization, and postoperative care are as described for Ureteroneocystostomy.

Intestinal Conduit (Ileal or Colon)

- *Indications:* urinary diversion, usually for vesicovaginal fistula; it is not suitable for primary closure (postradiation or tumor involvement).
- *Preoperative prep:* adequate renal evaluation. Have enterostomal nurse mark the abdomen for location of the stoma. Alternatively the umbilicus may be used. Avoid placing conduit in an abdominal crease with bending, as with colostomy.
- *Consent:* risks—ureteral stricture, hydronephrosis, ureteral leak, stoma necrosis. Alternatives—percutaneous nephrostomy, continent urinary diversion.
- *Description:* the procedure starts by transecting the ureters as near as possible to the bladder to allow for sufficient length. The distal end of the ureter may be trimmed later if it is ischemic after manipulation. Create a window in the mesentery of the sigmoid colon to allow for passage of the ureter to the opposite side; this is usually done below the inferior mesenteric artery. Prepare a segment of bowel for resection in the fashion as described for Small Bowel or Large Bowel Resection, earlier. The mesentery incisions are usually about 5 cm long, allowing for good vascularity of the conduit. The correct orientation of this segment to its natural fecal stream peristalsis is noted. The segment length should be 8 to 12 cm to avoid problems with hyperchloremic metabolic acidosis. Use nonpermanent suture to avoid stone formation. Place ureteral catheters (7 to 9 French) into renal pelvis. These stents are of the single J or Bandor variety. Suture them into ureter loosely with a 3-0 chromic to avoid premature expulsion of the catheter. Remove the distal suture line. Pass an

Anderson clamp through the distal opening to an area near the proximal suture line, and make a small incision. Place full-thickness 4-0 synthetic sutures circumferentially from the ureter to the colon segment. Anchor the periureteral tissue at the site to reduce tension on the suture line. Take care not to twist the ureter, which would compromise blood supply. Over the abdominal site, remove a core as described for Stoma Formation. Bring the conduit to the skin and suture it in a rosebud pattern. Place stay sutures near the conduit and the abdominal wall with 2-0 synthetic absorbable suture. Bring a drain through a separate wound and place it under the ureteral anastomoses. Then reconnect the bowel segments as mentioned earlier, and close the mesentery with 3-0 synthetic absorbable suture.

- *Postoperative care:* remove the drain when no output is noted. Excessive drain output should be sent for analysis of creatinine level; high levels (greater than serum creatinine) would indicate urinary leak. The stents are removed in about 14 days.

Ureteroileoneocystostomy

- *Indications:* intact bladder and normal kidney in a patient with long segment of stenosed ureter.
- *Consent:* same as for Ureteroneocystostomy.
- *Description:* prepare the proximal and distal ureteral segments by making longitudinal incisions to open the ureter. Measure and divide the ileal segment. It is important to maintain the axis of the peristaltic wave. Suture the proximal end of ileum with a 4-0 synthetic suture to the end of the ureter and over a ureteral stent, as previously described. Then reapproximate the bowel as for an Intestinal Conduit, described earlier. Place a drain under the ureteral anastomoses.
- *Postoperative care:* similar to that for Ureteroneocystostomy.

Continent Urostomy (Miami Type)

- *Indications, preoperative prep, consent:* similar to those for Intestinal Conduit, earlier. Patients should be good candidates (capable of self-catheterization) and motivated for the procedure.

- *Description:* prepare the ureters as for Intestinal Conduit, earlier. In this procedure, the ileum and ascending colon will become the bladder substitute and continence mechanism. Inspection of the vascular supply to the colon is critical, especially if a sigmoid resection has been performed as part of the procedure. The author prefers to leave the middle colic artery with the remaining colon for better vascularity of the distal segments. Transilluminate the right colic branches through the mesentery and choose a healthy vascular bowel segment; approximately 32 cm from the ileocecal valve. Similarly, choose a segment of ileum approximately 12 to 15 cm long. This segment may be trimmed after being placed in the anterior abdominal wall, if necessary, but the length is chosen to provide a straight line to the conduit. Redundant tissue makes postoperative catheterization difficult. Once the bowel segments have been prepared, detubularization of the colon is required. The easiest technique is to fold the colon along its antimesenteric side, so that the haustra are aligned, and place an absorbable stapler (polyglycolic acid) along this line; this procedure will detubularize the colon and divide it to make a pouch. If a stapler is not available, cut and hand sew the longitudinal muscles with a delayed absorbable suture. The pouch should be watertight. Bring the ureteral segments to the conduit as for an intestinal conduit. Because the internal conduit surfaces are visible, an antireflux mechanism may be utilized if desired (as described earlier). Fix the periureteral tissue to the conduit to remove tension from the ureters. Before closing the colon pouch, prepare the continence mechanism of the ileal segment. Continence is maintained because the narrower tube of the ileum as prepared, along with the ileal cecal valve, provide higher luminal pressures compared with the colon reservoir. Place a 16-French Foley into the ileum after removing the distal staple line. Then place a GIA-55 stapler along the long axis, antimesenteric side, hugging the Foley. Two or three cuts are required to trim off the excess muscularis. Place three permanent 3-0 sutures in a purse-string fashion at the ileal cecal location, taking care not to constrict too tightly and disrupt the ileo-colic arterial branches. Leave the Foley in situ after testing the ability to pass the catheter through the stoma. This will be used for postoperative irrigation. Bring the ureteral stents through a separate stab wound or through the ileal segment. Close the cecal incision. If an appendectomy has not been performed, it should be performed at this time. Place the conduit into position and fix with 2-0 synthetic absorbable sutures. Place a drain under the conduit, as previously mentioned. Bring the ileal segment through the skin and trim the excess length. Take care not to compromise the vascular supply to the ileum. Fix the stoma with rosebud sutures, as previously described. Pass the Foley catheter several times to ensure a straight passage to the reservoir. Place individual ureteral catheters on the collecting tube. Fix the drain with nonabsorbable sutures.

- *Postoperative care:* irrigate the reservoir every 4 to 6 hours for the first several days to clear mucus. The ureteral stents will be removed in about 14 days, along with the catheter shortly thereafter. It is important that irrigation (50 mL) be continued because mucous plugging is a frequent problem. Patients require frequent catheterization early on to determine their capacity and to avoid mucous plugging.

Cystoscopy

- *Indications:* evaluation of the bladder mucosa, placement of ureteral stents, biopsy.
- *Preoperative prep:* if done for staging purposes, review other radiographic materials.
- *Consent:* risks—bladder rupture (rare), trauma, bleeding, infection.
- *Description:* place the patient in the lithotomy position and perform an examination under anesthesia. Pass the obturator into the urethra and drain the urine. A sample may be taken

for cytology or culture, if necessary. Pass the 30-degree lens into the bladder. Inspect the ureteral orifices by angling the scope laterally and inferiorly as soon as the urethral-vesical junction is observed. Most difficulty is encountered by inserting the scope too far. Use a 70-degree lens to visualize the dome of the bladder. Make a general inspection and obtain biopsies of suspicious areas with a cystoscopic biopsy tool inserted through one of the operating channels. If a ureteral stent is to be placed, prepare a proper double J stent over a guide wire and the catheter. Place the guide wire into the ureteral orifice with the aid of the positioning arm of the cystoscope, and pass the guide wire to the renal pelvis. The placement catheter then pushes the stent through the cystoscope along the guide wire to the ureteral orifice and into the renal pelvis. Once the stent is in position, the guide wire and placing catheter are removed. Bleeding may be controlled with a rollerball or resectoscope.

- *Postoperative care:* occasionally, a three-way catheter may be placed for continuous irrigation.

Suprapubic Catheter

- Postoperative day (POD) 0: leave both urethral Foley and suprapubic catheter drains to gravity.
- POD 1: may discontinue urethral Foley if suprapubic catheter drains well.
- POD 4: may clamp suprapubic catheter for up to 2 hours.

Cystectomy (Anterior Exenteration)

- *Indications:* performed as part of an exenterative procedure for recurrent cancer; occasionally performed for severe bleeding or contraction following radiotherapy.
- *Consent:* risk—bleeding, infection. Requires a conduit.
- *Description:* transect the ureters and dissect the paravesical, parametrial, and Retzius' space. Resect the bladder (most often, a radical resection to include the pelvic tissue to the levator ani). Ligate and transect the vascular supply from the

internal iliac artery. Successive tissue ligation is made in the perivesical fat and fixed with delayed absorbable suture. The vagina and uterus is usually resected with the bladder and the lateral attachments of the uterosacral ligaments. Resect para-vaginal lymphovascular tissue free from the pelvic side wall. If only the bladder is to be removed, development of the vesicovaginal plane is progressively made with a lateral vascular attachment clipped or suture ligated. Transect or completely resect the urethra (if necessary for primary tumor indication) during the perineal phase of the operation. Tie the urethra with a 0 synthetic suture. Place a drain in the resection bed; if vascularity is compromised to the retained pelvic organs, fix an omental J flap to the pelvis. The planned urinary diversion is then completed.

RADIATION THERAPY *(Robert L. Coleman)*

Brachytherapy

- *Indications:* cervical cancer.
- *Preoperative prep:* know the external dose used, and have treatment planning films available.
- *Consent:* risk—uterine perforation, infection, thromboembolic events (during bed rest).
- *Description:* place the patient in the dorsal lithotomy. Perform examination under anesthesia to direct uterine placement. Grasp the cervix with a tenaculum, and sound the uterus. Document the axis and depth of the uterine cavity. Place a Foley catheter with radiopaque dye in the bladder. Place the proper uterine tandem (#1, 2, 3, or 4) in the uterus with the phlange fixed at the cervical interface. The ovoids are placed, and the largest possible diameter maintaining proximity with the cervix is selected and placed. Pack the system with triple sulfa cream around the vaginal packing gauze. Once the vagina and system is tightly packed, take an x-ray (both AP and lateral) to confirm placement. When the system is appropriate, approximate the labia around the system with #1 nylon

suture. Make a reference mark for the ovoids and the tandem on the adjacent thigh. If the system is the first tandem ovoid insertion for the patient, place radiopaque seeds at the external os to allow for comparison with the ovoids.

- *Postoperative care:* patients should be given a low-residue diet and constipating medication (e.g., Lomotil q.i.d.). Because patients will have bed rest for up to 72 hours, sequential pneumatic boots should be given. Check the system daily and compare with marks made intraoperatively.

RECONSTRUCTIVE SURGERY (*(Robert L. Coleman and Joseph T. Santoso)*

Y-plasty Flap (Rhomboid-Style)

- *Indications:* closure of vulvar defect from WLE.
- *Preoperative prep:* the planned flap transfer should be measured and undermined to allow for appropriate tissue mobilization.
- *Consent:* risks—the vulva will likely be distorted and may be cosmetically or functionally displeasing. Alternatives—primary closure, skin flap, rhomboid.
- *Description:* measure the vertical length from the apex of the wound (usually clitoral) to the base of vaginal margin (usually posterior fourchette); this constitutes the length of the superior full-thickness incision. This angle is acute (60 degrees) to the lateral margin of the resection field. Undermine the flap, taking particular care of the base of the flap, which constitutes the vascular supply to the skin. Mobilization lateral to the donor site is required to close the lateral attachments. Suture the flap into place with sutures or staples. Meticulous hemostasis is critical for the flap to take.
- *Postoperative care:* best results are obtained with limited shearing tension across the suture line. Ideally, patients should have 5 to 7 days of bed rest, but they are at increased thromboembolic risk and should wear lower extremities compression devices. Diet should be low residue, and constipating medication may be given, particularly for patients with large posterior flaps.

Z-plasty Flap

- *Indications, preoperative prep, consent:* postoperative care is similar to that for Y-plasty.
- *Description:* the flap is similar to the Y-plasty or rhomboid, but incisions are made from either apex of the wound at an acute angle. Mobilize tissue under each flap incision and bring it to the midline for approximation. Use synthetic sutures or staples to secure the flaps. Medial and lateral incisions are required with this incision and not as well suited for the vulva lesions encroaching the midline.

Gracilis Myocutaneous Flap

- *Indications:* closure of radical vulvar excision/vulvectomy or creation of neovagina following vaginal resection. The flap is myocutaneous and thick, making it a good choice for post-exenterative vaginal reconstruction.
- *Preoperative prep:* examination of the gracilis muscle and preparation of the leg to the knee.
- *Consent:* risks—wound breakdown, failure of graft to take, graft or skin devascularization. Alternatives—skin graft over omental J-plasty; small bowel vaginoplasty, vertical rectus abdominus myocutaneous (VRAM) flap.
- *Description: creation of the neovagina*—palpation of the gracilis muscle is made with the patient in low lithotomy position. Topographically, the muscle will lie below a line drawn from the pubic tubercle to the medial epicondyle of the femur. Make the skin paddle incision 6 cm from its tendinous insertion (labiocrural fold) and extend 12 cm in total length. The paddle below the line is 6 cm thick. Continue the skin incision deeply through the fascia. The proximal vascular supply comes from the medial circumflex femoral artery (a branch of the deep femoral artery). Take care to avoid traumatizing this neurovascular bundle, which generally lies 8 to 10 cm from the labiocrural fold. When the gracilis is encountered, a 2-cm distal muscle transection is made to allow for muscle contraction. Because the blood

supply to the skin comes from underneath the muscle, following flap mobilization fix the skin with a few absorbable sutures to its underlying fascia. This prevents shearing trauma to the skin. Harvest both sides in this manner if needed. Mobilize the tissue under the labiocrural fold to allow for tunneling of the graft to the vulva. Take care to ensure the vascular pedicle is not torsed. Once this is accomplished, suture the distal-most portion of the flap to the opposite side with absorbable sutures. Once an approximation of the skin is made, rotate the flap posteriorly to fill the vaginal cavity. Suture the hymenal remnant to the flap with absorbable sutures. Closure of the thigh is made by approximation of the fascia and placement of subcutaneous drains (e.g., 19-French Blake tubes). Close the skin sites with staples. *Closure of vulvar wound*—in this scenario, there frequently is no labiocrural fold. In this case, harvest the graft and rotate into place, trimming for confirmation, and suturing into place with synthetic material or staples, as previously described.

Vertical Rectus Abdominus Myocutaneous (VRAM) Flap

- *Indications, consent:* same as for the Gracilis Myocutaneous Flap, earlier.
- *Preoperative prep:* prepare abdominal wall up to the breasts.
- *Description:* locate the skin paddle at and above the level of the umbilicus, reaching through a midline incision. Carry the paddle down to the anterior rectus sheath and mobilize the skin overlying the lateral margins to expose the fascia. Cut a 5-cm wide strip of fascia just lateral to the linea alba. Continue the fascia harvest slightly above the skin paddle. Transect the rectus muscle cephalad and caudal, and roll the skin flap to construct it into a vaginal vault. Then rotate the flap 180 degrees and pass it through a posterior fascia caudal incision and into the pelvic cavity. Then reapproximate and close the fascial incisions. A mesh closure of the ab-

domen is occasionally necessary. Suture the neovagina into place.

Omental J-Flap

- *Indications:* neovagina, pelvic vascularity, pelvic sling.
- *Preoperative prep:* take care intraoperatively not to injure the vascular supply of the omentum.
- *Description:* the omentum is supplied by the right and left gastroepiploic vessels, and either of the vessels may be used to make the flap. However, division of the right vessel is performed most commonly. Dividing some of the omental branches of the right gastroepiploic artery makes a flap that is mobilized to the pelvis. The periphery is sutured to the pelvic inlet to make a sling. To make a neovagina form a cavity with absorbable suture. Harvest a skin flap, suture it around a condom-covered foam block, and insert it into the omental cavity. Approximate the labia loosely around the condom end.
- *Postoperative care:* this is left in place for 7 to 10 days. After that time, the foam/condom is removed. The patient will need to continue dilation for several months, otherwise the graft will undergo contraction.

Martius Flap (Bulbocavernosus Muscle Flap)

- *Indications:* vesicovaginal, rectovaginal fistula.
- *Description:* clear the fistula hole of scar tissue, and measure the size of the skin flap to cover the defect. Make the paddle slightly larger than the defect so that it will close. If the flap is to be rotated anteriorly, the paddle is often chosen at the dorsal location. If the flap is to be rotated posteriorly, the ventral skin paddle is made. Make a skin incision in the labia majora and dissect to the bulbocavernosus muscle, which is divided at the side of the skin paddle. Create a window under the labia minora, and bring the flap to the fistula where it is trimmed to cover the deflect. Close the donor site with delayed absorbable suture.

Skin Graft

- *Indications:* to cover granulating surface.
- *Description:* split-thickness (epidermis and part of the dermis) skin grafts, with open blood vessels on the underside, are able to survive in granulated/contaminated wounds. Cut the skin to a preselected dermis (0.012- to 0.018-inch or 0.3- to 0.45-mm thickness; adjust the dermatome blade to the sharp part of a #15 Bard-Parker blade). Extra skin may be stored at 4° C in saline with antibiotics. Equipment needed: Padgett dermatome (electrical), mineral oil, epinephrine solution, petroleum gauze, and mesher to perforate the graft.

  Preoperatively, give the routine preoperative antibiotics, shave the donor site, and wash the recipient site with Hibiclens (not Betadine). Prepare the recipient site by scraping it with a tongue depressor or scalpel until flat to the skin level (taking lots of granulation tissues). Measure graft size. Apply mineral oil to the donor site (usually lateral hip) to allow smooth movement of the dermatome during skin graft harvesting. Once the skin is obtained, mesh it at 1:1 to 1:3. Apply the graft to the donor site (be careful not to implant the skin graft in reverse), and use staples to immobilize it. Use puffed-up Kerlex over the graft.

- *Postoperative care:* cover the donor site with xerofoam and dressing. Use PCA for pain control. The next morning, open the donor site dressing. Keep the Xerofoam. Apply a heat lamp or fan for 20 minutes q.i.d. Xerofoam will peel off by itself in a few days. Immobilize the graft site with the same dressing for the next 7 days.

IV | SYNOPSIS OF TREATMENT MODALITIES AND INTERVENTIONS

Sara Crowder and Joseph T. Santoso

PREOPERATIVE CHECKLIST

Indications for Surgery

- Be clear about the indication for surgery and confirm that the right procedure is planned.
- Discuss the indications and options with the patient so she understands why the procedure is indicated.

Surgical Consent

The surgeon should prepare and review the consent with the patient. Consent should contain:

- All of the planned procedures.
- "Other indicated procedures" to cover unforeseen situations.
- Risks of the procedures: in general—pain, infection, bleeding, injury to surrounding organs (i.e., bowel, bladder, blood vessels, ureter, etc.), and need for repair; failure to cure problem, need for further treatment or procedures. Specifically— colostomy, lymphedema, pneumothorax, and perforation of the uterus, depending on the procedure.
- The possibility of a blood transfusion and accompanying risks. The risk of transmission of HIV is 1/500,000; of hepatitis B, 1/60,000; of hepatitis C, 1/100,000. Possible risk of yet undiscovered viruses.[1] See Appendix B.
- No guarantee: the results of the surgery cannot be guaranteed.

Document

Make sure the following is written in the history and physical examination section: "The risks, benefits, indications, options were discussed with the patient and informed consent was obtained. The patient and her family had no unanswered questions." Documentation of such discussion is a JCAHO requirement.

Patient Expectations

Review the type of incision, pain control, anticipated hospital stay, need for early ambulation, incentive spirometer use, visitation rules, and so forth.

Code Status/Living Will

This is a good time to discuss these issues and conform to your institution's documentation guidelines for admission.

Preoperative Studies

A. Laboratory studies:
   1. CBC.
   2. Chemistry/electrolytes panel.
   3. Liver function tests.
   4. Thyroid panel: if adequacy of replacement is unclear or symptomatic.
   5. Tumor markers should be obtained preoperatively, as applicable.

Marker	Indication
CA-125	Postmenopausal adnexal masses, suspected ovarian cancer, epithelial uterine cancer (see Chap. 2)
β-hCG, α-FP, LDH	Young women with suspected germ cell tumor
Inhibin	Suspected granulosa cell tumor
CEA, CA-19-9	If bowel cancer primary is suspected

B. Other studies:
   1. ECG: all patients 40 years of age or older; cardiac history; cardiac symptoms; prior exposure to cardiotoxic drugs (e.g., doxorubicin).

2. Chest x-ray—all patients 40 years of age or older; pulmonary history; pulmonary symptoms; newly diagnosed or suspected cancer; prior exposure to pulmonary toxic drugs (e.g., bleomycin).
3. Medical/cardiology clearance—patients with poorly controlled diabetes, hypertension, angina, thyroid, asthma or other chronic disease.
4. Pulmonary function tests—significant pulmonary history/symptoms or morbid obesity.
5. See also Preoperative Risk Assessment, later in this chapter.

C. Blood:
1. When large blood loss is anticipated, obtain type and cross-match for 2 U.
2. Otherwise, type and screen.

D. Bowel preparation (see also later discussion)
1. Reasons for bowel prep:

Reason	Example	Recommended Bowl Prep
Risk to bowel integrity	Ovarian debulking, GI cases, colostomy	Full bowel prep (see later discussion)
Need for visualization inside bowel or by manipulating bowel out of operative field	Laparoscopic lymphadenectomy, proctoscopy, colonoscopy	1-day bowel prep (see later discussion)
Need to keep a clean perineum postoperatively	Vulvectomy, radical local excision	1-day bowel prep (see later discussion)
Need to empty sigmoid colon for mobility/visualization	Radical hysterectomy, endometrial cases	Enemas in morning on day of surgery

E. Prophylactic antibiotics
   1. Cefotetan, 2 g IV on call to OR.
   2. If the patient is allergic to cephalosporins, could use clindamycin, 900 mg IV.
   3. See Bacterial Endocarditis Prophylaxis in Adults later in this chapter, under Perioperative Drug Management.
F. Other surgical orders: e.g., NPO after midnight, sequential compression device/TED hose.
G. OR coverage and equipment:
   1. Arrange scheduling with the OR, anesthesia, and any anticipated consultants.
   2. Equipment:
      a. Very obese patient—order Bookwalter or Omni retractor and a special OR table. Connecting two OR tables will not work because this will impair the surgeon's ability to operate well.
      b. Ovarian cases—consider ABC (argon beam coagulator) and CUSA (cavitronic ultrasound surgical aspirator) to maximize tumor debulking.
      c. Allen or "candy cane" stirrup, as needed.
      d. Fluoroscopic equipment and table for placement of mediport or hemaport to assess the location of the catheter tip.
H. Ostomy planning: Mark the colostomy or ileostomy site preoperatively. The guidelines for marking are as follows: Avoid skin folds. Request the patient to stand and bend over to identify the abdominal fold. Avoid clothing marks. Request the patient to identify where clothing fits. Best placement is generally at one-half to two-thirds the distance from the anterior superior iliac spine to the umbilicus. It should be where the patient can adjust it easily, usually medial to the nipple line.
I. Preoperative note: document the following in the patient's chart prior to surgery—that the consent is on the chart, the patient has no questions or new problems, and the results of any preoperative laboratory, x-rays, or other studies.

PREOPERATIVE RISK ASSESSMENT

ASA Classification—Assessment of Operative Risk[3]

ASA Class	Condition of Patient	Postoperative Mortality (%)
I	Normal, healthy	0.08
II	Mild to moderate systemic disease	0.27
III	Severe disease that limits activity but not incapacitating	1.8
IV	Incapacitating and life threatening	7.8
V	Moribund	9.4

Goldman Preoperative Cardiac Risk Assessment[4]

Category	Finding	Score
History	Age > 70 years	5
	MI within 6 months	10
Exam	S_3 gallop, JVD, or left heart failure	11
	Ventricular atrial stenosis	3
ECG	Nonsinus rhythm	7
	> 5 PVC/min	7
General (any one = 3 pts)	K < 3, HCO_3 < 20, BUN > 50, Cr > 3, Po_2 < 60, Pco_2 > 50, abnormal AST, chronically bedridden	3
Operation	Intraperitoneal, thoracic, or aortic	3
	Emergency	4
	Sum Total Points _____	
	Total Possible	53

The Goldman class is assigned based on the total points with the associated risk as outlined below:

Class	Points	Major Cardiac Complications (%)	Cardiac Death (%)
I	0–5	0.7	0.2
II	6–12	5	2
III	13–25	12	2
IV	> 25	22	56

RECENT MYOCARDIAL INFARCTION (MI)

Surgery should be postponed until 6 months after an MI, because the risk of reinfarction within 6 months is 2% to 5%.[5] This is compared with a baseline risk for American adults of about 0.2% risk of MI or cardiac death associated with general anesthesia and surgery.[6] In patients with cardiovascular symptoms, preoperative exercise testing will be valuable. If the patient has physical limitations (i.e., orthopedic fracture), a dipyridamole-thallium testing will mimic the coronary vasodilatory response associated with exercise. The thallium will bind to nonischemic cardiac muscle, thus highlighting old infarct versus transient ischemic area.

BOWEL PREPARATION

A. Mechanical preparation:
  1. Reduces total bacterial counts.
  2. Can add an antibiotic preparation, as described later.
      a. Whole gut lavage with polyethylene glycol (Golytely, Colyte, Nulytely):
        (1) One day before surgery:
            (a) Provide a clear liquid diet.
            (b) Have patient start taking Golytely at 9 A.M.
            (c) Give Golytely—PO or NG, chilled, at least 1 L/hour until rectal effluent is clear (usually requires 3 to 6 hours or 3 to 8 L).
            (d) Keep patient NPO after midnight.
            (e) Give enemas as needed in the morning on the day of surgery (enemas usually are not needed with adequate lavage).
      b. One-day bowel prep:
        (1) One day before surgery:
            (a) Provide a clear liquid diet.
            (b) Order magnesium citrate, 2 bottles—have patient start drinking at 9 A.M. (encourage to finish by noon).
            (c) At 6 P.M. take Ducolox PO 2–4 tablets at once.
            (d) Keep patient NPO after midnight.
            (e) Give enemas as needed in the morning on day of surgery.

B. Antibiotic preparation:
1. Reduces bacterial concentration and alters flora.
2. The antibiotic tablets are poorly absorbed, and thus are active in the gut lumen.
3. Should be given in conjunction with a mechanical bowel prep the day before surgery (for 8 A.M. start time):
   a. Neomycin sulfate, 1 g PO at 1 P.M., 2 P.M., and 11 P.M.
   b. Erythromycin base, 1 g PO at 1 P.M., 2 P.M., and 11 P.M.
   c. Some clinicians use metronidazole, 500 mg, in place of erythromycin base.
C. Inpatient bowel prep: In patients who are severely malnourished, elderly, or frail, consider admission for IV fluid hydration and monitoring of electrolytes during bowel preparation.

DVT PROPHYLAXIS

Treatment of deep venous thrombosis/pulmonary embolism (DVT/PE) and heparin protocol are discussed in Chap. 22.

Options for DVT and PE Prophylaxis

Type	Order	Risk
Heparin	5000 U SC 2 hours prior to surgery, then q 8–12 h until ambulatory	Increases minor bleeding or hematoma
Low-molecular-weight heparin	Dalteparin, 2500 U SC q 24 h started 2 hours prior to abdominal surgery	Less bleeding and heparin-induced thrombocytopenia/thrombocytosis risks than unfractionated heparin[7]
Dextran 40 or 70	500 mL IV during surgery; 500 mL IV postoperatively until the next day (8 A.M.), then 500 mL IV (75 mL/h) daily for 3–5 days	Anaphylactic reaction, 0.1%–0.25%, can induce excessive renal diuresis (caution in hypovolemic patient)
Compression device	Should be worn prior to general anesthesia	Minimal, mainly discomfort

PERIOPERATIVE DRUG MANAGEMENT

Aspirin

- Stop 2 weeks prior to surgery (as platelet life span is about 7 days).
- May use heparin supplement for patients with unstable angina or coronary artery disease.

Antidepressant

- Stop MAO inhibitors and tricyclics 1 week before surgery.

Steroid-Dependent Patient

- Defined as greater than 40 mg prednisone for 1 week, or 7.5 mg when taken chronically. Chronic use of prednisone can result in steroid dependency.
- Give 100 mg IV hydrocortisone in the evening before and on the morning of surgery.

Postoperative Taper

POD	Hydrocortisone	Prednisone Equivalent
0	100 mg IV q 8 h	37.5 mg PO q 12 h
1	100 mg IV q 8 h	37.5 mg PO q 12 h
2	80 mg IV q 8 h	30 mg PO q 12 h
3	60 mg IV q 8 h	22.5 mg PO q 12 h
4	40 mg IV q 8 h	15 mg PO q 12 h
5	20 mg IV q 8 h	7.5 mg PO q 12 h

POD = postoperative day.

- Discontinue or resume preoperative maintenance dose.

Cardiovascular Medications

- Continue nitrates, beta-blockers, calcium channel blockers, and clonidine to prevent rebound hypertension.
- Can be taken with a sip of water the morning of surgery.

NIDDM Patients

- Convert long-acting drugs to short-acting ones (e.g., chlor-propamide or glyburide to tolbutamide).
- Keep patient NPO after midnight.
- Administer regular insulin at 6 A.M.
- Postoperatively: resume patient's IV medications and sliding scale regular insulin.
- Check serum glucose in the recovery room and every 6 hours.

Sliding Scale Insulin

Glucose Level	Action
< 70	Call MD and give 50 mL of $D_{50}W$
70–249	0 insulin
250–299	2 U regular insulin SQ
300–349	4 U regular insulin SQ
350–400	6 U regular insulin SQ
> 400	8 U and call MD

- Next day, add extra insulin given in the past 24 hours, divide it by 4, and then add that amount to the previous q.i.d. dose.

IDDM Patients (Minor Surgery)

- Keep NPO after midnight and start IV lactated Ringer's solution (LR) with 20 mEq KCl at 100 mL/hour.
- Give half NPH and half regular insulin dose SQ at 6 A.M.
- Postoperatively: continue half of daily dose until the patient resumes the ADA diet or TPN.

IDDM Patients (Major Surgery)

- Postoperatively: order insulin drip, 1 U/hour, check blood glucose hourly times 6, then every 4 hours times 4, then every 6 hours times 4. Adjust the insulin drip to maintain blood glucose between 100 and 200.
- Give IV fluid without glucose for a day or two and check blood glucose every 6 hours.

Birth Control Pill

- Stop 1 month prior to surgery, as it doubles the risk of thromboembolism compared with nonusers.[8]
- Hormone replacement therapy may continue as long as patient is given prophylactic measures (SQ heparin or sequential compression device), as the increase in absolute risk is small.[9]

Heparin (Unfractionated)

- Stop 4 hours prior to surgery. Half-life of heparin is about 90 minutes. In a bleeding emergency, use protamine to reverse heparin. One milligram of protamine antagonizes approximately 100 U of heparin dose.
- Give half calculated dose of protamine initially to minimize hypotension; maximum overall dose is 50 mg.

Warfarin

- Stop warfarin 2 days before surgery and restart heparin infusion. May give 5 mg vitamin K PO or IM or IV to lower PT/INR (international normalized ratio) to a safe level in 4 hours and to a normal level in 24 hours.
- In an emergent reversal case, use 2 to 4 U of fresh frozen plasma.
- Postoperatively, restart heparin 12 to 24 hours after surgery. Warfarin then may be restarted on POD 2 (to prevent skin necrosis related to warfarin) concurrent with heparin infusion. (See the heparin protocol in Chap. 22.)

Bacterial Endocarditis Prophylaxis in Adults

- Give ampicillin, 2 g + gentamicin, 1.5 mg/kg IM/IV (120 mg maximum) within 30 minutes of the procedure.
- If the patient is allergic to penicillin, substitute ampicillin with vancomycin, 1 g IV, over 1 to 2 hours.
- For minor procedures, give amoxicillin, 2 g PO (or ampicillin 2 g IV) within 30 minutes.

- If the patient is allergic to penicillin, use clindamycin, 600 to 900 mg PO/IV.[10]

Patient-Controlled Analgesia (PCA)

- See Chap. 20 discussion of pain control measures.

Ulcer Prophylaxis

- Give ranitidine, 150 mg in 250 mL D_5W at an IV rate of 10 mL/hour.
- Alternately, use cimetidine, 900 mg in 250 mL D_5W at an IV rate of 10 mL/hour. If creatinine level is higher than 2 mg/dL, decrease the rate to 5 mL/hour.
- Another option is sucralfate, 1 g PO/NG every 4 to 6 hours.
- *Note:* warfarin increases the half-life of H_2 blockers.

Hypothyroidism

- Patients on adequate supplementation can tolerate a few days without their usual medications when necessary to keep NPO.
- Patients should stay on their usual dose until the evening before surgery.

Hyperthyroidism

- If untreated, patients are at risk for thyroid storm.
- Treatment can be given for urgent procedures with propranolol, propylthiouracil, and potassium iodide to prevent storm (see Chap. 17).

SURGICAL DRAINS/LINES

G-Tube (Gastric Tube)

- Indication: to release pressure on the stomach caused by bowel obstruction, or for feedings.
- With PEG (percutaneous G tube), can start feeding the next day if desired.

- For open procedures, wait a few more days for return of bowel function. Incidental dislodgement of the tube usually occurs on POD 3. Leave drainage to gravity—not to wall suction.

Chest Tube

- Used for pneumothorax, hemothorax, or pleural effusion.
- Attach to a pleuravac at 20 cmH_2O. Obtain a chest x-ray daily.
- For pneumothorax, continue wall suction for 2 days, then water seal for at least 1 day. Keep water sealed until the output is less than 100 mL/24 hour before pulling out the tube. For hemothorax or pleural effusion, place on suction for 1 day, then water seal. Pull out the tube when the output is less than 100 mL/24 hour. To remove, ask the patient to take a deep breath and bear down (Valsalva maneuver), and remove the tube at the end of the inspiration. Apply an occlusive bandage (petroleum jelly gauze) rapidly to cover the chest opening. Obtain a chest x-ray after water seal and after discontinuing the tube.

Jackson Pratt or Blake (JP, Closed Drain)

- Drain to bulb suction. May discontinue if intra-abdominal JP output is less than 50 mL/24 hours. It can also be placed subcutaneously in an obese patient for about 2 days to prevent seroma formation.
- For groin wounds after inguinal LAD, leave in place until output is less than 10 mL/24 hours. Be sure to "strip" the tubing daily to prevent any blockage from clots.

Abramson (Open/Sumped Drain, Large Drain)

- Drain to low wall suction.
- Ideal to evacuate large amount of fluid from the abdominal/pelvic cavity or for abscess pockets.

Penrose (Passive) Drain

- For large bleeding or drainage. Place a stoma bag to collect drainage and pull ("crack") the drain 1 to 2 cm/day out from the wound.
- Not usually recommended as it is easily infected.

Tenckhoff Catheter/Intraperitoneal Port-a-cath

- Irrigate with 500 U heparin in 15 mL sterile NS q.i.d. for 3 days.
- Then, irrigate once a week.

NG Tube

- Attach to continuous (not intermittent) low wall suction (as all of them are sump drains).
- Replace 1 mL NG drainage with 1 mL of D5 ½ NS + 20 mEq KCl/L intravenously.
- Routine usage of an NG tube postoperatively after bowel anastomosis does not protect anastomosis.[11]

Standard CVP Line

- Requires daily flushing with heparin.
- Use it as long as there are no signs of infection (erythema, pus, fever).
- In burn or immunosuppressed patients, change the line every 3 days.

Peripherally Inserted Central Venous Catheter (PICC)

- Placed antecubitally.
- Because it's lumen has a small diameter, it requires extensive local care and daily flushing.

Hickman Catheter

- Usually a subclavian catheter that is skin-tunneled to exit through skin. It requires daily flushing and may last for a few months.

- If the catheter is clogged with blood clot, use urokinase as follows: make up 5000 U/mL of urokinase solution. Inject 1 mL of the solution and follow with 3 mL of NaCl. Allow it to stay in catheter for 1 hour. Then try to draw back again.

Mediports/Hemaport/Port-a-cath

- Subcutaneously inserted tunneled lines that enter a central vein. It is accessed in a sterile manner using a special bent needle (Huber needle). It requires flushing once a month.
- If it does not draw back, consider irrigation with urokinase, as previously described for Hickman catheter.
- If there is a concern about catheter patency, inject Hypaque contrast under fluoroscopic examination.

Baker's Tube

- Used to keep the small bowel patent.

Ureteral Stent (6 French)

- When used after ureteral anastomosis, leave in place for 2 weeks. Obtain an IVP to confirm patency of the ureter. The stent, then, may be pulled out via cystoscope.
- For patency in relieving hydronephrosis, the stent may need to be changed every 3 months or 1 year (depending on the type of stent).

Percutaneous Nephrostomy Tube (PCN)

- Placed to relieve obstructive hydronephrosis.
- Can be placed by an interventional radiologist.
- Give prophylactic antibiotics prior to the procedure as many patients will develop infection.

Admission Order

Admit to Gyn-Oncology	
Diagnosis:	Admit for surgery . . .
Condition:	Stable/Fair/Guarded
Vital signs:	Per routine (or q 4 h)
Allergy:	
Activity:	Ad lib
Nursing:	Daily weight, strict I & Os
	Place sequential compression device (SCD) + TED hose on call to OR
	Call MD for T > 38.5° C, 90/60 > BP > 160/105, Pulse > 110, RR > 28
Diet:	Clear liquid then NPO after midnight
IV:	TKO then start D5 1/2 NS + 20 Meq KCl 100 mL/hour at midnight
Med:	1. H_2 blocker of choice
	2. Bowel prep—see earlier discussion
	3. Diphenhydramine, 25 to 50 mg IV q 6 h prn insomnia
	4. Cefotetan, 2 g IV on call to OR
	5. Promethazine, 25 mg IV q 6 h prn nausea/vomiting
Labs:	CBC, chemistry, LFTs, Mg, β-hCG, UA, CA-125, T & S, ECG, chest x-ray (Pa + lateral)

Preop by anesthesia, any other needed consults

Postop Order (ICU Admission)

Admit to Gyn-Oncology (first call: Dr. Resident; second call: Dr. Attending Physician)	
Diagnosis:	Condition: Activity: Allergy: Diet:
Vital signs	q 15 min × 4, then q 30 min × 4, then per ICU routine
Swan-Ganz catheter:	Chest x-ray to confirm placement
	Obtain CVP, PaOP, CI, SVI, SVR q 1 h × 4, then q 4 hr
	Obtain Do_2, Vo_2, MVo_2 q 6 h
IV:	D_5 NS + 20 Meq KCl at _____ mL/h
Ventilator	Pressure-controlled—SIMV, rate 12, TV 750,

setting:	PS 5, PEEP 5; FiO_2 100%, then wean it to < 50% to keep O_2 sat > 95% or PaO_2 > 90 mmHg
Nursing:	Daily weight, strict I & Os Call MD for T ≥ 38.5° C, 90/60 > BP > 160/105, pulse > 110, RR > 28, UO < 30 mL/h, excessive bleeding TED and SCD all the time except when walking
Meds:	1. H_2 blocker of choice

     2. Diphenhydramine, 25–50 mg IV q 6 h prn insomnia

     3. Potassium sliding scale:

K < 2.5	Give 40 mEq KCl IV, call MD, get ECG
2.5 < K < 3	Give 30 mEq KCl IV
3 < K ≤ 3.5	Give 20 mEq KCl IV
3.6 < K < 5.4	No K supplement
K > 5.5	Get ECG and call MD

     4. Calcium sliding scale (normal ionized Ca 1.12–1.23 mmol/L); if ionized Ca < 1.1, give 1 amp $CaCl_2$

     5. Phosphate (normal 2.7–4.5 mg/dL); if PO_4 <1, give 5 mg/kg of elemental phosphorus IV over 6 hours; 1 > PO_4 > 2, give 2.5 mg/kg phosphorus over 6 hours; recheck phosphate level in 6 hours

     6. Mg level (normal: 1.3–2.1 mEq/L): if Mg level < 1.3, give 2 g $MgSO_4$ IV; recheck level in 6 hours

     7. Morphine, 1–8 mg IV q 1 h prn pain if MAP > 70

     8. Versed/lorazepam, 1–2 mg IV q 1 h prm anxiety if MAP > 70

     9. Compazine, 10 mg IV q 6 h prn nausea

Lab:	Chest x-ray in recovery room to check line placement and/or endotracheal tube Once patient arrives in ICU, obtain CBC, chem 7, PT/INR, PTT (if concern about ongoing bleeding, obtain serial hemoglobin q 4 h × 6), ionized Ca, Mg levels

     CBC and chem 7, q 8 h × 2, then b.i.d.
     ABGs b.i.d. and prn ventilator changes
     Chem 20, Mg, ionized calcium, phosphate q Tuesday and Thursday
     Chest x-ray q A.M., drains

REFERENCES

1. Schreiber GB, Busch MP, Kleinman SH, Korelitz JJ: The risk of transfusion-transmitted viral infections. The Retrovirus Epidemiology Donor Study. N Engl J Med 334:1685, 1996.
2. Narr BJ: Preanesthetic evaluation, in *Critical Care Medicine—Perioperative Management,* MJ Murray, DB Coursin, RG Pearl, DS Prough (eds). Philadelphia, Lippincott-Raven, 1997, pp 11–18.
3. Vacanti CJ, Van Houten RJ, Hill RC: A statistical analysis of the relationship of physical status to postoperative mortality in 68,388 cases. Anesth Analg 49:564, 1970.
4. Goldman L: Cardiac risks and complications of noncardiac surgery. Ann Intern Med 98:504, 1983.
5. Averette HE, Janicek MF: Perioperative care and critical care, in *Principals and Practice of Gynecologic Oncology,* WJ Hoskins, CA Perez, RC Tony (eds). Philadelphia, Lippincott-Raven, 1997, p 277.
6. Goldman L: Cardiac risks and complications of noncardiac surgery. Ann Intern Med 98:504, 1983.
7. Warkentin TE, Levine MN, Hirsh J, Horsewood P, Roberts RS, Gent M, Kelton JG: Heparin-induced thrombocytopenia in patients treated with low-molecular-weight heparin or unfractionated heparin. N Engl J Med 332:1330, 1995.
8. Vessey M, Mand D, Smith A, Yeates D: Oral contraceptives and venous thromboembolism: Findings in a large prospective study. BMJ 292:526, 1986.
9. Jick H, Derby LE, Myers MW, Vasilakis C, Newton KM: Risk of hospital admission for idiopathic venous thromboembolism among users of postmenopausal oestrogens. Lancet 348:981, 1996.
10. Anonymous: Antimicrobial prophylaxis in surgery. Med Lett Drugs Therapeut 41:75, 1999.
11. Colvin DB, Lee W, Eisenstat TE, Rubin RJ, Salvati EP: The role of nasointestinal intubation in elective colonic surgery. Dis Colon Rectum 29:295, 1986.

*Joseph T. Santoso
and Robert L. Coleman*

TREATMENT PRINCIPLES AND APPROACHES

Chemotherapy has a narrow therapeutic window. Potential complications from chemotherapy range from drug reaction to death. Consequently, administration of chemotherapy requires more intensive preparation than other drug prescriptions.

Before giving chemotherapy, we recommend going over the following checklist:

- The cancer diagnosis must be confirmed histologically.
- The chemotherapy agents must be appropriate for the diagnosis (see Table 26–1).
- The patient must be healthy enough to stand up to the rigors of chemotherapy (GOG performance status of 0, 1, or 2 and an estimated survival of $\geq$ 3 months).
- Laboratory results should be adequate (WBC $\geq$ 3000 [ANC > 1500]), platelets $\geq$ 100,000. AST, ALT, GGT, LDH, and alkaline phosphatase $\leq$ 3 times normal. Bilirubin must be $\leq$ 1.5 times normal. Creatinine $\leq$ 2 mg/dL or creatinine clearance $\geq$ 50 mL/min.
- Finally if the patient's body surface area (BSA) is more than 2, the chemotherapy dose is usually limited to a BSA of 2.

During chemotherapy, treatment is modified or stopped when the cancer is cured, the cancer is resistant to chemotherapy, or the chemotherapy side effects become intolerable. Therefore, before beginning chemotherapy, the cancer should be evaluated and identified as one of the following categories:

- *Complete response* (*CR*): a complete disappearance of all clinical evidence of tumor, including normalization of the CA-125 value, determined by two observations at least 4 weeks apart.
- *Partial response* (*PR*): a greater than 50% decrease in the sum of the product of measured lesions, determined by two

observations not less than 4 weeks apart. No simultaneous increase in the size of any lesion or the appearance of new lesions may occur. Nonmeasurable lesions must remain stable or regress to be included in this category.

- *Stable disease* (*SD*): a steady state of response less than PR, or progression less than PD, lasting at least 4 weeks. No new lesions.
- *Progressive disease* (*PD*): an unequivocal increase of at least 50% in the product of the measured lesion. New lesions also constitute PD.

Elimination and degradation of chemotherapy occur mainly via the kidney or liver. Most drugs require substantial dose reductions or termination when these organs are compromised. If the laboratory criteria in the checklist are not met, delaying the next chemotherapy for 1 week and then reducing the dose by 25% to 50% are usually recommended. An exception is in the treatment of germ cell tumors where drug intensity has to be maintained, even if it means requiring granulocyte-stimulating factor.

Tumors grow exponentially due to the disruption in the regulation of programmed cell death (apoptosis), not because of rapid proliferation. As the tumor grows larger, the rate of growth slows (Gompertzian growth). However, the tumor burden increases rapidly at the end stage of disease. A tumor will have generally undergone 30 doubling times before being clinically detectable (1-cm size, 1 g, or 10^9 cells); it takes only two doubling times for a 1-cm tumor to reach 4 cm.

Chemotherapy acts by first-order kinetics (killing a constant fraction of cells exposed to the drug rather than a constant number). A single chemotherapy agent can be curative only by producing a high log kill ($> 99\%$) and repetitive therapy. Multiagent chemotherapy is generally favored over single-agent therapy, because the additive cell kill capabilities through alternate mechanisms (e.g., cell cycle) and non–cross resistant characteristics can produce a higher log kill.

Dose intensity plays a minor role in gynecologic tumors. Although retrospective studies on highly chemotherapy-sensitive tumors (e.g., seminoma, germ cell tumor, acute leukemia) have suggested that higher dose intensity gives a better response rate, this effect is less clear in other solid tumors, such as breast and ovarian. The ultimate dose intensity regimens are bone marrow transplantations. Currently, no data have conclusively demonstrated that marrow ablative strategies have improved progression-free or overall survival. In studies involving cisplatin,[1] carboplatin, and others, increased dosage showed little difference in response rate but did increase toxicity. Consequently, most clinicians have now reduced cisplatin from 100 to 50 mg/m^2 and carboplatin AUC from 7.5 to 4–6 in treating ovarian cancers.

SETTINGS FOR CHEMOTHERAPY

- *Induction:* given when no alternative treatment is available.
- *Adjuvant:* used after initial surgical or radiation therapy to minimize recurrence.
- *Salvage:* used after recurrence of refractory tumor after previous chemotherapy.
- *Chemosensitive:* given concurrently with radiation to increase radiosensitivity.
- *Neoadjuvant:* given prior to definitive treatment (surgery or radiation) to reduce tumor burden.

EXAMPLES OF CHEMOTHERAPY AND OTHER RELATED AGENTS (IN ALPHABETICAL ORDER)

Altretamine (Hexamethylmelamine, Hexalen)

- *Indications:* second-line therapy in cisplatin-resistant ovarian cancer with limited activity. Overall response rate was 10%, with 21% experiencing grades 3 to 4 nausea and vomiting.[2]
- *Dose:* 260 mg/m^2 day PO for 14 days, followed by 14 days without drugs. Taking standard antiemetics (i.e., prochlorperazine [Compazine]) and chemotherapy pills at night significantly reduces nausea. It is dispensed as a 50-mg capsule.
- *Toxicity:* mild myelosuppression and nausea/vomiting.
- *Mechanism:* unknown.

Amifostine (Ethiol)

- *Indications:* to reduce cisplatin toxicity.
- *Dose:* 740 mg/m^2 IV over 15 minutes once a day, 30 minutes before cisplatin.
- *Toxicity:* hypotension during infusion, dizziness, hiccups, sneezing, and flushing.
- *Mechanism:* free radical scavenger.

Bleomycin (Blenoxane)

- *Indications:* germ cell and sex cord stromal tumors (as part of BEP), recurrent cervical cancer, and pleurodesis.
- *Dose:* 20 to 30 U/m^2 mixed in 50 to 100 D_5W or normal saline given through IV for 30 minutes weekly. Intrapleural dose is 60 U/m^2.
- *Toxicity:* dark discoloration on the hands, tongue, and skin may occur, as well as fever, in 50% of patients; chemotherapy may continue. Warn patients not to scratch the skin to avoid skin hyperpigmentation. Myelosuppression is minimal, but pulmonary fibrosis is dose-limiting and occurs in up to 1% of patients receiving cumulative doses greater than 200 U/m^2 and up to 10% in patients receiving more than 300 U/m^2. Discontinue bleomycin if there is a 50% decrease in vital capacity or diffusion capacity of carbon monoxide or if there are fine lung rales or skin discoloration on examination. Reduce the dose in renal insufficiency, because up to 70% of bleomycin is excreted by the kidney (if serum creatinine is 2 to 2.5, reduce by 50% of full dose; if serum creatinine is 2.5 to 4, reduce by 75% of full dose).
- *Mechanism:* a cell-cycle phase-specific antibiotic acts mainly on G_2- and M-phases by breaking DNA bonds.

Carboplatin (Paraplatin)

- *Indications:* carboplatin is as effective as cisplatin in ovarian cancer (primary tumor, salvage setting).[3,4] However, carboplatin as part of a multiagent chemotherapy regimen was less effective than cisplatin in two trials of male nonseminoma germ cell tumors. It is suspected this difference was due to the fractionation schemes employed. In recurrent cervical carcinoma, carboplatin has a 15% overall response rate.[5] It has not been widely used in endometrial or sarcoma tumors.

- *Dose:* Area under the curve (AUC) is chosen (4 to 7.5). In most GOG studies, AUC is 6 to 7.5 when combined with paclitaxel, because paclitaxel offers a platelet-sparing effect of unknown mechanism. In most cases, AUC 4 to 5 provides adequate response with the least toxicity.[6] Dose of carboplatin = AUC (mg/mL × min) × [GFR (mL/min) + 25]. GFR (glomerular filtration rate) is estimated by 24-hour urine collection or by serum creatinine (Cockcroft-Gault or Jellife methods). Premedications and postmedications are similar to cisplatin, but do not require hydration or magnesium supplement. It is mixed in 50 to 250 mL D_5W or normal saline infused by IV over 30 minutes and given every 3 to 4 weeks.
- *Toxicity:* carboplatin is more myelosuppressive (mainly thrombocytopenia) but less nephrotoxic and neurotoxic than cisplatin. Clinical response and myelosuppression correlate to the area under the carboplatin plasma disappearance concentration versus time curve.
- *Mechanism:* this alkylating agent intercalates DNA, causing strand breaks.

Chlorambucil (Leukeran)

- *Indications:* persistent ovarian cancer or trophoblastic diseases.
- *Dose:* 0.2 mg/kg/day PO every 2 to 3 weeks as part of MAC regimen.
- *Toxicity:* leukopenia, thrombocytopenia, nausea, and vomiting. Alopecia, anemia, and pulmonary fibrosis are rare. The drug is metabolized mostly by the liver.
- *Mechanism:* alkylating agent similar to cyclophosphamide.

Cisplatin (Platinol, CDDP)

- *Indications:* ovarian, gestational trophoblastic, endometrial, vaginal, and cervical tumors, as well as increased tumor radiosensitivity.
- *Dose:* for ovarian cancer and recurrent cervical or endometrial cancers, 50 to 75 mg/m^2 mixed in 250 mL of normal saline or D$_5$W given by IV at the rate 1 mg/minute or less every 3 weeks. In a chemoradiation regimen for cervical cancer, cisplatin is given at 40 mg/m^2 IV once a week for 6 weeks, or 50 to 75 mg/m^2 IV every 3 weeks.
- *Toxicity:* cisplatin damages the renal tubule and causes loss of magnesium and sodium. Consider adding 2 g magnesium sulfate IV or magnesium gluconate, 500-mg tablets, 2 to 8 tablets/day. Ototoxicity starts with loss of high-pitched sounds. Neurotoxicity may be either sensory or motor and starts with tingling and numbness in the toes and fingers, which may be permanent. Neurosensory toxicity has been described as "stocking-glove" in its distribution and can be accentuated by other neurotoxic agents (such as paclitaxel, mitomycin-C, vincristine). Neuromotor toxicity is less common, but is caused by cumulative treatment and can be disabling. Leukopenia is usually mild and is lowest at 2 weeks, with recovery in approximately 3 weeks. Other toxicities include hepatotoxicity, loss of taste, thrombophlebitis on extravasation, and mild alopecia. Some toxicity can be reduced with amifostine. Premedications include generous hydration before and after cisplatin, serotonin antagonists, and dexamethasone. Nausea and vomiting are severe with doses of 75 mg/m^2 or higher. Incidence of delayed emesis range from 20% to 90%, with maximal intensity on days 2 and 3 after chemotherapy. Patients should be discharged with metoclopramide in combination with 4 mg of dexamethasone PO every 8 hours for 4 days. Serotonin antagonists are not more effective than other less-expensive antiemetics in delayed emesis. Adverse effects of antiemetics include extrapyrami-

dal symptoms with metoclopramide (6%) and headache with granisetron (8%).[7]

- *Cautions:* if combined with paclitaxel for ovarian cancer, paclitaxel should be given before cisplatin to reduce toxicity. Furthermore, paclitaxel should be administered over 24 hours (versus a 3-hour infusion) to minimize neurotoxicity. A 3-hour infusion with cisplatin results in 20% grade 3/4 neurotoxicity.[8] An alternative is to administer a 3-hour paclitaxel infusion, followed by carboplatin (although for carboplatin, the sequence is less important).
- *Mechanism:* similar to that for carboplatin.

Cyclophosphamide (Cytoxan, Neosar, Endoxan)

- *Indications:* ovarian cancer, trophoblastic diseases.
- *Dose:* if used in combination with carboplatin (AUC 5), the cyclophosphamide dose equals 600 mg/m^2 given by mouth, IV push, or IV infusion in 100 mL of normal saline over 30 minutes.
- *Toxicity:* nausea and vomiting begin 6 to 10 hours after administration. The leukopenia nadir (time of lowest WBC count) appears at 8 to 12 days. Other signs of toxicity include hemorrhagic cystitis, hemorrhagic colitis, and alopecia. Hemorrhagic cystitis usually occurs at high doses (50 to 60 mg/kg) and can be prevented by generous hydration and mesna (see later discussion of Ifosfamide). The drug is metabolized in the liver and requires activation to be cytotoxic.
- *Mechanism:* alkylating agent.

Dactinomycin (Cosmogen, Actinomycin-D)

- *Indications:* ovarian tumors, trophoblastic diseases, and pleurodesis (to fuse pleural lining). It is not active in endometrial carcinoma (GOG 129E).
- *Dose:* 1 to 2 mg/m^2 every 3 weeks mixed with 50 mL of D$_5$W or normal saline IV over 30 minutes.
- *Toxicity:* nausea/vomiting, mucositis, and pancytopenia,

which occur in about 7 to 10 days. It can cause hyperpigmentation and severe extravasation.
- *Mechanism:* a cell-cycle phase-nonspecific antibiotic that intercalates DNA, therefore inhibiting DNA transcription and RNA translation.

Dexrazoxane (Zinecard)

- *Indications:* cardiomyopathy prophylactic in patients receiving cumulative dose of greater than 300 mg/m^2 of doxorubicin.
- *Dose:* 10 mg dexrazoxane for every 1 mg of doxorubicin infused over 30 minutes.
- *Toxicity:* mild myelosuppression.
- *Mechanism:* acts as chelating agent to interfere with free radical generation.

Doxorubicin (Adriamycin, Rubex)

- *Indications:* carcinosarcoma, endometrial, ovarian, and cervical tumors.
- *Dose:* 50 to 60 mg/m^2 mixed in 50 to 100 mL D$_5$W or normal saline (NS) given through a central line for 30 minutes, every 3 weeks.
- *Toxicity:* myelosuppression, nausea, vomiting, radiation recall, alopecia, severe extravasation reaction, and stomatitis. Because it is excreted in the bile and metabolized mainly by the liver, cholestasis (high bilirubin value) may delay doxorubicin clearance and increase toxicity. A cumulative dose of 500 mg/m^2 has less than a 1% risk of cardiomyopathy (11% risk for doses between 501 and 600 mg/m^2; 30% risk for doses greater than 600 mg/m^2). The risk is higher in older patients and in patients with a history of chest radiation, and is reduced by using dexrazoxane. The patient requires a prechemotherapy cardiac ejection fraction more than 50% (normal value: 40% to 60%).
- *Mechanism:* this antibiotic inhibits topoisomerase II (an enzyme involved in the uncoiling of DNA), binding directly to DNA and generating free radicals. The last mechanism ex-

plains why cardiac muscles are susceptible to damage, as they are low in catalase enzyme, which neutralizes free radicals. It is not cell-cycle phase-specific, but acts maximally during the S-phase.

Doxorubicin—Liposomal (Doxil)

- *Indications:* endometrial adenocarcinoma, carcinosarcoma, and recurrent ovarian cancers.
- *Dose:* 40 to 50 mg/m^2 IV every 4 weeks. For doses of less than 90 mg, dilute in 250 mL D_5W. Infuse the initial dose over 2 to 3 hours (not more than 1 mg/min); the subsequent dose can then be infused over 1 hour. For doses of 90 mg or higher, dilute in 500 mL of D_5W, infuse the initial dose over 3 to 4 hours, and infuse the subsequent dose over 2 hours.
- *Toxicity:* similar to free doxorubicin with the exception of a possible decrease in cardiotoxicity and an increase in palmar-plantar erythrodysthesia (PPE) or hand-foot syndrome (painful erythema, peeling, and occasional blisters of the skin at pressure points). The cause of PPE is unknown. PPE usually occurs after 2 to 3 cycles of Doxil and is found in 37% of ovarian cancer patients treated with Doxil. Management of PPE starts with prompt detection of early symptoms (tingling sensation, burning, redness, or other skin changes), and treatment involves increasing the dose interval (delay for 1 to 2 weeks). Similar dose may be continued unless the symptoms were severe, in which case a 25% dose reduction may be recommended at the next dose. The day before and 5 days after Doxil infusion, patients should avoid tight clothing, pressure or friction on skin, hot water bath/shower, sun exposure, or vigorous activities (exercise, gardening). One pretreatment strategy using steroids has been successful. Prednisone 8 mg, is given on day 1 b.i.d. and continued through day 5 of subsequent cycle. On day 6, 4 mg b.i.d. is given, and on day 7, 4 mg is given. A reduced rate of PPE has also been observed with prednisone 10 mg given with dose administration. Anecdotal reports describe benefits with topical DMSO or oral vi-

tamin B_6 (pyridoxine) in decreasing the incidence and severity of PPE.

Initial infusion may provoke symptoms similar to those of a rapid lipid infusion, such as lower back pain, flushing, chest tightness, shortness of breath, and hypotension. These symptoms are usually self-limiting and can be managed by stopping the Doxil infusion and reinstituting infusion 30 minutes later at a slower rate. Pretreatment with antihistamine and steroids does not prevent the symptoms but may decrease the intensity once symptoms occur.

Finally, mucositis can be minimized by avoiding hot beverages and spicy foods for 24 hours before and 72 hours after Doxil infusion, maintaining good oral hygiene, various swish-and-swallow regimens (see Chap. 14), oral lysine (up to 2 g every 6 hours).

- *Mechanism:* encapsulation in polyethylene glycol liposomes reduces doxorubicin clearance by the reticuloendothelial system and prolong the duration of the drug in the plasma.

Epoetin (Epo, Epogen, Procrit)

- *Indications:* chemotherapy, zidovudine, or renal-induced anemia. Contraindicated in hypertension.
- *Dose:* 150 U/kg or 10,000 U SC or IV three times a week. Check ferritin levels (should be > 100 mg/mL). Administer iron and folate supplement. Check hemoglobin (Hb), reticulocyte count, and blood pressure weekly until the Hb stabilizes (Hb goal is 12 g/dL), then monthly. Increase erythropoietin to 20,000 U three times a week if the increase in hemoglobin is less than 1 g/dL. Discontinue this therapy if, after an additional 4 weeks of therapy at the higher dose level, the Hb increase is still less than 1 g/dL. About one-third of gynecologic oncology patients are resistant to erythropoietin.[9] Once the target hemoglobin is reached, the maintenance dose must be individualized (usually 25 to 50 U/kg SC, three times a week) and may be doubled with persistent anemia. Alternative dosing is 40,000 U SC once a week.

- *Toxicity:* hypertension, rashes.
- *Mechanism:* induces erythropoiesis.

Etoposide (Vepesid, VP-16)

- *Indications:* used to salvage epithelial ovarian cancer, but it is not effective in advanced cervical cancer. Also used in trophoblastic disease and ovarian germ cell/stromal cell tumors.
- *Dose:* 50 mg/m^2/day PO for 14 to 21 days, followed by 7 to 14 days of rest (for cisplatin-resistant ovarian cancer); 100 mg/m^2/day for 5 days (in combination with cisplatin and bleomycin for germ cell tumors); 100 mg/m^2/day for 2 days (part of EMA for trophoblastic diseases). IV infusion should be given as a 0.2- to 0.4-mg/mL solution in D$_5$W or NS for at least 30 minutes. It is cleared by the kidney and requires dose reduction if the kidneys are impaired (25% and 50% dose reduction for creatinine clearance of 10 to 50 mL/min and 10 mL/min, respectively). Etoposide is available by mouth (50-mg tablet) or IV. The oral dose is usually twice the IV dose.
- *Toxicity:* myelosuppression, mild nausea/vomiting, alopecia, and acute myelogenous leukemia (2% when total dose is > 2000 mg/m^2).
- *Mechanism:* this alkylating agent inhibits DNA topoisomerase II.

Fluorouracil (5-FU, Effudex, Adrucil)

- *Indications:* radiation sensitizer in cervical cancer, recurrent ovarian cancer, vaginal dysplasia (5% cream).
- *Dose:* 500 to 1000 mg/m^2 IV infused over a 24-hour period for 4 to 5 days, every 3 weeks, given concurrently with pelvic radiation. Topically, 5% 5-FU cream is used for vaginal intraepithelial neoplasia (1.5 g intravaginal once a week for 10 weeks).
- *Toxicity:* nausea/vomiting, mucositis, diarrhea, anorexia, and bone marrow depression (nadir at 10 to 14 days). When applied topically, fluorouracil may cause severe vaginal mucosa or vulvar ulceration.

- *Mechanism:* this antimetabolite mimics pyrimidine and inhibits the enzyme thymidylate synthase.

Gemcitabine (Gemzar)

- *Indication:* recurrent ovarian cancer.
- *Dose:* 800 to 1500 mg/m^2 IV infused over 1 hour weekly for 2 weeks out of a 3-week cycle.
- *Toxicity:* myelosuppression—leukopenia, neutropenia, thrombocytopenia, GI toxicity, rash, diarrhea, stomatitis.
- *Mechanism:* nucleoside analog similar to 5-FU.

Granulocyte Colony–Stimulating Factor (Filgrastim, Neupogen)

- *Indications:* to reduce neutropenic complications in the following situations: (1) *Primary prophylaxis*—for patients who are expected to have a febrile neutropenia incidence of more than 40% or high-risk patients (i.e., preexisting neutropenia, open wounds, active tissue infection, poor performance status, advanced cancer, etc.). (2) *Secondary prophylaxis*—to decrease febrile neutropenia and neutropenic duration after a documented occurrence in an earlier cycle. However, if data supporting maintenance of chemotherapy dose intensity are absent, physicians should consider dose reduction instead of using GCSF. (3) *Therapeutic use*—combined with antibiotics in treating febrile neutropenia with poor prognostic factors (neutrophil counts $<$ 100/μL with pneumonia, sepsis, fungal infection or neutrophil counts $<$ 500/μL without clinical improvement after 2 to 3 days of antibiotics).
- *Dose:* 5 μg/kg SC once a day; stop when neutrophils are 1500/μL or higher.
- *Toxicity:* bone pain that is usually responsive to NSAIDs.
- *Mechanism:* stimulate WBC production.

Ifosfamide (Ifex)

- *Indications:* first-line treatment for advanced or recurrent cervical cancer; second-line treatment for advanced ovarian cancer; first-line treatment for high-grade endometrial stromal sarcoma[10]; first-line treatment for carcinosarcoma.[11]

- *Dose:* 1 to 1.2 g/m^2/day mixed with 2 to 3 L of normal saline/m^2/day for 5 days of infusion, given every 3 weeks. Mesna (Mesnex, Mesnum) is added as 20% of the ifosfamide dose, given just before, and 4 and 8 hours after ifosfamide. Thus, the total mesna dose is 60% of the ifosfamide dose. The last dose of mesna may be given in pill form so the patient may go home earlier. Mesna can also be given as a continuous infusion together with ifosfamide.

- *Toxicity:* structure and side effects are similar to those of cyclophosphamide. Hydration and mesna infusion can reduce the incidence of hemorrhagic cystitis from acrolein metabolite. Chloracetaldehyde metabolite can predispose the patient to lethargy, confusion, and seizure and be exacerbated by hypoalbuminemia. Ifosfamide is relatively contraindicated with an albumin level below 3. Other toxicities are myelosuppression, nausea/vomiting, alopecia, and transient elevated liver enzymes.

- *Mechanism:* same as for Cyclophosphamide, earlier. This alkylating agent's different spectrum of activity compared with cyclophosphamide results from the interval dosing highlighting cell cycle effects.

Interleukin 11 (IL-11, Oprelvekin, Neumega)

- *Indication:* to stimulate platelet production.
- *Dose:* 50 μg/kg SC once a day. Start 24 hours after the end of chemotherapy. Stop when platelets are 50,000/μL or higher.
- *Toxicity:* edema, dyspnea, pleural effusion, arrhythmias.
- *Mechanism:* stimulates megakaryocyte progenitor cell production and maturation.

Medroxyprogesterone Acetate (Provera, Depo-Provera)

- *Indication:* adenocarcinoma of the cervix or endometrium.
- *Dose:* 150 mg PO/day or 400 mg IM/weekly for endometrial hyperplasia; 200 mg/day for advanced, persistent, and recurrent

endometrial carcinoma; 100 mg/day for low-grade endometrial stromal sarcoma; and 160 mg/day for breast cancer. Medroxyprogesterone is commercially available by mouth (2.5-, 5-, 10-mg tablet) and IM injection (100 mg/mL and 400 mg/mL).

- *Toxicity:* menstrual changes, weight gain, nausea/vomiting, hypercalcemia, depression, and headache.
- *Mechanism:* induces apoptosis through progesterone receptor activation.

Megestrol Acetate (Megace, Megestrol)

- *Dose* (*indication*): 160 mg/day (for endometrial hyperplasia), 800 mg/day (for advanced, persistent, recurrent endometrial carcinoma), and 480 to 1600 mg/day (for appetite stimulants). Megestrol is commercially available as 20- to 40-mg tablets and as an elixir of 40 mg/mL.
- *Toxicity:* similar to that of Medroxyprogesterone Acetate, earlier.
- *Mechanism:* induces apoptosis through progesterone receptor activation.

Melphalan (Alkeran)

- *Indications:* ovarian and endometrial cancer.
- *Dose:* 0.2 mg/kg daily for 5 days, repeated every 4 weeks. Can be given by mouth or IV as a solution of 2 mg/mL in NS for 30 minutes or longer. Oral absorption is erratic (25% to 90%) and is significantly affected by drugs that alter the L-amino acid transport system, such as doxorubicin, indomethacin, tamoxifen citrate, and chlorpromazine.
- *Toxicity:* myelosuppressive; recovery can be slow, taking 6 to 8 weeks. Uncommon side effects include nausea (treat with standard antiemetics), alopecia, and hypotension. Prolonged duration of chemotherapy (12 months; dose > 600 mg) is associated with a 10% chance of developing a secondary malignancy (mostly acute nonlymphocytic leukemia) within 10 years.
- *Mechanism:* alkylating agent.

Methotrexate (Mexate, Folex, Abitrexate, Rheumatrex)

- *Indications:* ectopic pregnancy, trophoblastic diseases, cervical and recurrent ovarian cancers.
- *Dose:* various dosages (see Chap. 10); 50 to 100 mg/m^2 IV push in ovarian cancer.
- *Toxicity:* nausea, vomiting, stomatitis, diarrhea, myelosuppression, hepatotoxicity, pulmonary fibrosis, and dermatologic complications. More than 90% of methotrexate is cleared renally. The dose should be reduced in patients with renal compromise. Toxic levels can be reduced by hydration and alkalization of urine (50 mEq $NaHCO_3$ in 250 mL of D_5W IV over 1 hour to maintain urine pH > 7.5). Patients with a fluid collection cavity (i.e., ascites, theca-lutein cysts, pleural effusion) can store methotrexate in the fluid and release it to systemic circulation, causing dangerously high blood levels.

  Methotrexate levels can be followed sequentially in patients with substantial toxicity. When treating for rescue, much higher doses of leucovorin (50 to 100 mg/m^2) should be administered until the level falls below 50 nm. Leucovorin, which bypasses the site of methotrexate action by directly supplying tetrahydrofolate, is used to rescue normal cells from drug toxicity. Twenty-four hours after the initiation of high-dose methotrexate, the patient receives leucovorin 15 mg/m^2 PO every 6 hours for a total of 12 doses. For most patients, detectable methotrexate should disappear within 24 hours at standard doses for ectopic pregnancy and trophoblastic diseases.
- *Mechanism:* a folate antagonist that inhibits dihydrofolate reductase, which supplies one carbon fragment for purine synthesis. Thus, it inhibits both DNA and RNA synthesis by imitating a purine analog.

Mitomycin (Mitomycin-C, Mutamycin)

- *Indication:* cervical cancer.
- *Dose:* 10 to 20 mg/m^2 bolus in free-flowing IV line every 6 to 8 weeks. Total accumulated doses should not exceed 50

mg/m^2. Use a lower dose when giving with other agents, such as 5-FU. Incompatible when mixed with bleomycin.
- *Toxicity:* myelosuppression, fatigue, and mild nausea. Alopecia, dermatitis, anemia, paresthesias, and pneumonitis are rare.
- *Mechanism:* alkylating agent.

Mitoxantrone (Novantrone, DHAD, DHAQ)

- *Indication:* ovarian cancer.
- *Dose:* 12 mg/m^2 mixed in 50 mL D$_5$W or NS given by IV for 30 minutes every 3 weeks or 10 mg/m^2 in 2 L fluid every week intraperitoneally. Cardiac ejection fraction must be normal before using this drug.
- *Toxicity:* nausea/vomiting or diarrhea. It may cause "Smurf" syndrome (blue colored bowel and sclera). It inhibits topoisomerase II and is less cardiotoxic than doxorubicin.
- *Mechanism:* this alkylating agent inhibits topoisomerase II.

Paclitaxel (Taxol)

- *Indications:* ovarian, endometrial, cervical tumors; carcinosarcoma; nonsquamous advanced/recurrent cervical cancer[12]; carcinosarcoma; and breast cancers. It has little activity in leiomyosarcoma.
- *Dose:* 175 mg/m^2 for 3-hour dosing (with increase in allergic reaction) or 135 mg/m^2 for 24-hour dosing (more myelosuppressive toxicity). Another alternative that is currently being studied is weekly paclitaxel, used for various cancers, at 80 mg/m^2. In ovarian cancer, increasing paclitaxel from 175 mg/m^2 to 250 mg/m^2 did not alter survival.[12] Myelosuppression is less severe when cisplatin is given immediately after paclitaxel.[13] To reduce neurotoxicity, paclitaxel is infused for 24 hours and followed with cisplatin, *or* paclitaxel is infused for 3 hours and followed with carboplatin. Giving a 3-hour infusion of paclitaxel after cisplatin caused a 20% increase in grade 3 and 4 neurotoxicity.[14] Neurotoxicity is dose-dependent and reversible within 24 hours unless paclitaxel is used in combination with cisplatin.

- *Toxicity:* myelosuppression, transient neurotoxicity (stocking-glove distribution), bone pain, and complete but reversible alopecia. Bradycardia, vomiting, and diarrhea are rare. In a salvage setting using a 3-hour versus 24-hour paclitaxel infusion, the 3-hour dosing is less myelosuppressive but more neurotoxic.[15] Paclitaxel premedications are dexamethasone, 20 mg IV; diphenhydramine, 50 mg IV; and cimetidine, 300 mg IV, 30 minutes before paclitaxel infusion. This premedication protocol reduces the incidence (1% to 3%) of type I hypersensitivity reaction (dyspnea, wheezing, rashes, hypotension). These patients can be reinduced with paclitaxel by slowing the infusion rate.[16] Paclitaxel is also safe in patients with ischemic heart disease, but the risk is unknown in patients with conduction defect.[17] In treating recurrent endometrial carcinoma, doxorubicin should be infused first, followed by 24-hour paclitaxel infusion. Toxicity is higher if given in reverse sequence (both paclitaxel and doxorubicin are metabolized in the liver). Paclitaxel is given first then followed with carboplatin when used in combination.
- *Mechanism:* stabilizes microtubules (contrary to vinca alkaloids, which inhibit microtubule polymerization).

Tamoxifen (Novaldex)

- *Indications:* adenocarcinoma of the endometrium, cervix, recurrent ovarian cancer, breast cancer.
- *Dose:* 20 mg PO b.i.d. for advanced recurrent endometrial, cervical, or ovarian adenocarcinoma and 10 mg PO b.i.d. for breast cancer. Prolonged therapy is advised since the effect is cytostatic, not cytocidal.
- *Toxicity:* mild nausea, menstrual irregularity, and endometrial cancer.
- *Mechanism:* this estrogen antagonist binds reversibly to estrogen receptors and reduces estrogen-mediated transcription, which leads to accumulation of cells in the G0/G1-phase and cell cycle arrest.

Taxotere (Docetaxel)

- *Indications:* ovarian and breast cancers.

- *Dose:* 80 to 100 mg/m^2 IV for 1 hour every 3 weeks, 12 mg/m^2/day for 5 days IV for 1 hour every 3 weeks; it can be mixed in 250 mL of D$_5$W or NS.
- *Toxicity:* similar to those of paclitaxel except for significant edema. Steroids (dexamethasone, 8 mg b.i.d. PO) are administered 24 hours prior to therapy and continued for 3 to 5 days posttherapy to reduce edema. Taxotere is a semisynthetic analog of paclitaxel prepared from the needles of the European yew tree.
- *Mechanism:* similar to that of Paclitaxel, earlier. However, data from recent breast trials suggests that paclitaxel-resistant patients may respond to this agent upon retreatment. It may also be active in recurrent ovarian cancers. The mechanism is unknown but may be related to differential binding to the tubulin tau receptor.

Thiotepa (Tespa, TSPA)

- *Indication:* ovarian cancers.
- *Dose:* 30 to 35 mg/m^2 IV bolus every week for 4 weeks. It can be administered directly into cavity spaces (intrathecal, intravesical, intraperitoneal, etc.).
- *Toxicity:* extremely myelosuppressive when used in combination with other agents, such as cisplatin. Other rare toxicities are nausea, alopecia, and pulmonary fibrosis.
- *Mechanism:* alkylating agents.

Topotecan (Hycamtin)

- *Indication:* recurrent ovarian carcinomas.
- *Dose:* 1.0 to 1.5 mg/m^2/day IV for 5 days every 3 weeks. Use lower dose (1.0 mg/m^2) in heavily pretreated patients. It is primarily cleared by the kidneys and requires dose reduction in renal impairment (creatinine clearance of 20 to 40 mL/min equals 0.75 mg/m^2/day). Oral dosage equals 2.3 mg/m^2/day for 5 days every 3 weeks (under study).

- *Toxicity:* nausea/vomiting, myelosuppression, fatigue, diarrhea, and mild alopecia.
- *Mechanism:* a topoisomerase I inhibitor that inhibits uncoiling of DNA during its synthesis.

Vinblastine (Velban, VLB, Velsar, Alkaban)

- *Indications:* cervical, ovarian, and trophoblatic tumors.
- *Dose:* 6 to 10 mg/m^2 every 2 to 4 weeks; mix in 50 mL or more of D$_5$W IV for 96 hours or longer of infusion through a central venous catheter.
- *Toxicity:* severe myelosuppression (*hint:* vin**bl**astine—**bl**ood), extravasation. Nausea and neurotoxicity are rare.
- *Mechanism:* this vinka alkaloid inhibits the assembly of the microtubules.

Vincristine (Oncovin, Vincasar PFS, VCR, Leurocristine)

- *Indications:* cervical, ovarian, and trophoblatic tumors.
- *Dose:* 0.5 to 1.4 mg/m^2 every 1 to 4 weeks; mix in 50 mL or more of D$_5$W IV for 96 hours or longer of infusion through a free-flowing IV line.
- *Toxicity:* neurotoxic and causes peripheral neuropathy (i.e., constipation), depression, insomnia, and convulsions (especially in the elderly). Excreted in the bile. Relatively contraindicated with abnormal liver function tests.
- *Mechanism:* similar to vinblastine.

Vinorelbine (Navelbine, NVB)

- *Indication:* cervical cancer (experimental).
- *Dose:* 30 mg/m^2/week IV mixed in 100 mL of D$_5$W or NS and infused over 20 minutes through a free-flowing IV. Oral dose is 80 mg/m^2/week.
- *Toxicity:* myelosuppression, nausea/vomiting, mild alopecia, and rare neurotoxicity.
- *Mechanism:* nucleoside analog; the mechanism is not exactly known.

TABLE 26–1. Recommended Chemotherapy in Gynecologic Oncology

Cancer	Primary treatment	Second-line treatment
Primary ovarian cancer	Surgical debulking + paclitaxel and platinum (carboplatin or cisplatin)	Topotecan, doxil/doxorubicin, altretamine, ifosfamide, etoposide, tamoxifen
Recurrent ovarian cancer	Reinduction with platinum and/or paclitaxel if patient has not received platinum in > 6 mo	Topotecan, doxil/doxorubicin, altretamine, ifosfamide, etoposide, tamoxifen
Ovarian germ cell and sex cord stromal tumors	Surgery ± adjuvant BEP (bleomycin + etoposide + cisplatin)	BEP reinduction or vincristine, altretamine, cyclophosphamide (VAC)
Primary endometrial cancer	TAH-BSO ± adjuvant radiation	Doxorubicin + cisplatin
Recurrent endometrial cancer	Doxorubicin + cisplatin	Paclitaxel, megestrol acetate, medroxyprogesterone acetate, tamoxifen
Uterine sarcoma	Surgical debulking ± adjuvant radiation (only to reduce local recurrence)	Ifosfamide for carcinosarcoma; doxorubicin for leiomyosarcoma; progestin for low-grade endometrial stromal sarcoma (ESS), ifosfamide for high-grade ESS
Early cervical cancer (up to stage IIA)	Radical hysterectomy + lymphadenectomy ± adjuvant radiation	Radiation ± chemosensitizing agents (5-fluorouracil and/or cisplatin)
Advanced cervical cancer	Radiation ± chemosensitizing agent (cisplatin, 5-fluorouracil)	Cisplatin ± ifosfamide; paclitaxel; carboplatin
Recurrent cervical cancer	If initially treated with surgery, administer radiation; perform pelvic exenteration if patient was treated initially with radiation	Cisplatin ± ifosfamide ± bleomycin; paclitaxel; topotecan; vinorelbine; carboplatin
Vulvar cancer	Surgery ± adjuvant radiation	Radiation ± chemotherapy
Trophoblastic disease	Methotrexate or dactinomycin	EMACO (etoposide, methotrexate, actinomycin, cyclophosphamide, Oncovin [vincristine])
Choriocarcinoma	EMACO	EMA-EP (EP = etoposide and platinum)

274

EXAMPLES OF CHEMOTHERAPY PROTOCOLS

Carboplatin + Paclitaxel Protocol (Outpatient Setting)

A. Indications: ovarian, endometrial, carcinosarcoma.

B. Orders:

    1. Prechemotherapy laboratory studies: CBC with differential, serum creatinine, liver function tests.

    2. Premedicate 30 minutes before paclitaxel with the following: diphenhydramine, 50 mg IV; cimetidine, 300 mg IV; dexamethasone, 20 mg IV; ondansetron, 8 to 16 mg IV. Then give paclitaxel, 175 mg/m^2 IV in 3 hours.

    3. Follow with carboplatin AUC, 4 to 7.5 mg/m^2 mixed in 250 mL of NS IV infused over 30 minutes.

TABLE 26–2. Emetogenic Potential (mg/m^2 of BSA) of Chemotherapy Agents

Level	% Emesis	Agents
5	> 90	Cisplatin $\geq$ 50, cyclophosphamide > 1500, dacarbazine
4	60–90	Carboplatin, cisplatin < 50, cyclophosphamide > 750 and $\leq$ 1500, doxorubicin > 60, methotrexate > 1000
3	30–60	Cyclophosphamide < 750, cyclophosphamide oral, doxorubicin 20–60, altretamine, ifosfamide, methotrexate 250–1000
2	10–30	Taxotere, etoposide, fluorouracil < 1000, gemcitabine, methotrexate > 50 and < 250, paclitaxel
1	< 10	Bleomycin, methotrexate < 50, vinblastine, vincristine

Modified from Hesketh PJ, et al: J Clin Oncol 15:103, 1997.

TABLE 26–3. Antiemetic Guidelines for Adults

	Regimen
Low emetogenicity (level 1): does not require standard premedications	Metoclopramide, 20 mg PO q 8 h prn ± dexamethasone, 20 mg PO q 8 h prn
Moderate emetogenicity (level 2): does not require 5-HT$_3$ antiemetics	Metoclopramide, 20 mg PO premed; then q 6–8 h prn ± diphenhydramine, 25 to 50 mg PO premed; then q 6–8 h prn ± dexamethasone, 20 mg PO premed ± lorazepam 1 mg PO q 4–6 h prn
High emetogenicity (level 3–5)	Ondansetron, 8 mg (0.15 mg/ kg) IV premed ± dexamethasone, 20 mg IV premed ± metoclopramide, 20 mg (0.5 mg/kg) IV premed *or* Dolasetron, 100 mg (1.8 mg/ kg) PO premed ± dexamethasone, 20 mg PO premed ± metoclopramide, 20 mg PO premed
Delayed regimen (all level 3–5 regimens should receive)	Metoclopramide, 20 mg IV/PO q 8 h ± dexamethasone, 8 mg IV/PO b.i.d. ± lorazepam, 1 mg IV/PO q 4–6 h prn × 3 days except cisplatin- or carboplatin-containing regimens; × 5 days if cisplatin or carboplatin

Cisplatin + Paclitaxel Protocol (Inpatient Setting)

A. Indications: ovarian, endometrial, carcinosarcoma.
B. Orders:
    1. Prechemotherapy laboratory studies: CBC with differential, creatinine, liver function tests, magnesium.

2. Premedicate 30 minutes before paclitaxel with the following: diphenhydramine, 50 mg IV; cimetidine, 300 mg IV push; dexamethasone, 20 mg IV. Then give paclitaxel, 135 mg/m^2 IV for 24 hours.

3. Prior to paclitaxel completion, increase IV NS to 500 mL/hour for 2 hours, then decrease the IV rate back to 125 mL/hour. Once urine output is 100 mL/hour or higher, follow with cisplatin.

4. Premedicate 30 minutes prior to cisplatin with dexamethasone, 20 mg IV and ondansetron, 8 to 16 mg IV.

5. Follow with cisplatin, 50 to 75 mg/m^2 mixed in 250 mL of NS IV at equal or less than 1 mg/min.

6. After cisplatin, give another 1000 mL of NS infused over 2 to 3 hours.

Cisplatin Chemoradiation Protocol (Outpatient Setting)

A. Indications: cervical cancer—concurrent with radiation.
B. Orders:
   1. Prechemotherapy laboratory studies: CBC with differential, creatinine, liver function tests, magnesium.
   2. Premedicate 30 minutes prior to cisplatin with dexamethasone, 20 mg IV; ondansetron, 8 to 16 mg IV; and 750 mL of NS in 2 to 3 hours by IV.
   3. Follow with cisplatin, 40 mg/m^2 mixed in 250 mL of NS IV at equal to or less than 1 mg/min.
   4. After cisplatin, give another 750 mL of NS infused over 2 to 3 hours.

Cisplatin + Doxorubicin Protocol (Inpatient Setting)

A. Indications: cervical cancer—concurrent with radiation.
B. Orders:
   1. Prechemotherapy laboratory studies: CBC with differential, creatinine, liver function tests, magnesium, echocardiogram to check cardiac ejection fraction.
   2. Premedicate 30 minutes before doxorubicin with dexamethasone, 20 mg IV and ondansetron, 8 to 16 mg IV. Then give doxorubicin, 50 to 60 mg/m^2 IV in 3 hours.

3. Prior to cisplatin, give 1000 mL IV of NS in 2 to 3 hours, then decrease the IV rate back to 125 mL/hour. Once urine output is 100 mL/hour or higher, follow with cisplatin.

4. Administer cisplatin, 50 to 75 mg/m^2 mixed in 250 mL of NS IV at equal or less than 1 mg/min.

5. After cisplatin, give another 1000 mL of NS infused over 2 to 3 hours.

Doxil or Doxorubicin Protocol (Outpatient Setting)

A. Indications: leiomyosarcoma, endometrial and recurrent ovarian cancers.

B. Orders:

1. Prechemotherapy laboratory studies: CBC with differential, creatinine, liver function tests, echocardiogram to check cardiac ejection fraction.

2. Premedicate 30 minutes before doxorubicin with dexamethasone, 20 mg IV and ondansetron, 8 to 16 mg or 0.15 mg/kg IV.

3. Then give doxorubicin, 50 to 60 mg/m^2 IV over 30 minutes or Doxil, 40 to 50 mg/m^2 over 2 to 3 hours (initial Doxil dose) or over 1 hour in subsequent doses.

4. Schedule it usually after 3 to 4 weeks.

Topotecan Protocol (Outpatient Setting)

A. Indications: recurrent ovarian cancer.

B. Orders:

1. Prechemotherapy laboratory studies: CBC with differential, creatinine, liver function tests.

2. Premedicate 30 minutes before topotecan with metoclopramide, 20 mg PO every 8 hours prn $\pm$ dexamethasone, 20 mg IV.

3. Then give topotecan, 1.0 to 1.5 mg/m^2/day IV over 30 minutes for 5 days.

Ifosfamide Protocol (Inpatient Setting)

A. Indications: carcinosarcoma, ovarian cancer.

B. Orders:
   1. Prechemotherapy laboratory studies: CBC with differential, creatinine, liver function tests.
   2. Premedicate several hours before ifosfamide with 1 L of NS IV over a few hours. Then, 30 minutes before ifosfamide, give dexamethasone, 20 mg IV; ondansetron, 8 to 16 mg IV; and mesna, 120 mg/m^2 in 50 mL NS IV over 15 minutes infusion (this 120 mg/m^2 of mesna is given only on the first day of ifosfamide infusion).
   3. Then infuse ifosfamide, 1.2 to 1.5 g/m^2/day mixed with mesna, 1.2 to 1.5 g/m^2/day in 2 to 3 L of NS infused over 24 hours for 5 days (give only 1.2 g ifosfamide if the patient has a prior history of radiation therapy).
   4. Daily urinalysis is needed to rule out hematuria.

Methotrexate Protocols

There are various regimens with varying effectiveness.
A. Indications: nonmetastatic or low-risk metastatic gestational trophoblastic diseases
B. Orders (5-day regimen—outpatient setting)
   1. Methotrexate, 0.4 mg/kg body weight IV or IM (maximum dose: 25 mg/day) daily for 5 days.
   2. Treatment course is repeated as often as toxicity permits, usually every 14 days (9-day window). β-hCG is obtained weekly. Prechemotherapy laboratory studies include WBC, platelets, creatinine, and liver function tests (AST, ALT). A successful treatment is determined by 3 weekly β-hCGs of less than 5.
   3. This therapy has a remission rate of 89.3%.[18]
C. Orders (combination of IM and PO—outpatient setting)
   1. Same as previously noted, with the patient beginning the IM dose as stated earlier followed by 4 days of oral dosage. Remission is defined as 3 consecutive weekly β-hCG levels of less than 5 mIU/mL following the last course of oral methotrexate.
   2. Remission rate in this study was 83.8%. Major toxicity

was mucositis (40.5%). Febrile neutropenia was only 2.7%.[19]

D. Orders (GOG weekly regimen—outpatient setting)
   1. Methotrexate, 20 to 50 mg/m^2 body surface area IM weekly.
   2. This regimen is more convenient to the patient, but the remission rate is only 74%.[20]
E. Orders (methotrexate and folinic acid rescue—inpatient setting).[21]

Day	Time	Follow-up Test and Therapy
1	8 A.M.	CBC, platelet count, AST
	4 P.M.	Methotrexate, 1.0 mg/kg IV
2	4 P.M.	Folinic acid, 0.1 mg/kg IV
3	8 A.M.	CBC, platelet count, ALT
	4 P.M.	Methotrexate, 1.0 mg/kg IV
4	4 P.M.	Folinic acid, 0.1 mg/kg IV
5	8 A.M.	CBC, platelet count, ALT
	4 P.M.	Methotrexate, 1.0 mg/kg IV
6	4 P.M.	Folinic acid, 0.1 mg/kg IV
7	8 A.M.	CBC, platelet count, ALT
	4 P.M.	Methotrexate, 1.0 mg/kg IV
8	4 P.M.	Folinic acid, 0.1 mg/kg IV

Dactinomycin Protocols

There are various regimens with varying effectiveness.

A. Indications: nonmetastatic or low-risk metastatic gestational trophoblastic diseases.
B. Orders ("convenient" protocol—outpatient setting)
   1. Dactinomycin, 1.25 mg/m^2 via IV push once every 2 weeks.
   2. Results of one study showed 94% patients went into remission with an average 4.4-treatment course.[22]
C. Orders ("traditional" protocol—outpatient setting)
   1. Dactinomycin, 12 μg/kg/day IV for 5 days.

2. Laboratory workup includes CBC, platelet count, and AST daily. Follow-up tests include CBC, platelet count, AST three times weekly for 2 weeks, then as needed. Subsequent course—with response, re-treat at same dose; without response, add 3 μg/kg to the initial dose.

EMACO Protocol

A. Indications: high-risk metastatic gestational trophoblastic diseases, choriocarcinoma.

B. Give these chemotherapeutic agents on days 1, 2, and 8 and repeat on days 15, 16, 22, and so forth.

Course 1 (EMA)	Regimen
Day 1	Etoposide, 100 mg/m^2 IV infusion in 20 mL of NS over 30 min; dactinomycin, 0.5 mg via IV push; methotrexate, 100 mg/m^2 via IV push followed by a 200-mg/m^2 IV infusion over 12 hours
Day 2	Etoposide, 100 mg/m^2 IV infusion in 200 mL of NS over 30 min; actinomycin-D, 0.5 mg IV push; folinic acid, 15 mg IM or PO q 12 h for 4 doses beginning 24 hours after the start of methotrexate
Course 2	
Day 8	Vincristine (Oncovin), 1.0 mg/m^2 via IV push; cyclophosphamide, 600 mg/m^2 IV in NS

REFERENCES

1. McGuire WP, Hoskins WJ, Brady MF, et al: Assessment of dose-intensive therapy in suboptimally debulked ovarian cancer: a Gynecologic Oncology Group study. J Clin Oncol 13:1589, 1995.
2. Markman M, Blessing JA, Moore D, et al: Altretamine (hexamethylmelamine) in platinum-resistant and platinum-refractory ovarian cancer: a Gynecologic Oncology Group phase II trial. Gynecol Oncol 69:226, 1998.
3. Eisenhauer EA, ten Bokkel Huinink WW, Swenerton KD, et al: European-Canadian randomized trial of paclitaxel in relapsed ovarian cancer: high-dose versus low-dose and long versus short infusion. J Clin Oncol 12:2654, 1994.

4. OZOLS RF, GREER B, BAERGEN R, REED E: A phase III randomized study of cisplatin and paclitaxel (24-hour infusion) versus carboplatin and paclitaxel (3-hour infusion) in optimal stage III epithelial ovarian carcinoma [abstract]. ASCO 18:356a, 1999 (Abstr. 1373).

5. WEISS GR, GREEN S, HANNIGAN EV, et al: A phase II trial of carboplatin for recurrent or metastatic squamous carcinoma of the uterine cervix: a Southwest Oncology Group study. Gynecol Oncol 39:332, 1990.

6. JODRELL DI, EGORIN MJ, CANETTA RM, et al: Relationships between carboplatin exposure and tumor response and toxicity in patients with ovarian cancer. J Clin Oncol 10:520, 1992.

7. GEBBIA V, TESTA A, VALENZA R, et al: Oral granisetron with or without methylprednisolone versus metoclopramide plus methylprednisolone in the management of delayed nausea and vomiting induced by cisplatin-based chemotherapy. Cancer 76:1821, 1995.

8. CONNELLY E, MARKMAN M, KENNEDY A, et al: Paclitaxel delivered as a 3-hr infusion with cisplatin in patients with gynecologic cancers: unexpected incidence of neurotoxicity. Gynecol Oncol 62:166, 1996.

9. DEMETRI GD, KRIS M, WADE J, et al: Quality-of-life benefit in chemotherapy patients treated with epoetin alfa is independent of disease response or tumor type: results from a prospective community oncology study. J Clin Oncol 16:3412, 1998.

10. SUTTON G, BLESSING JA, PARK R, et al: Ifosfamide treatment of recurrent or metastatic endometrial stromal sarcomas previously unexposed to chemotherapy: a study of the Gynecologic Oncology Group. Obstet Gynecol 87:747, 1996.

11. SUTTON GP, BLESSING JA, ROSENSHEIN N, et al: Phase II trial of ifosfamide and mesna in mixed mesodermal tumors of the uterus (a Gynecologic Oncology Group study). Am J Obstet Gynecol 161(2):309, 1989.

12. ROSE PG, BLESSING JA, GERSHENSON DM, MCGEHEE R: Paclitaxel and cisplatin as first-line therapy in recurrent or advanced squamous cell carcinoma of the cervix: a Gynecologic Oncology Group study. J Clin Oncol 17(9):2676, 1999.

13. ROWINSKY EK, GILBERT MR, MCGUIRE WP, et al: Sequences of Taxol and cisplatin: a phase I and pharmacologic study. J Clin Oncol 9:1692, 1991.

14. CONNELLY E, MARKMAN M, KENNEDY A, ET AL: Paclitaxel delivered as a 3-hr infusion with cisplatin in patients with gynecologic cancers: unexpected incidence of neurotoxicity. Gynecol Oncol 62:166, 1996.

15. EISENHAUER EA, TEN BOKKEL HUININK WW, SWENERTON KD, ET AL: European-Canadian randomized trial of paclitaxel in relapsed ovarian cancer: high-dose versus low-dose and long versus short infusion. J Clin Oncol 12:2654, 1994.

16. MARKMAN M, KENNEDY A, WEBSTER K, ET AL: Paclitaxel-associated hypersensitivity reactions: experience of the gynecologic oncology program of the Cleveland Clinic Cancer Center. J Clin Oncol 18:102, 2000.

17. PEREZ EA: Paclitaxel and cardiotoxicity. J Clin Oncol 16:3481, 1998.

18. LURAIN JR, ELFSTRAND EP: Single-agent methotrexate chemotherapy for the treatment of nonmetastatic gestational trophoblastic tumors. Am J Obstet Gynecol 172:574, 1995.

19. BARTER JF, SOONG SJ, HATCH KD, ET AL: Treatment of nonmetastatic gestational trophoblastic disease with sequential intramuscular and oral methotrexate. Gynecol Oncol 33:82, 1989.

20. HOMESLEY HD, BLESSING JA, RETTENMAIER M, ET AL: Weekly intramuscular methotrexate for nonmetastatic gestational trophoblastic disease. Obstet Gynecol 72:413, 1988.

21. BERKOWITZ RS, GOLDSTEIN DP, BERNSTEIN MR: Methotrexate infusion and folinic acid in the primary therapy of nonmetastatic gestational trophoblastic tumors. Gynecol Oncol 36:56, 1990.

22. PETRILLI ES, TWIGGS LB, BLESSING JA, ET AL: Single-dose actinomycin D treatment for nonmetastatic GTD. Cancer 60:273, 1987.

Synopsis of Radiation Oncology

Sandra Hatch

RADIATION BIOLOGY

A. As energy is absorbed from radiation, excitation or ionization may occur.[1]

B. Ionizing radiation may be classified as electromagnetic (photons, x-rays, gamma ray) or particulate (electrons).[1]

C. Radiation may be further classified as directly or indirectly ionizing.[1]

D. In general, x-rays are indirectly ionizing because the damage created is a consequence of depositing energy in the tissues as they pass through the body, creating a chain of events.[1]

E. Chain of events of indirect action of x-rays:

An absorbed incident x-ray photon
↓
Conversion to a fast moving electron (e^-)
↓
Production of an ion radical
↓
Production of a free radical
↓
Chemical changes from the breakage of bonds
↓
Biological effects[1]

F. The critical target of the radiation is the DNA in chromosomes and the nuclear membrane.[1]

G. Radiation-induced damage and incorrect repair may lead to aberrations in chromosomes and chromatids. These aberrations lead to cell death, which occurs at the next attempted mitosis.[1]

H. Cells in the late G_2/M phase of their cell cycle are the most sensitive to radiation; those in S phase are the most resistant.[1]

I. The absence or presence of oxygen dramatically alters the biologic effect of x-rays. To be effective, oxygen must be present during the lifetime of the free radicals involved in the indirect action of x-rays.

J. The tumor's radiosensitivity is influenced by the 4 Rs of radiation biology:
   1. Repair: ability to repair sublethal damage.
   2. Redistribution: more cancer cells become sensitive to radiation.
   3. Repopulation of normal cells: decrease injury to normal organs.
   4. Reoxygenation: radioresistant in hypoxic tumor cells.[1]

K. Increasing the number of daily treatments (fractions) and extending overall treatment time allows normal cells and tumor cells the opportunity to repair radiation-induced damage through repair, cell division, and repopulation while allowing reoxygenation of hypoxic tumor cells, which are radioresistant.

L. The overall treatment time for which the treatment may be protracted is limited by repopulation of the tumor cells.

M. The Patterns of Care Study for Cervical Cancer has reported a significant adverse effect on survival and pelvic control with prolongation of the total radiation treatment time for stage III squamous cell carcinoma of the cervix.[2,3]

TOXICITY ASSOCIATED WITH RADIATION TREATMENT

A. Tumors often recur because of the inability to give a tumoricidal dose without excessive damage to the surrounding normal tissue; this is referred to as the therapeutic ratio.[1,4–8]

B. Tissue damage is considered the result of parenchymal cell depletion caused by mitotic-linked death.[6]

C. Radiation toxicities are divided into two categories: acute effects and late effects.[1,4–8]

D. The acute effects that occur during therapy and typically resolve within 1 to 2 months following completion of treatment are due to transient suppression of cell proliferation in rapidly replicating tissues.[1,4–8]

1. The severity of acute reactions depends on the radiation dose delivered per unit time (weekly dose rate) and the regenerative capacity of the tissues irradiated.[1,4–8]
2. The volume of tissue irradiated will influence the rate of recovery.[1,4–8]
3. Acute side effects may be enhanced by the addition of chemotherapy, the presence of malnutrition, and the use of tobacco.[1,4–6]

E. Late effects and their severity are dose limiting in radiation delivery.[1,4–8]

   1. The clinical significance of late toxicity is affected by the following:
      a. Radiation quality and quantity: type and energy of radiation used, dose per treatment or fraction size, total dose, volume treated, dose rate.
      b. Radiosensitivity or tolerance of the tissue irradiated.
      c. Administration of additional therapies: surgery, chemotherapy.
      d. Age and medical condition of the patient: elderly, children, diabetes, hypertension, anemia, obesity, cachexia.
      e. Co-existent medical problems that may enhance damage; systemic lupus, inflammatory bowel disease.
      f. Individual genetic factors that may enhance cellular radiosensitivity: ataxia-telangiectasia.
      g. Prior or co-existent infections: pelvic inflammatory disease, tubo-ovarian abscess, peritonitis.[1,4–8]

   2. Models used to describe the mechanism of induction of long-term complications include:
      a. Depletion of very slowly proliferating "stem" cells beyond their functional reserve.
      b. Depletion of cells with nonproliferating function (i.e., CNS).
      c. Functional or structural damage to blood vessels.
      d. Combination of parenchymal cell depletion and vascular damage.
      e. Inflammatory reaction and endogenous cytokine production.[1,4–8]

3. Although the total dose of radiation is important, the amount of radiation delivered in a single fraction is the predominant treatment-related factor in determining late effects.[1,4,6–8]

F. Both the fraction size and overall treatment time determine the response of acutely responding tissues.[1,2,4,6–8]

RADIATION PHYSICS

A. A quantity of radiation is sometimes referred to in roentgens, rads, or gray.
   1. Roentgen (R): unit of exposure; related to the ability of x-rays to ionize air.
   2. Rad: unit of absorbed dose; corresponds to an energy absorption of 100 ergs/g.
   3. Gray (Gy): new term for the unit of absorbed dose; corresponds to an energy absorption of 1 joule/kg.
   4. One Gray = 100 Rad.
   5. One centigray (cGy) = 1/100th of a Gray (Gy) = 1 Rad.[9]
B. External beam radiation:
   1. The majority of external beam radiation (high-energy x-rays or photons) is delivered using a treatment machine called a linear accelerator (LINAC).
   2. A LINAC can produce x-ray (photon) or electron beams of different energies.
   3. Cobalt machines were previously used in the treatment of gynecologic cancers. This practice is now discouraged due to the findings of the Patterns of Care Study of Cervical Cancer, which reported the use of LINACS to be associated with a lower recurrence rate (14% compared with 21% with Cobalt machines, $P = .02$.[2]
   4. Before beginning radiation with external beam, the area to receive radiation treatment must be carefully defined by a procedure called simulation.
   5. A simulator uses a diagnostic x-ray unit (usually fluoroscopy guidance) to mimic a treatment machine setup in its geometrical, mechanical, and optical properties.

By visualizing internal structures, treatment areas (fields) may be accurately positioned and these parameters recorded for daily treatment use. Films are taken and customized shielding or blocking is designed. Some simulators are equipped with a tomography attachment to allow CT images at designated intervals within the treatment fields (ports) designed. Alternatively, some centers use a CT scanner for simulation or for obtaining further anatomic detail.

6. The information obtained from simulation, history, physical examination, and staging evaluation are used in a process called treatment planning. There are many commercially available planning systems to assist in the design of treatment delivery. These plans are analyzed for the best approach that maximizes dose to the treatment and tumor volume while sparing the surrounding tissues. The treatment volume is then shaped to exclude as much of the surrounding normal tissue as possible. This may be accomplished by using custom-made cerrobend blocks, multileaf collimators (MLC), and jaws that may be opened or closed independently of one another.

C. Brachytherapy:

1. Brachytherapy is the use or implantation of sealed radioisotopes to deliver radiation over a short distance or range.

2. Atoms with the same atomic number but different atomic mass are called isotopes.[9]

3. Certain atoms have excess energy in their nuclei; therefore, they are considered to exist in an excited state, characterized by an unstable nucleus. The nucleus will spontaneously emit particles and energy in order to reach a stable state. This is referred to as radioactive decay, and the atoms undergoing this process are radionuclides.[9]

4. Radioactive material is measured in curies (Ci), where 1 Ci = 3.7×10^{10} atoms disintegrating per second (3.7×10^{10} Bq).[9]

5. Radioisotopes disintegrate into stable isotopes at a decreasing rate. The rate of decay and quantity present at any one time is described by a formula known as the radioactive decay law, where a quantity known as half-life ($T_{1/2}$) of a radioisotope is the time required for a quantity of radioactivity to be reduced to one-half its original value. Half-life is measured in periods of time from seconds to years.[9]

6. The energy emitted during this decay process is used in radiation implants to deliver radiation to a tumor volume.

7. An important principle in brachytherapy is that the dose of radiation from a point source varies as the square of the distance from that source. In fact, the dose varies more rapidly in the first cm than in the second or third cm. Therefore, a higher dose of radiation may be delivered to the target volume with a rapid fall off of the dose sparing surrounding normal tissues. However, the effect of this inverse square law does not allow for dose uniformity, and dose gradients do occur.[9]

8. Cesium-137 (^{137}Cs) and iridium-192 (^{192}Ir) are the most commonly used radionuclides for brachytherapy of gynecologic cancers. (See Table 27-1).

9. Interstitial and intracavitary are the most commonly used techniques. Typically, gynecologic implants are temporary and afterloading. The choice of one technique over the other is based on the area to be implanted, the anatomy, the volume of tumor to be covered, as well as overall accessibility.

TABLE 27–1. Radionuclides for Gyn Brachytherapy

Nuclide	Symbol	Half-life	Average energy (MeV)	Exposure (Rcm^2/ mCi h)
Cesium-137	^{137}Cs	30.0 years	Gamma: 0.662	3.32
Iridium-192	^{192}IR	74.0 days	Gamma: 0.316	4.69

From Hilaris BS, Nori D, Anderson LL.[10]

10. There are several designs of applicators for this pur-
    pose which hold the sources in a fixed configuration.
    One system is a tandem and ovoids (colpostats). The
    Fletcher-Suit tandem and ovoid system is constructed
    from stainless steel with hollow handles that allows the
    sources to be loaded following insertion of the appli-
    cator. The loading at a later time minimizes exposure
    of the medical staff to the radioactive sources; this
    technique is referred to as afterloading.

11. A dosimetric system refers to a set of rules governing
    a certain applicator type, radioisotope, and distribution
    of the sources in the applicator to deliver a defined
    dose to a treatment region. Some of these systems are
    the Stockholm, Paris, Manchester, MDACC (Fletcher),
    and Washington University (Perez). Our discussion is
    limited to the Manchester and Fletcher systems.

12. Manchester system:
    a. Standardizes treatment with predetermined doses and
       dose rates directed to certain fixed points in the pelvis.
    b. The fixed points A and B were selected on the the-
       ory that the dose in the paracervical triangle re-
       flected normal tissue tolerance and not the dose to
       the bladder, rectum, or vagina.
    c. The paracervical triangle was described as a pyra-
       mid-shaped area with its base resting on the lateral
       vaginal fornices and its apex curving around the an-
       teverted uterus.
    d. This is the concept of point A, defined as 2 cm lat-
       eral to the central canal of the uterus and 2 cm from
       the mucous membrane of the lateral fornix in the
       axis of the uterus.
    e. Point A is felt to correlate with the point where the
       ureter and the uterine artery cross; it is taken as a
       point from which to assess dose in the paracervical
       tissues.
    f. Point B was located 5 cm from the midline at the
       level of point A and was thought to correlate to the
       location of the obturator lymph nodes.[9,11–14]

13. Fletcher system:
    a. The primary prescription parameter in the Fletcher system is tumor volume with prescription rules based on mg-h and maximum time, taking into account the total external beam dose and the calculated dose.
    b. Calculated bladder and rectal doses are noted and may sometimes limit the implant duration. After adding the dose from the external beam treatments, the point dose calculations to the bladder are kept at below 75 to 80 Gy and the rectum at below 70 to 75 Gy. The total amount of mg-Radium-equivalent cesium-137 is multiplied by the duration of the implant in hours to calculate mg-Ra-eq-h.
    c. Mg-Ra-eq-h provide an estimate of the internal dose to the pelvis from the implant and are usually limited to less than 6500 after 40 to 45 Gy external beam to the pelvis.
    d. The tandem should be positioned in the axis of the pelvis, equidistant from the sacral promontory and pubis and the lateral sidewalls to avoid overdosage to the bladder, sigmoid, or ureter. The tandem should bisect the ovoids on the AP film and bisect their height on the lateral films.[13]
14. The limitation of the point A system is that no one point is representative of the volume implanted. Points A and B are still widely used, with definition interpreted differently at varying institutions. Also there is no consensus on conversion of mg-Ra-eq-h to dose rate at point A. Therefore in 1985, the ICRU recommended that radioactive sources be specified in "reference air kerma rate." This is the kerma (kinetic energy released in a medium) rate to air, in air, at a reference distance of 1 m, corrected for air attenuation and scattering. The total reference air kerma is then the sum of the products of the reference air kerma rate and the duration of the application for each source. Specifications of an in-

tracavitary application in terms of a reference dose rate curve (isodose line) were suggested.[11]

15. An interstitial implant is the insertion of brachytherapy sources in the form of needles, wires, seeds, or seed-containing ribbons into the tumor volume in a pattern dictated by the distribution rules of a specific system, for example, Patterson-Parker, Quimby, Paris, or the computer system. Many templates are commercially available. An example is the Syed/Neblett template. The template is made from 2 Lucite plates joined by screws that, when tightened, secure up to 38 afterloading, hollow stainless steel needles with an additional 6 needles that may be inserted within the vaginal obturator in the event that a tandem is not used. After obtaining computerized dosimetry, iridium sources on individual ribbons are loaded into each needle.

16. The preceding systems are considered low-dose rate systems (LDR) and were developed during a time before remote afterloading techniques were available. These systems have now become available as remote afterloading techniques that enhance radiation protection of the medical staff and public.

17. High-dose rate (HDR) is also used in some centers for the treatment of gynecologic cancers. There are differing opinions regarding its use. The ICRU defines HDR as a dose rate greater than 12 Gy/hour. Several models have evolved to estimate the dose rate correction factor when correlating HDR doses with conventional LDR. Multiple treatment schemes and fractionation doses exist.[11–15]

REFERENCES

1. HALL EJ: *Radiobiology for the Radiologist,* 3rd ed. Philadelphia, Lippincott, 1988.
2. HANKS GE: Patterns of Care Study of Carcinoma of the Cervix. *Patterns of Care Newsletter,* American College of Radiology, Philadelphia, 1990–1991, No. 1.
3. LANCIANO RM, et al: The influence of treatment time on outcome for squamous cell cancer of the uterine cervix treated with radia-

tion: A Patterns-Of-Care Study. Int J Rad Onc Bio Phys 25:391, 1993.

4. HALL EJ: Radiobiology in clinical radiation therapy, in 41st Annual Scientific Meeting for Therapeutic Radiology and Oncology, Refresher Course No. 203C, November 2, 1999, San Antonio, Texas.

5. MOSS WT, COX JD: *Radiation Oncology Rationale, Technique, and Results,* 6th ed. Toronto, Mosby, 1989.

6. KAANDERS, JHAM, ANG KK: Early reactions as dose-limiting factors in radiotherapy. Sem Rad Oncol 4:55, 1994.

7. ROSEN EM: Biologic basis of radiation sensitivity: Part 1. Factors governing radiation tolerance. Oncology April:543, 2000.

8. EMAMI B, et al: Tolerance of normal tissue to therapeutic irradiation. Int J Rad Onc Bio Phys 21:111, 1991.

9. KHAN FM: *The Physics of Radiation Therapy,* 2nd ed. Baltimore, Williams & Wilkins, 1994.

10. HILARIS BS, NORI D, ANDERSON L: *Atlas of Brachytherapy.* New York, McMillan, 1988.

11. International Committee on Radiation Units and Measures (ICRU) Report No. 38: Dose and Volume Specification for Reporting Intracavitary Therapy in Gynecology.

12. LEVITT SH, KHAN FM, POTISH RA: *Levitt and Tapley's Technological Basis of Radiation Therapy: Practical Clinical Applications.* Philadelphia, Lea & Febriger, 1992.

13. EIFEL PJ: Carcinoma of the cervix, in 41st Annual Scientific Meeting for Therapeutic Radiology and Oncology, Refresher Course No. 314, November 2, 1999, San Antonio, Texas.

14. ERICKSON B: Intracavitary application in the treatment of cancer of the cervix: Low, medium and high dose rate. ASTRO Review Course.

15. PETEREIT, DG: High dose rate brachytherapy for carcinoma of the cervix, in 41st Annual Scientific Meeting for Therapeutic Radiology and Oncology; Refresher Course No. 404, November 2, 1999, San Antonio, Texas.

Joseph T. Santoso

OUTLINE FOR READING ECGs

A. Determine rate (normal: 60 to 100): Rate determination QRS peak—300, 150, 100, 75, 60, 50. For bradycardia, find the 6-second interval (30 large boxes) and multiply the number of QRS by 10. One small box = 0.04 seconds. One large box (5 small boxes) = 0.2 seconds.

B. Determine rhythm (scan tracing for abnormal waves, pauses, and irregularities):
   1. Check P wave for every QRS and check for QRS after every P wave.
   2. Measure PR interval (normal ≤ 0.2 seconds): rule out AV block.
   3. Measure QRS interval: rule out bundle branch block.

C. Determine axis deviation: vector of lead I and aVF (normal: −30 to 120 degrees): see the figure below.

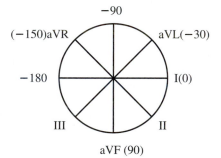

D. Determine the presence of hypertrophy:
   1. Atrial enlargement: look at the P wave in leads II and V1.
   2. Ventricular hypertrophy: look at QRS in all leads (see the figure at the top of page 295).

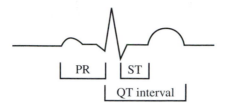

CRITERIA FOR MYOCARDIAL INFARCTION (IN CHRONOLOGICAL APPEARANCE)

- First, the T wave peaks then inverts (symmetrically).
- This is followed by ST-segment elevation (J point elevation is normal).
- Finally, the Q wave appears.
- ST depression is a reciprocal change picked up by a distant lead; the location of infarction is still associated by ST elevation.

CRITERIA FOR LOCALIZING THE INFARCTION

- Anterior leads infarction: V_1 to V_4 (occlusion of the left anterior descending artery).
- Lateral leads infarction: aVL, I, V_5, V_6 (occlusion of the left circumflex artery).
- Inferior leads infarction: II, III, aVF (occlusion of the right coronary artery).
- aVR lead is not informative (just ignore).
- Posterior infarction: reciprocal changes in V_1, V_2 (ST depression, tall R wave).

CRITERIA FOR SIGNIFICANT Q WAVES

- Q wave greater than 0.04 seconds in duration.
- Depth of Q wave one-third or more the height of the R wave in the same QRS complex

CRITERIA FOR NON-Q WAVE INFARCTION

- T-wave inversion.
- ST-segment depression ($\geq$ 1 mm depression) for more than 48 hours in an appropriate clinical setting.

CRITERIA FOR AV BLOCK

A. First degree: PR interval greater than 0.2 seconds.
B. Second degree:
   1. Mobitz type I (Wenckebach): progressive prolongation of PR followed by a dropped QRS.
   2. Mobitz type II: all-or-nothing conduction. QRS is dropped without PR prolongation.
C. Third degree: atria and ventricles beat by independent pacemakers.
D. Place pacemaker for Mobitz type II and third-degree heart block. Other AV block can be observed if not symptomatic.

CRITERIA FOR BUNDLE BRANCH BLOCK (BBB; DIAGNOSED BY LOOKING AT THE WIDTH AND CONFIGURATION OF QRS)

A. Criteria for right BBB:
   1. QRS complex widened more than 0.12 seconds.
   2. RSR in leads V_1 and V_2 (rabbit ears) with ST-segment depression and T-wave inversion.
   3. Reciprocal changes in leads V_5, V_6, and aVL.
B. Criteria for left BBB:
   1. QRS complex widened more than 0.12 seconds.
   2. Broad or notched R wave with prolonged upstroke in leads I, aVL, V_5, and V_6, with ST-segment depression and T-wave inversion.
   3. Reciprocal changes in V_1 and V_2.
   4. Left axis deviation may be present.

CRITERIA FOR ATRIAL HYPERTROPHY

- Right atrial: increased amplitude in the first person of the P wave; possible right axis deviation.

- Look at the P wave in lead II (tallest) and lead V_1 (biphasic right/left).
- Left atrial: increased P-wave duration; no significant axis deviation.

CRITERIA FOR VENTRICULAR HYPERTROPHY

A. Right ventricular hypertrophy:
1. Right axis deviation of more than 100 degrees.
2. Ratio of R-wave amplitude to S-wave amplitude is greater than 1 in V_1 and less than 1 in V_6.
B. Left ventricular hypertrophy:
1. R-wave amplitude in V_5 or V_6 plus S-wave amplitude in V_1 or V_2 is greater than 35 mm (this may not apply to patients less than 35 years old—thin chest leads to high voltage).
2. Presence of strain (asymmetric ST depression and T inversion): significant hypertrophy, most often seen in leads with tall R waves (ventricular dilation/failure).

MISCELLANEOUS ECG CHANGES

- Hyperkalemia: peaked T, PR prolongation and flattening P → QRS widening → sine wave → ventricular fibrillation.
- Hypokalemia: ST depression → T-wave flattening → U-wave → atrial fibrillation.
- Hypercalcemia: shortened QT, prolonged PR.
- Hypocalcemia: prolonged QT, decreased ST interval.
- Digitalis: therapeutic level associated with ST and T-wave changes.
- Chronic obstructive pulmonary diseases: Low voltage, right axis deviation, poor R-wave progression, and right ventricular hypertrophy with strain.
- Acute pulmonary embolism: right ventricular hypertrophy with strain, right BBB, S1Q3 (large S wave in lead I and a deep Q wave in lead III). Sinus tachycardia and atrial fibrillation are the most common arrhythmias.

Joseph T. Santoso

INDICATIONS FOR INTUBATION

- Hypercarbia.
- Hypoxemia.
- Airway protection.

VENTILATOR "BUTTONS"

A. To oxygenate: F_{IO_2} and positive end-expiratory pressure (PEEP).
B. To ventilate: rate and tidal volume.
C. Airflow control:
   1. Pressure control: tidal volume is limited by preset pressure (usually ≤ 40 cm). This is the preferred mode as it reduces the risk of barotrauma to the alveoli. Close monitoring needs to be done because the delivered tidal volume may change with changes in lung compliance.
   2. Volume control: delivers the preset tidal volume regardless of pressure. May risk barotrauma, but requires less work in monitoring tidal volume.
D. Modes:
   1. Assist control (AC): give the assigned tidal volume and any extra inhalation will be given the same amount of tidal volume. This mode is uncomfortable and is used mainly for very sick patients.
   2. Intermittent mandatory ventilation (IMV): give the assigned tidal volume as previously, but any extra inhalation by the patient will only provide her own tidal volume. This mode is more comfortable and offers less risk of hyperventilation. Synchronization to patient's respiratory motion is called SIMV.
   3. Pressure support (PS): additional pressure is triggered by inhalation to a preset pressure. This is used to overcome ET tube resistance or weaning.

4. Continuous positive airway pressure (CPAP): commonly used for weaning.

POSTOPERATIVE VENTILATION ORDER

- Set F_{IO_2} to 100% during transport to the ICU, then wean rapidly to keep O_2 saturation at 95% or greater.
- Mode: SIMV.
- Airflow control is pressure control, if possible. If not available, may use volume control for most patients with the exception of severe ARDS.
- Rate: 12 breaths/min; tidal volume: 10 mL/kg ideal body weight.
- PEEP: 5 cm, pressure support (PS): 5 cm.
- Obtain ABGs on arrival to the ICU and after every ventilator change.
- Obtain a daily chest x-ray while the patient is intubated.

GOALS WHILE THE PATIENT IS ON A VENTILATOR

- Keep F_{IO_2} less than 50% to reduce absorptive atelectasis.
- Keep peak inspiratory pressure below 40 cm to reduce barotrauma to alveoli.
- Extubate as soon as possible.

PROBLEMS WHILE ON A VENTILATOR

A. Hypoxemia:
   1. Increase F_{IO_2} or PEEP, or both, to improve oxygenation.
   2. Rule out pulmonary causes (pneumothorax, pneumonia, ARDS, right main bronchus intubation, mucous plug) or cardiac causes (MI, congestive heart failure, poor contractility, low preload, etc.), or a combination of cardiopulmonary causes.
B. Hypercarbia:
   1. Increase tidal volume or ventilation rate, or both.
   2. Rule out pulmonary or cardiac causes, as previously noted, versus a decrease in respiratory drive (caused by injury to central nervous system).

C. Agitation:
  1. Rule out pain, anxiety, and alcohol withdrawal versus hypoxemia.
  2. Hypoxemia may induce agitation and vice versa.
  3. If reversible etiologies have been ruled out, administering haloperidol, 0.5 to 5 mg IV or IM, may sedate the patient without decreasing respiratory drive.

TIMING TO WEAN FROM THE VENTILATOR

- When underlying disease is resolving.
- Clinically stable: negative fluid balance, Fio_2 less than 40%, alert, minimal airway secretion.

WAYS TO WEAN

- There are various rituals (CPAP, PS, IMV, etc.) that use different kinds of indices. The most popular is the shallow breathing index (ratio of respiratory rate/Fio_2), which predicts successful extubation with a ratio of less than 100.
- The most accurate is to T-tube the patient and measure her spontaneous respiratory rate.[1] If the patient continues to be comfortable on spontaneous breathing with the T-tube, she can usually be extubated. Some clinicians also order ABGs before and after extubation. This practice is not necessary if an O_2 saturation monitor is available and the patient continues to be comfortable, with stable vital signs.

REFERENCE

1. ESTEBAN A, FRUTOS F, TOBIN MJ, ALIA I, SOLSONA JF, VALVERDU I, FERNANDEZ R, DE LA CAL MA, BENITO S, TOMAS R, ET AL: A comparison of four methods of weaning patients from mechanical ventilation. N Engl J Med 332:345, 1995.

GOAL

To provide nutrition to stop catabolism, rebuild lean tissue, and improve the immune system and wound healing.

ENERGY REQUIREMENT

A. Patient's nutrition consists of carbohydrates, protein, and fat.
B. Calculating the daily caloric energy requirement:
  1. Difficult way: Harris Benedict equation × stress factor, indirect calorimetry.
  2. Simple way: for most patients, 25 to 30 kcal/kg/day. Hypermetabolic patients need 35 kcal/kg/day.
C. Protein requirement: 1 to 1.5 g/kg/day of protein.
D. Fat requirement: at least 4% of calories should come from essential fatty acids (linolenic acid) to prevent dermatitis. Because fat is caloric-dense (9 kcal/gm), it can be used to supply calories with less volume. Maximal allowance is 2.5 g/kg/day. Most ICU patients are given fat, which contributes to 10% to 20% of total calories.

IDEAL BODY WEIGHT DETERMINATION (GIVES AN AMOUNT ±10% OF IDEAL BODY WEIGHT)

- Male—106 lb for the first 5 feet, then add 6 lb per additional inch.
- Female—100 lb for the first 5 feet, then add 5 lb per additional inch.
- Then multiply by the conversion factor of 1 kg/2.2 lb.

NUTRITIONAL ASSESSMENT

A. Initial assessment:
  1. Baseline nutritional reserve.

2. Temporal course of illness:
   a. Patient will recovery quickly (e.g., C-section).
   b. Recovery will take a while (e.g., bowel resection, wound dehiscence).
   c. Patient will not recover (e.g., terminal cancer).
3. Nutritional demands of the illness:
   a. Hypermetabolic (e.g., early sepsis).
   b. Low demand (e.g., MI, stroke).

B. Follow-up assessment:
   1. Nitrogen balance = (protein intake/6.25) − (24-hour urea nitrogen in urine + 4 g).
   2. Subjective global assessment: a clinical assessment using the history and physical examination.
   3. Prognostic nutritional index (PNI): an objective assessment predicting the % risk of complication from malnutrition: low risk (PNI < 40%), intermediate (PNI of 40% to 49%), and high risk (PNI > 50%). It is calculated as follows: 158% − 16.6 (alb in g/100 mL) − 0.78 (triceps skinfold in mm) − 0.2 serum transferrin in mg/dL − 5.8 delayed skin hypersensitivity (DSH). DSH represents cutaneous delayed hypersensitivity (mumps, streptokinase-streptodornase, candida). It is graded as 0 (nonreactive), 1 (< 5-mm induration), or 2 (≥ 5-mm induration).
   4. Indirect calorimetry: the most accurate method, but expensive and time consuming. Resting energy expenditure (almost like basal energy requirement) is calculated as follows: (3.9 [oxygen consumption] + 1.1 [CO_2 production]) × 1440 minutes.

NUTRITIONAL SUPPLEMENT TIMING

- Types of nutritional supplements are listed in Table 30-1.
- Most healthy adults can be NPO for 7 to 10 days.
- Postpyloric (tip of feeding tube in duodenum) enteral feeding is tolerated by most patients even at postoperative day (POD) 1 to 2.

TABLE 30–1. Types of Nutritional Supplementation

Types	Benefits	Risks
Oral	Cheapest, comfortable	Aspiration, low intake
Enteral feeding	Most natural, cheaper, possibly prevents bacteria translocation	Aspiration, diarrhea, uncomfortable nasal tube, unable to reach caloric goal
TPN	Easy to use, comfortable for patient, reaches caloric goal easily	Electrolyte abnormalities, expensive, infection, pneumothorax, hypercarbia, cholecystitis

- Malnourished patients need to start as soon as possible. (*Note:* Chronic malnutrition leads to water retention.) Early refeeding must be performed slowly to prevent fluid overload (CHF, edema).

ENTERAL FEEDING ORDER

- Calculate caloric needs (i.e., 30 kcal/kg/day × 70 kg body weight = 2100 kcal/day). Use Osmolite HN (approximately 1 kcal/mL), which means 2100 mL/day. Osmolite HN usually has enough protein and fat already premixed. If additional protein is needed, give Promod.
- Decide to proceed with bolus/stomach feeding (start 50 mL every 3 hours and increase gradually to goal) or continuous/postpyloric feeding (2100 mL/24 hours).
- Check chest x-ray for tube placement before feeding (ideally, the tip of the tube is postpyloric).
- In patients at high risk for aspiration, use a feeding tube with an NG tube to suction. Also, feed the patient during the day, elevate the head of the bed, and decrease sedation.

• Laboratory studies: chem 20 twice a week, record I&O volume, and daily weight.

ENTERAL FEEDING: COMPLICATIONS AND SOLUTIONS

A. Enteral formula on NG aspirate or high gastric residual (1000 mL or more in 12 hours):
   1. Stop the tube feeding, attach the NG tube to wall suction, and restart the feeding if the NG aspirate is clear.
   2. If the problem persists, the tube may not be postpyloric (check the x-ray).
B. Low enteral intake (< 75% of daily caloric goal):
   1. Rule out ileus, tube feeding formula in the NG aspirate, emesis, or feeding-related diarrhea (i.e., not caused by drugs or infection).
   2. Stop the enteral feeding and attempt to solve the underlying problem. Leave the patient NPO for approximately 12 hours, then feed. If the problem persists, consider TPN.
C. Severe diarrhea (5 or more loose stools or > 750 mL of stool volume in 24 hours):
   1. Rule out possible etiologies: stop medications that promote diarrhea (theophylline, magnesium-containing antacids, antibiotics, ascorbic acid).
   2. Send for *Clostridium difficile* toxin assay or ova-parasite culture, as indicated.
   3. Decrease the rate of infusion or strength of the enteral formula.
   4. Can give Kaopectate (30 mL b.i.d. or t.i.d. for 48 hours). Avoid Lomotil or paregoric initially. If diarrhea persists and no infectious etiologies are found, reduce the feeding rate by 50% and use Lomotil (10 mL per NG q.i.d.) or paregoric (1 mL of opium/100 mL of formula) for 24 hours.
   5. If this noninfectious diarrhea continues for 4 or more days, stop the enteral feeding and start TPN until the diarrhea resolves.

D. Obstructed feeding tube:
   1. Use Coke, meat tenderizer, or cranberry juice to digest the obstructed material in the feeding tube; wait, then retry.
   2. Do not reinsert the feeding tube stylet as it can perforate the tube and injure esophagus.

WRITING TPN ORDERS

A. Determine fluid (30 mL/kg/day) and caloric requirements (30 kcal/kg/day). These nonprotein calories come from glucose solution (70% of calorie) and fat (30%).
B. Determine protein requirement (1 to 1.5 g/kg/day). Keep calorie-nitrogen ratio at 150:1 (i.e., 1 g of nitrogen or 6.25 g of protein for each 150 kcal). This is the required calorie-to-nitrogen ratio to prevent nitrogen loss in critically ill patients. In contrast, a normal diet has a ratio of 1:300.
C. Choose the appropriate amino acid/dextrose solution to meet the preceding specifications.
D. The maximal fat allowance per day is 2.5 g/kg/day.
E. Add electrolyte requirements: Na (1 to 2 mEq/kg/day), K (1 to 2 mEq/kg/day), Cl (1 to 2 mEq/kg/day), Ca (0.2 to 0.3 mEq/kg/day), Mg (0.35 to 0.45 mEq/kg/day), phosphorus (variable) starts with 10 mmol/1000 kcal.
F. Add multivitamins, trace elements, heparin (1000 U/L), or any other additional medications (regular insulin, 20 U; Tagamet, 300 mg/L; HCl, 100 mEq/L to adjust pH).
G. Monitor laboratory values:
   1. Obtain baseline chem 20, CBC, and lipid panel before TPN is started.
   2. Once TPN is started:
      a. Check fingerstick blood glucose q.i.d. (keep blood glucose at 100 to 200).
      b. Chem + 7, Mg, Ca, PO_4 daily until values are stable (about 3 days).
      c. Lipid panel twice a week, then discontinue if triglyceride is stable.

H. Special situations:
   1. Hepatic failure: delete aromatic amino acids which serve as neurotransmitter precursor. They may exacerbate hepatic encephalopathy.
   2. Renal failure: delete nonessential amino acids.
I. For example: A patient with an ideal body weight of 100 kg needs TPN.
   1. Her daily caloric requirement is approximately 100 kg × 30 kcal/kg, which is equal to 3000 kcal/day. Her volume requirement is usually about the same as her caloric requirement, which is 3000 mL/day.
   2. Caloric energy comes from three sources: protein, fat, and carbohydrate. Each gram of protein gives 4 kcal, 1 g of fat gives 9 kcal, and 1 g of carbohydrate gives 3.4 kcal.
   3. Since we decided that her daily protein requirement is 1.5 g/kg body weight, she needs 150 g protein. The most common protein solution has a 10% concentration (i.e., 10 g of protein in 100 mL solution). Thus, the daily requirement of 150 g of protein will generate 600 kcal (i.e., 150 g × 4 kcal/g) and requires a volume of 1500 mL (i.e., 150 g × 100 mL/10 g protein).
   4. About 20% of her daily caloric requirement will be given in the form of fat, which is 600 kcal (i.e., 20% × 3000 kcal/day). Because most fat solutions contain 2 kcal/mL, her fat requirement will have a volume of 300 mL.
   5. The rest of her daily caloric requirement, which is 1800 kcal (i.e., 3000 − 600 − 600), will come from sugar solution. This calorie value is equivalent to about 529 g of carbohydrate (i.e., 1800 kcal × 1 g carbohydrate/3.4 kcal). The most commonly used carbohydrate solution is D70 (i.e., 70% carbohydrate, or 70 g per 100 mL solution). Thus, we need a volume of D70 of 756 mL.
   6. So far, we have achieved a total caloric goal of 3000 kcal/day by getting 600 kcal from protein, 600 kcal from fat, and 1800 kcal from carbohydrate, with a total volume of 2556 mL (i.e., 1500 mL of protein + 300 mL of

fat + 756 mL of D70). As her total daily volume requirement is 3000 mL, we need to add 444 mL of water. Usually, we add electrolytes, heparin, and insulin.

7. Her nonprotein calorie requirement is 2400 kcal (from carbohydrate and fat). She gets 150 g of protein, which is equal to 24 g of nitrogen (150 × 6.25 g nitrogen/1 g of protein). Thus, her nitrogen to nonprotein calorie ratio is 2400/24 = 100.

STOPPING TPN

TPN infusion increases endogenous insulin. Abrupt interruption of TPN may cause hypoglycemia. Two ways to discontinue TPN are:

- Cut the infusion rate to half. Then stop TPN 6 hours later and check glucose.
- Stop TPN and substitute with $D_{10}W$ at 100 mL/hour for 6 hours then stop. The use of $D_{10}W$ IV can prevent hypoglycemia in a patient whose central line has accidentally pulled out.

SPECIAL CASES

- Terminal cancer: consider not giving TPN.
- Renal failure: keep the nitrogen supply at 1 to 1.3 g/kg/day; do not provide fat-soluble vitamins (A, D, E, K); may use more essential amino acid.
- Respiratory failure: use a higher percentage of fat (RQ 0.7) than carbohydrates (RQ 1) to supply calories. In general, use fewer calories (the excess will be converted to fat [RQ 1.3]). RQ stands for respiratory quotient and is equal to the amount of CO_2 produced for each mole of O_2 consumed.
- Preoperative TPN for 7 to 10 days reduces morbidity in severely malnourished patients.
- Early (within 48 hours postoperatively) enteral feeding reduces morbidity in most patients.

V | **APPENDICES**

GENERAL TRANSFUSION RECOMMENDATION

Packed Red Blood Cells (PRBC)

In most adults, the indications are anemia (HB < 7 g/dL), symptomatic anemia, or acute, severe blood loss. In a patient who is hypotensive from blood loss, start giving 1 unit PRBC when 2 L of crystalloid does not stabilize blood pressure. In this situation, keep giving 1 unit PRBC for each liter of crystalloid transfused.

Fresh Frozen Plasma (FFP)

It contains all clotting factors. Give FFP when PT is greater than 18 seconds and/or PTT is greater than 54 seconds, for massive blood transfusion, or DIC. The dose of FFP is calculated based on patient body weight. The initial recommendation is 10 to 15 mL/kg. One unit of FFP is about 220 mL. It takes about 30 minutes for FFP to thaw. Thus, call the blood bank early in anticipation of delay for thawing the FFP.

Cryoprecipitate

Indicated mainly for fibrinogen replacement. For most surgery, the fibrinogen level should be greater than 100 mg/dL to assure clotting capability. One unit of cryoprecipitate contains 250 mg of fibrinogen and should increase fibrinogen levels by 10 to 15 mg/dL. The initial recommended order is 1 unit of cryoprecipitate for every 10 kg of body weight.

Platelets

Indicated when platelet count is less than 100,000 for major surgery or less than 10,000 to 20,000 in spontaneous thrombocytopenia. Some clinical judgment is needed here as patients with symptomatic bleeding may require platelets in higher count. The initial recommended order is 1 unit of single donor platelets, as it reduces the infectious risk compared with random donor platelets. See Table A–1 for differences in these two types of platelets.

TABLE A–1. Summary of Blood Components

Product (vol in mL)	Content	Indications	Risks	Comments
PRBC (250)	Red cells	Blood loss	Infection	Increase hematocrit 3% per unit
Whole blood (500)	All components WBC and platelet, are non-functional	Massive blood loss	Infection and volume overload	Consider component therapy
WBC-poor RBC (approx. 300)	Mostly RBC, WBC $< 5 \times 10^{6-8}$	History of febrile reaction, to prevent alloimmunization, for paroxysmal nocturnal hemoglobinuria	Infection	May not be readily available
Frozen PRBC (180)	RBC, no platelets or plasma	Long-term storage for patients with rare antibody	Infection	Expensive, not for emergency use
Platelets—random donor (50)	$> 5.5 \times 10^{10}$ platelets/U	Bleeding due to low platelet count	Infection, Rh immunization	Increase 5000–8000 platelets/U

continued

TABLE A–1. (*Continued*)

Product (vol in mL)	Content	Indications	Risks	Comments
Platelet—single donor, pheresis (300)	$> 3 \times 10^{11}$ platelets/U	Bleeding due to low platelet count	Lower risk of infection, Rh immunization	Equivalent to 6–8 U of regular platelets
Cryoprecipitate (40)	Fibrinogen, factors VIII and XIII, and von Willebrand's factor	Factor deficiency, Von Willebrand, fibrinogen deficiency, DIC	Infection	Use desmopressin for Von Willebrand type 1
Fresh frozen plasma (200), jumbo FFP (600)	Plasma, all coagulation factors	DIC, factor deficiency, warfarin reversal, massive transfusion	Infection	Not to be used for volume expansion or nutritional support; jumbo FFP = 3 FFPs with less infection
Albumin 5% (250)	Albumin, some globulins	Volume expansion	No infection	Expensive

Table A–2. Risk of Transfusion per Unit of Blood

Infection Type	Risk[a]
Hepatitis C	1:103,000
Hepatitis B	1:63,000
HIV	1:493,000
HTLV I/II	1:641,000
Bacterial/parasite	< 1:1,000,000

[a]According to Schrieber GB, Busch MP, Kleinman SH, Korelitz JJ: The risk of transfusion-transmitted viral infections. N Engl J M 334:1685, 1996.

B | NCI Toxicity Criteria

TABLE B–1. NCI Toxicity Criteria

Adverse Event	0	1	2	3	4
			Grade		
			Allergy/Immunology		
Allergic reaction/ hypersensitivity (including drug fever)	None	Transient rash, drug fever < 38° C (< 100.4° F)	Urticaria, drug fever ≥ 38° C (≥ 100.4° F), and/or asymptomatic bronchospasm	Symptomatic bronchospasm, requiring parenteral medication(s), with or without urticaria; allergy-related edema/angioedema	Anaphylaxis

Note: Isolated urticaria, in the absence of other manifestations of an allergic or hypersensitivity reaction, is graded in the DERMATOLOGY/SKIN category, later

			Auditory/Hearing		
Inner ear/hearing	Normal	Hearing loss on audiometry only	Tinnitus or hearing loss, not requiring hearing aid or treatment	Tinnitus or hearing loss, correctable with hearing aid or treatment	Severe unilateral or bilateral hearing loss (deafness), not correctable

continued

TABLE B-1. (*Continued*)

Adverse Event	0	1	2	3	4
			Grade		
			Blood/Bone Marrow		
Hemoglobin (Hb)	WNL	< LLN–10.0 g/dL	8.0–< 10.0 g/dL	6.5–< 8.0 g/dL	< 6.5 g/dl
Leukocytes (total WBC)	WNL	< LLN–3000/μL	≥ 2000–< 3000/μL	≥ 1000–< 2000/μL	< 1000/μL
Neutrophils/ granulocytes (ANC/AGC)	WNL	≥ 1500–< 2000/μL	≥ 1000–< 1500/μL	≥ 500–< 1000/μL	< 500/μL
Platelets	WNL	< LLN–75,000/μL	≥ 50,000–< 75,000/μL	≥ 10,000–< 50,000/μL	< 10,000/μL
			Cardiovascular (General)		
Cardiovascular/ arrhythmia— other (specify)	None	Asymptomatic, not requiring treatment	Symptomatic, but not requiring treatment	Symptomatic, and requiring treatment of underlying cause	Life-threatening (e.g., arrhythmia associated with CHF, hypoten-sion, syncope, shock)
Cardiac— ischemia/ infarction	None	Nonspecific T-wave flattening or changes	Asymptomatic, ST- and T-wave changes suggesting ischemia	Angina without evidence of infarction	Acute, MI

	Normal				
Cardiac left ventricular function	Normal	Asymptomatic decline of resting ejection fraction of > 10% but < % of baseline value; shortening fraction > 24% but < 30%	Asymptomatic but resting ejection fraction below LLN for laboratory or decline of resting ejection fraction > 20% of baseline value; < 24% shortening fraction	CHF responsive to treatment	Severe or refractory CHF or requiring intubation
Cardiac troponin T (cTnT)	Normal	≥ 0.03–< 0.05 ng/mL	≥ 0.05–< 0.1 ng/mL	≥ 0.1–< 0.2 ng/mL	≥ 0.2 ng/mL
Edema	None	Asymptomatic, not requiring therapy	Symptomatic, requiring therapy	Symptomatic edema limiting function and unresponsive to therapy or requiring drug discontinuation	Anasarca (severe generalized edema)
Hypertension	None	Asymptomatic, transient increase by > 20 mmHg (diastolic) or to > 150/100[a] if previously WNL; not requiring treatment	Recurrent or persistent or symptomatic increase by > 20 mmHg (diastolic) or to > 150/100[a] if previously WNL; not requiring treatment	Requiring therapy or more intensive therapy than previously	Hypertensive crises

Note: For pediatric patients, use age- and sex-appropriate normal values > 95th percentile ULN.

continued

TABLE B–1. (*Continued*)

Adverse Event	0	1	2	3	4
			Grade		
Hypotension	None	Changes, but not requiring therapy (including transient orthostatic hypotension)	Requiring brief fluid replacement or other therapy but not hospitalization; no physiologic consequences	Requiring therapy and sustained medical attention, but resolves without persisting physiologic consequences	Shock (associated with acidemia and impairing vital organ function due to tissue hypoperfusion)

Also consider syncope (fainting).

Notes: Angina or MI is graded as cardiac—ischemia/infarction in the CARDIOVASCULAR (GENERAL) category, earlier. For pediatric patients, systolic BP 65 mmHg or less in infants up to 1 year and 70 mmHg or less in children older than 1 year of age, use two successive or three measurements in 24 hours.

| Thrombosis/embolism | None | — | Deep vein thrombosis, not requiring anticoagulant therapy | Deep vein thrombosis, requiring anticoagulant therapy | Embolic event including pulmonary embolism |

Constitutional Symptoms

Fatigue (lethargy, malaise, asthenia)	None	Increased fatigue over baseline, but not altering normal activities	Moderate (e.g., decrease in performance status by 1 ECOG level or 20% Karnofsky or Lansky scale or causing difficulty performing some activities)	Severe (e.g., decrease in performance status by ≥ 2 ECOG levels or 40% Karnofsky or Lansky scale or loss of ability to perform some activities)	Bedridden or disabling
Fever (in the absence of neutropenia, where neutropenia is defined as AGC < 1.0 × 10^9/L)	None	38.0–39.0° C (100.4–102.2° F)	39.1–40.0° C (102.3–104.0° F)	> 40.0° C (> 104.0° F) for < 24 hours	> 40.0° C (>104.0° F) for > 24 hours

Also consider allergic reaction/hypersensitivity.
Note: the temperature measurements listed above are oral or tympanic.

Weight gain	< 5%	5–< 10%	10–< 20%	≥ 20 %	—

Also consider vomiting, dehydration, diarrhea.

continued

TABLE B–1. (Continued)

Adverse Event	Grade				
	0	1	2	3	4
Dermatology/Skin					
Alopecia	Normal	Mild hair loss	Pronounced hair loss	—	—
Hand-foot skin	None	Skin changes or dermatitis without pain (e.g., erythema, peeling)	Skin changes with pain, not interfering with function	Skin changes with pain, interfering with function	—
Pigmentation changes (e.g., vitiligo)	None	Localized pigmentation changes	Generalized pigmentation changes	—	—
Pruritus	None	Mild or localized, relieved spontaneously or by local measures	Intense or widespread, relieved spontaneously or by systemic measures	Intense or widespread and poorly controlled despite treatment	—
Radiation dermatitis	None	Faint erythema or dry desquamation	Moderate to brisk erythema or a patchy moist desquamation, mostly confined to skin folds and creases; moderate edema	Confluent moist desquamation > 1.5-cm diameter and not confined to skin folds; pitting edema	Skin necrosis or ulceration of full-thickness dermis; may include bleeding not induced by minor trauma or abrasion

	None	Requiring no medication	Requiring PO or topical treatment or IV medication or steriods for < 24 hours	Requiring IV medication or steroids for ≥ 24 hours	—
Urticaria (hives, welts, wheals)	None	Requiring no medication	Requiring PO or topical treatment or IV medication or steriods for < 24 hours	Requiring IV medication or steroids for ≥ 24 hours	—
Wound—infectious	None	Cellulitis	Superficial infection	Infection requiring IV antibiotics	Necrotizing fasciitis
Wound—noninfectious	None	Incisional separation	Incisional hernia	Fascial disruption without evisceration	Fascial disruption with evisceration
Hot flashes/flushes	None	Mild or no more than 1 per day	Moderate and greater than 1 per day	—	—
SIADH (syndrome of inappropriate antidiuretic hormone)	Absent	—	—	—	—
Gastrointestinal					
Anorexia	None	Loss of appetite	Oral intake significantly decreased	Requiring IV fluids	Requiring feeding tube or parenteral nutrition
Ascites (nonmalignant)	None	Asymptomatic	Symptomatic, requiring diuretics	Symptomatic, requiring therapeutic paracentesis	Life-threatening physiologic consequences

continued

TABLE B–1. (Continued)

Adverse Event	Grade				
	0	1	2	3	4
Colitis	None	—	Abdominal pain with mucus and/or blood in stool	Abdominal pain, fever, change in bowel habits with ileus or peritoneal signs, and radiographic or biopsy documentation	Perforation or requiring surgery or toxic megacolon

Also consider hemorrhage/bleeding with grade 3 or 4 thrombocytopenia; hemorrhage/bleeding without grade 3 or 4 thrombocytopenia; melena/GI bleeding; rectal bleeding/hematochezia; hypotension.

Adverse Event	Grade				
	0	1	2	3	4
Constipation	None	Requiring stool softener or dietary modification	Requiring laxatives	Obstipation requiring manual evacuation or enema	Obstruction or toxic megacolon
Dehydration	None	Dry mucous membranes and/or diminished skin turgor	Requiring IV fluid replacement (brief)	Requiring IV fluid replacement (sustained)	Physiologic consequences requiring intensive care; hemodynamic collapse

Also consider diarrhea, vomiting, stomatitis/pharyngitis (oral/pharyngeal mucositis), hypotension.

Diarrhea patients without colostomy	None	Increase of < 4 stools/day over pretreatment	Increase of 4–6 stools/day, or nocturnal stools	Increase of > 7 stools/day or incontinence; or need for parenteral support for dehydration	Physiologic consequences requiring intensive care; or hemodynamic collapse
Diarrhea patients with colostomy	None	Mild increase in loose, watery colostomy output compared with pretreatment	Moderate increase in loose, watery colostomy output compared with pretreatment, but not interfering with normal activity	Severe increase in loose watery colostomy output compared with pretreatment, interfering with normal activity	Physiologic consequences requiring intensive care; or hemodynamic collapse
Dyspepsia/heartburn	None	Mild	Moderate	Severe	—
Dysphagia, esophagitis, odynophagia (painful swallowing)	None	Mild dysphagia, but can eat regular diet	Dysphagia, requiring predominantly pureed, soft, or liquid diet	Dysphagia, requiring IV hydration	Complete obstruction (cannot swallow saliva) requiring enteral or parenteral nutritional support, or perforation

Note: if the adverse event is radiation-related, grade *either* under dysphagia-esophageal related to radiation *or* dysphagia-pharyngeal related to radiation.

Ileus (or neuroconstipation)	None	—	Intermittent, not requiring intervention	Requiring non-surgical intervention	Requiring surgery

continued

TABLE B-1. (Continued)

Adverse Event	0 Normal	1 Mild	Grade 2 Moderate	3	4
Mouth dryness	Normal	Mild	Moderate		
Nausea	None	Able to eat	Oral intake significantly decreased	No significant intake, requiring IV fluids	—
Proctitis	None	Increased stool frequency, occasional blood-streaked stools or rectal discomfort (including hemorrhoids) not requiring medication	Increased stool frequency, bleeding, mucous discharge, or rectal discomfort requiring medication; anal fissure	Increased stool frequency/diarrhea requiring parenteral support; rectal bleeding requiring transfusion; or persistent mucous discharge, necessitating pads	Perforation, bleeding, or necrosis or other life-threatening complication requiring surgical intervention (e.g., colostomy)
Stomatitis/pharyngitis (oral/pharyngeal mucositis)	None	Painless ulcers, erythema, or mild soreness in the absence of lesions	Painful erythema, edema, or ulcers, but can eat or swallow	Painful erythema, edema, or ulcers requiring IV hydration	Severe ulceration or requires parenteral or enteral nutritional support or prophylactic intubation
Taste disturbance (dysgeusia)	Normal	Slightly altered	Markedly altered	—	—

324

	None	1 episode in 24 hours over pretreatment	2-5 episodes in 24 hours over pretreatment	> 6 episodes in 24 hours over pretreatment; or need for IV fluids	Requiring parenteral nutrition; or physiologic consequences requiring intensive care; hemodynamic collapse
Vomiting	None	1 episode in 24 hours over pretreatment	2-5 episodes in 24 hours over pretreatment	> 6 episodes in 24 hours over pretreatment; or need for IV fluids	Requiring parenteral nutrition; or physiologic consequences requiring intensive care; hemodynamic collapse

Also consider dehydration.

Hemorrhage					
Hemorrhage/bleeding with grade 3 or 4 thrombocytopenia	None	Mild without transfusion	—	Requiring transfusion	Catastrophic bleeding requiring major non-elective intervention
Hemorrhage/bleeding without grade 3 or 4 thrombocytopenia	None	Mild without transfusion	—	Requiring transfusion	Catastrophic bleeding requiring major non-elective intervention
Hemorrhage/bleeding associated with surgery	None	Mild without transfusion	—	Requiring transfusion	Catastrophic bleeding requiring major non-elective intervention

Note: Expected blood loss at the time of surgery in not graded as an adverse event.

continued

TABLE B–1. (Continued)

Adverse Event	Grade 0	1	2	3	4
Petechiae/purpura (hemorrhage/bleeding into skin or mucosa)	None	Rare petechiae of skin	Petechiae or purpura in dependent areas of skin	Generalized petechiae or purpura of skin or petechiae of any mucosal site	—
Rectal bleeding/hematochezia	None	Mild without transfusion medication	Persistent, requiring medication (e.g., steriod suppositories) and/or break from radiation treatment	Requiring transfusion	Catastrophic bleeding requiring major non-elective intervention
Vaginal bleeding	None	Spotting, requiring < 2 pads per day	Requiring > 2 pads per day, but not requiring transfusion	Requiring transfusion	Catastrophic bleeding requiring major non-elective intervention
Hepatic					
Alkaline phosphatase	WNL	> ULN–2.5 × ULN	> 2.5–5.0 × ULN	> 5.0–20.0 × ULN	> 20.0 × ULN
Bilirubin	WNL	> 2–< 3 mg/100 mL	> 3–< 6 mg/100 mL	> 6–< 15 mg/100 mL	> 15 mg/100 mL
GGT	WNL	> ULN–2.5 × ULN	> 2.5–5.0 × ULN	> 5.0–20.0 × ULN	> 20.0 × ULN
Hypoalbuminemia	WNL	< LLN–3 g/dL	> 2–< 3 g/dL	< 2 g/dL	—

326

SGOT (AST) (serum glutamic oxaloacetic transaminase)	WNL	> ULN–2.5 × ULN	> 2.5–5.0 × ULN	> 5.0–20.0 × ULN	> 20.0 × ULN
SGPT (ALT) (serum glutamic pyruvic transaminase)	WNL	> ULN–2.5 × ULN	> 2.5–5.0 × ULN	> 5.0–20.0 × ULN	> 20.0 × ULN

Infection/Febrile Neutropenia

Catheter-related infection	None	Mild, no active treatment	Moderate, localized infection, requiring local or oral treatment	Severe, systemic infection, requiring IV antibiotic or anti-fungal treatment, or hospitalization	Life-threatening sepsis (e.g., septic shock)
Febrile neutropenia (ANC, 1.0 × 109/L, fever > 38.5° C)	None	—	—	Present	Life-threatening sepsis (e.g., septic shock)
Infection without neutropenia	None	Mild, no active treatment	Moderate, localized infection, requiring local or oral treatment	Severe, systemic infection, requiring IV antibiotic or anti-fungal treatment, or hospitalization	Life-threatening sepsis (e.g., septic shock)

continued

TABLE B-1. *(Continued)*

Adverse Event	Grade				
	0	1	2	3	4
			Lymphatics		
Lymphatic	Normal	Mild lymphedema	Moderate lymphedema requiring compression; lymphocyst	Severe lymphedema limiting function; lymphocyst requiring surgery	Severe lymphedema limiting function with ulceration
			Metabolic/Laboratory		
Acidosis (metabolic or respiratory)	Normal	pH < normal, but ≥ 7.3	—	pH < 7.3	pH > 7.3 with life-threatening physiologic consequences
Alkalosis (metabolic or respiratory)	Normal	pH > normal, but ≥ 7.5	—	pH > 7.5	pH > 7.5 with life-threatening physiologic consequences
Amylase	WNL	> ULN-1.5 × ULN	> 1.5-2.0 × ULN	> 2.0-5.0 × ULN	> 5.0 × ULN
Hypercalcemia	WNL	> ULN-11.5 mg/dL	> 11.5-12.5 mg/dL	> 12.5-13.5 mg/dL	> 13.5 mg/dL
Hyperglycemia	WNL	> ULN-160 mg/dL	> 160-250 mg/dL	> 500 mg/dL	—
Hyperkalemia	WNL	> ULN-5.5 mmol/L	> 5.5-6.0 mmol/L	> 6.0-7.0 mmol/L	> 7.0 mmol/L
Hyper-magnesemia	WNL	> ULN-3.0 mg/dL > ULN-1.23 mmol/L	—	> 3.0-8.0 mg/dL > 1.23-3.30 mmol/L	> 8.0 mg/dL > 3.30 mmol/L
Hypernatremia	WNL	> ULN-150 mmol/L	> 150-155 mmol/L	> 155-160 mmol/L	> 160 mmol/L

Hypocalcemia	WNL	< LLN–8.0 mg/dL < LLN–2.0 mmol/L	7.0–< 8.0 mg/dL 1.75–< 2.0 mmol/L	6.0–< 7.0 mg/dL 1.5–< 1.75 mmol/L	< 6.0 mg/dL < 1.5 mmol/L
Hypoglycemia	WNL	< LLN–5.5 mg/dL < LLN–3.0 mmol/L	40–< 55 mg/dL 2.2–< 3.0 mmol/L	30–< 40 mg/dL 1.7–< 2.2 mmol/L	< 30 mg/dL < 1.7 mmol/L
Hypokalemia	WNL	< LLN–3.0 mmol/L	—	2.5–< 3.0 mmol/L	< 2.5 mmol/L
Hypo-magnesemia	WNL	< LLN–1.2 mg/dL < LLN–0.5 mmol/L	0.9–< 1.2 mg/dL 0.4–< 0.5 mmol/L	0.7–< 0.9 mg/dL 0.3–< 0.4 mmol/L	< 0.7 mg/dL < 0.3 mmol/L
Hyponatremia	WNL	< LLN–130 mmol/L	—	120–< 130 mmol/L	< 120 mmol/L
Hypo-phosphatemia	WNL	< LLN–2.5 mg/dL < LLN–0.8 mmol/L	> 2.0–< 2.5 mg/dL > 0.6–< 0.8 mmol/L	> 1.0–< 2.0 mg/dL > 0.3–< 0.6 mmol/L	< 1.0 mg/dL < 0.3 mmol/L
Musculoskeletal					
Muscle weakness (not due to neuropathy)	Normal	Asymptomatic with weakness on physical exam	Symptomatic and interfering with function, but not interfering with activities of daily living	Symptomatic and interfering with activities of daily living	Bedridden or disabling
Myositis (inflammation/damage of muscle)	None	Mild pain, not interfering with function	Pain interfering with function, but not interfering with activities of daily living	Pain interfering with function and interfering with activities of daily living	Bedridden or disabling

continued

TABLE B-1. (*Continued*)

Adverse Event		Grade			
	0	1	2	3	4
Osteonecrosis (avascular necrosis)	None	Asymptomatic and detected by imaging only	Symptomatic and interfering with function, but not interfering with activities of daily living	Symptomatic and interfering with activities of daily living	Symptomatic or disabling
Neurology					
Ataxia (incoordination)	Normal	Asymptomatic but abnormal on physical exam, and not interfering with function	Mild symptoms interfering with function, but not interfering with activities of daily living	Moderate symptoms interfering with activities of daily living	Bedridden or disabling
CNS cerebrovascular ischemia	None	—	—	Transient ischemic event or attack (TIA)	Permanent event (e.g., cerebral vascular accident)
Confusion	Normal	Confusion or disorientation or attention deficit of brief duration; resolves spontaneously with no sequelae	Confusion or disorientation or attention deficit interfering with function, but not interfering with activities of daily living	Confusion or delirium interfering with activities of daily living	Harmful to others or self; requiring hospitalization

Delusions	Normal	—		Present	Toxic psychosis
Depressed level of consciousness	Normal	Somnolence or sedation not interfering with function	Somnolence or sedation interfering with function, but not interfering with activities of daily living	Obtundation or stupor; difficult to arouse; interfering with activities of daily living	Coma
Dizziness/lightheadedness	None	Not interfering with function	Interfering with function, but not interfering with activities of daily living	Interfering with activities of daily living	Bedridden or disabling
Extrapyramidal/involuntary movement/restlessness	None	Mild involuntary movements not interfering with function	Moderate involuntary movements interfering with function, but not interfering with activities of daily living	Severe involuntary movements or torticollis interfering with activities of daily living	Bedridden or disabling
Insomnia	Normal	Occasional difficulty sleeping not interfering with function	Difficulty sleeping interfering with function, but not interfering with activities of daily living	Frequent difficulty sleeping, interfering with activities of daily living	—

Note: This adverse event is graded when insomnia is related to treatment. If pain or other symptoms interfere with sleep do *not* grade as insomnia.

continued

331

TABLE B–1. (Continued)

Adverse Event	Grade				
	0	1	2	3	4
Memory loss	Normal	Memory loss not interfering with function	Memory loss interfering with function, but not interfering with activities of daily living	Memory loss interfering with activities of daily living	Amnesia
Mood alteration—anxiety, agitation	Normal	Mild mood alteration not interfering with function	Moderate mood alteration interfering with function, but not interfering with activities of daily living	Severe mood alteration interfering with activities of daily living	Suicidal ideation or danger to self
Mood alteration—depression	Normal	Mild mood alteration not interfering with function	Moderate mood alteration interfering with function, but not interfering with activities of daily living	Severe mood alteration interfering with activities of daily living	Suicidal ideation or danger to self

332

	Normal	Mild	Moderate	Severe	Danger to self
Mood alteration—euphoria	Normal	Mild mood alteration not interfering with function	Moderate mood alteration interfering with function, but not interfering with activities of daily living	Severe mood alteration interfering with activities of daily living	Danger to self
Neuropathy—motor	Normal	Subjective weakness but no objective findings	Mild objective weakness interfering with function, but not interfering with activities of daily living	Objective weakness interfering with activities of daily living	Paralysis
Neuropathy—sensory	Normal	Loss of deep tendon reflexes or paresthesia (including tingling) but not interfering with function	Objective sensory loss or paresthesia (including tingling), interfering with function, but not interfering with activities of daily living	Sensory loss or paresthesia interfering with activities of daily living	Permanent sensory loss that interferes with function
Seizure(s)	None	—	Seizure(s) self-limited and consciousness is preserved	Seizure(s) in which consciousness is altered	Seizures of any type that are prolonged, repetitive, or difficult to control (e.g. status epilepticus, intractable epilepsy)

continued

TABLE B–1. (*Continued*)

Adverse Event	Grade				
	0	1	2	3	4
Speech impairment (e.g., dysphasia or aphasia)	Normal	—	Awareness of receptive or expressive dysphasia, not impairing ability to communicate	Receptive or expressive dysphasia, impairing ability to communicate	Inability to communicate
Tremor	None	Mild and brief or intermittent but not interfering with function	Moderate tremor interfering with function, but not interfering with activities of daily living	Severe tremor interfering with activities of daily living	—
Ocular/Visual					
Dry eye	Normal	Mild, not requiring treatment	Moderate or requiring artificial tears	—	—
Tearing (watery eyes)	None	Mild: not interfering with function	Moderate: interfering with function, but not interfering with activities of daily living	Interfering with activities of daily living	—

	Normal	—	Symptomatic and interfering with function, but not interfering with activities of daily living	Symptomatic and interfering with activities of daily living	—
Vision—blurred vision					
Pain					
Abdominal pain or cramping	None	Mild pain not interfering with function	Moderate pain: pain or analgesics interfering with function, but not interfering with activities of daily living	Severe pain: pain or analgesics severely interfering with activities of daily living	Disabling
Arthralgia (joint pain)	None	Mild pain not interfering with function	Moderate pain: pain or analgesics interfering with function, but not interfering with activities of daily living	Severe pain: pain or analgesics severely interfering with activities of daily living	Disabling
Bone pain	None	Mild pain not interfering with function	Moderate pain: pain or analgesics interfering with function, but not interfering with activities of daily living	Severe pain: pain or analgesics severely interfering with activities of daily living	Disabling

continued

TABLE B–1. (Continued)

Adverse Event	Grade				
	0	1	2	3	4
Chest pain (non-cardiac and nonpleuritic)	None	Mild pain not interfering with function	Moderate pain: pain or analgesics interfering with function, but not interfering with activities of daily living	Severe pain: pain or analgesics severely interfering with activities of daily living	Disabling
Dysmenorrhea	None	Mild pain not interfering with function	Moderate pain: pain or analgesics interfering with function, but not interfering with activities of daily living	Severe pain: pain or analgesics severely interfering with activities of daily living	Disabling
Dyspareunia	None	Mild pain not interfering with function	Moderate pain interfering with sexual activity	Severe pain preventing sexual activity	—
Headache	None	Mild pain not interfering with function	Moderate pain: pain or analgesics interfering with function, but not interfering with activities of daily living	Severe pain: pain or analgesics severely interfering with activities of daily living	Disabling

Myalgia (muscle pain)	None	Mild pain not interfering with function	Moderate pain: pain or analgesics interfering with function, but not interfering with activities of daily living	Severe pain: pain or analgesics severely interfering with activities of daily living	Disabling
Neuropathic pain (e.g., jaw pain, neurologic pain, phantom limb pain, postinfectious neuralgia, or painful neuropathies)	None	Mild pain not interfering with function	Moderate pain: pain or analgesics interfering with function, but not interfering with activities of daily living	Severe pain: pain or analgesics severely interfering with activities of daily living	Disabling
Pelvic pain	None	Mild pain not interfering with function	Moderate pain: pain or analgesics interfering with function, but not interfering with activities of daily living	Severe pain: pain or analgesics severely interfering with activities of daily living	Disabling

continued

TABLE B-1. *(Continued)*

Adverse Event	Grade				
	0	1	2	3	4
Pleuritic pain	None	Mild pain not interfering with function	Moderate pain: pain or analgesics interfering with function, but not interfering with activities of daily living	Severe pain: pain or analgesics severely interfering with activities of daily living	Disabling
Rectal or perirectal pain (proctalgia)	None	Mild pain not interfering with function	Moderate pain: pain or analgesics interfering with function, but not interfering with activities of daily living	Severe pain: pain or analgesics severely interfering with activities of daily living	Disabling
Tumor pain (onset of exacerbation of tumor pain due to treatment)	None	Mild pain not interfering with function	Moderate pain: pain or analgesics interfering with function, but not interfering with activities of daily living	Severe pain: pain or analgesics severely interfering with activities of daily living	Disabling

Adult respiratory distress syndrome (ARDS)	Absent	—	—	—	Present
Apnea	None	—	—	Present	Requiring intubation
Cough	Absent	Mild, relieved by nonprescription medication	Requiring narcotic antitussive	Severe cough or coughing spasms, poorly controlled or unresponsive to treatment	—
Dyspnea (shortness of breath)	Normal	—	Dyspnea on exertion	Dyspnea at normal level of activity	Dyspnea at rest or requiring ventilator support
Pleural effusion (nonmalignant)	None	Asymptomatic and not requiring treatment	Symptomatic, requiring diuretics	Symptomatic, requiring O_2 or therapeutic thoracentesis	Life-threatening (e.g., requiring intubation)
Pneumonitis/pulmonary infiltrates	None	Radiographic changes but asymptomatic or symptoms not requiring steroids	Radiographic changes and requiring steroids or diuretics	Radiographic changes and requiring O_2	Radiographic changes and requiring assisted ventilation
Pneumothorax	None	No intervention required	Chest tube required	Sclerosis or surgery required	Life-threatening

339

continued

TABLE B–1. (Continued)

Adverse Event	0	1	2	3	4
			Allergy/Immunology		
Pulmonary fibrosis	None	Radiographic changes, but asymptomatic or symptoms not requiring steroids	Requiring steriods or diuretics	Requiring O_2	Requiring assisted ventilation
			Renal/Genitourinary		
Bladder spasms	Absent	Mild symptoms not requiring intervention	Symptoms requiring antispasmodic	Severe symptoms requiring narcotic	—
Creatinine	WNL	$>$ ULN–1.5 $\times$ ULN	$>$ 1.5–3.0 $\times$ ULN	$>$ 3.0–6.0 $\times$ ULN	$>$ 6.0 $\times$ ULN
Note: Adjust to age-appropriate levels for pediatric patients.					
Dysuria (painful urination)	None	Mild symptoms requiring no intervention	Symptoms relieved with therapy	Symptoms not relieved despite therapy	—
Fistula or GU fistula (e.g., vaginal, vesicovaginal)	None	—	—	Requiring intervention	Requiring surgery

Incontinence	None	With coughing, sneezing, etc.	Spontaneous, some control	No control (in the absence of fistula)	—
Operative injury to bladder and/or ureter	None	—	Injury of bladder with primary repair	Sepsis, fistula, or obstruction requiring secondary surgery; loss of one kidney; injury requiring anastomosis or reimplantation	Septic obstruction of both kidneys or vesicovaginal fistula requiring diversion
Renal failure	None	—	—	Requiring dialysis, but reversible	Requiring dialysis and irreversible
Ureteral obstruction	None	Unilateral, not requiring surgery	—	Bilateral, not requiring surgery	Stent, nephrostomy tube, or surgery
Urinary electrolyte wasting	None	Asymptomatic, not requiring treatment	Mild, reversible and manageable with oral replacement	Reversible but requiring IV replacement	Irreversible, requiring continued replacement

Also consider acidosis, bicarbonate, hypocalcemia, hypophosphatemia.

continued

341

TABLE B-1. (*Continued*)

Adverse Event	Grade				
	0	1	2	3	4
Sexual/Reproductive Function					
Irregular menses (change from baseline)	Normal	Occasionally irregular or lengthened interval, but continuing menstrual cycles	Very irregular, but continuing menstrual cycles	Persistent amenorrhea	—
Libido	Normal	Decrease in interest	Severe loss of interest	—	—
Vaginal dryness	Normal	Mild	Requiring treatment and/or interfering with sexual function, dyspareunia	—	—

LLN = lower limit of normal; NCI = National Cancer Institute; ULN = upper limit of normal; WNL = within normal limits.
Adapted Common Toxicity Criteria from the National Cancer Institute, http://ctep.info.nih.gov.

C | Formulas

SUMMARY OF FORMULAS (ALL FOR ADULT FEMALE)

Cardiovascular

Parameter	Symbol	Formula	Normal values
Mean right atrial pressure	CVP	Measured	0–8 mmHg
Mean pulmonary wedge pressure	Pao or PW	Measured	6–12 mmHg
Mean arterial pressure	MAP	(Systolic + 2 diastolic) : 3	80–100 mmHg
Cardiac output	CO	Stroke volume × heart rate	4–5 L/min
Cardiac index	CI	CO/body surface area	2.5–3.5 L/min/m^2
Stroke volume	SV	CO/heart rate	50–100 mL/beat
Stroke volume index	SVI	SV/body surface area	40–50 mL/beat/m^2
Systemic vascular resistance	SVR	$\dfrac{(MAP - CVP) \times 80}{CO}$	800–2000 dynes/sec/cm^{-5}
Oxygen delivery	Do$_2$	(1.39 × Hb × O$_2$ sat% × CO) + (Pao$_2$ × 0.0031)	600–1400/mL O$_2$/min (500 mL O$_2$/min/m^2)
Oxygen consumption	Vo$_2$	[(Sao$_2$ − Smvo$_2$) × Hb × 1.39 × CO] : 10	180–280 mL O$_2$/min (110–160 mL/min/m^2)
Ejection fraction	EF	SV/end ventricular diastolic volume	40–60%
Mixed venous O$_2$	Svo$_2$	Measured	> 70%

Pulmonary/Blood Gas

Pressure Alveolar–arterial (A–a) O$_2$ Gradient (normal value: 5–20 mmHg) PAo$_2$ − Pao$_2$.

$Pao_2 = Pio_2 - Paco_2/0.8$ (21% × 760 mmHg).

$Pao_2 =$ this value you get from your ABGs.

Renal

Creatinine Clearance (normal value: > 75 mL/min)

Method	Formula
Cockroft–Gault	$\dfrac{\text{(Weight in kg) (140} - \text{age)} \times 0.85}{\text{(72) (Stable serum creatinine in mg/dL)}}$
Jellife	$\dfrac{(98 - [0.8\ (\text{Age} - 20)] \times 0.9}{\text{Serum creatinine in mg/dL}}$
Measured (24-hour urine collection)	$= \dfrac{\text{U cr} \times \text{U vol} \times 1.73}{\text{Serum creatine} \times \text{time} \times \text{BSA}}$

BSA = body surface area; U cr = urine creatinine in mg/dL; U vol = urine volume in mL for 24 hours; time = minutes.

Fractional Excretion of Sodium (FENA)

$$\frac{\text{Urine Na}}{\text{Serum Na}} \times \frac{\text{Serum creatinine}}{\text{Urine creatinine}} \times 100.$$

Electrolytes

Albumin-Corrected Serum Calcium (mg/dL)

Serum calcium (mg/dL) + 0.8 (4 − Serum albumin in g/dL).

Anion Gap (normal value: 8–12 mEq mmol/L)

$(Na + K) - (Cl + HCO_3)$.

Osmolality (normal 270–290 mosm/kg)

$[Na(mEq/L) \times 2] + [glu\ (mg/dL)/18] + [BUN\ (mg/dL)/2.8]$.

Total Body Water

Body weight in kg × 60%.

Water Deficit

$$\frac{0.6 \times \text{Weight in kg} \times \text{Serum Na}}{140 - 1}.$$

Or, Weight in kg × 0.6 × (1 − [$\frac{\text{Normal osm}}{\text{Observed osm}}$]).

Excess Water

[Total body water − (Actual serum Na/Desired serum Na)] × Total body water.

Nutrition

Nitrogen Balance

$\frac{\text{Protein intake (g)}}{0.625}$ − (24-hour urine urea nitrogen + 4 g).

Prognostic Nutritional Index (% risk)

158% − 16.6 (albumin in g/100 mL) − 0.78 (tricep skinfold in mm) − 0.2 (serum transferrin in mg/dL) − 5.8 (delayed skin hypersensitivity).

- Where delayed hypersensitivity consists of mumps, streptokinase, streptodornase, *Candida.*
- Graded as 0 (nonreactive), 1 (< 5-mm induration), or 2 (≥ 5-mm induration).
- Interpretation: well-nourished (PNI < 40); mildly malnourished (PNI 40–49); severely malnourished (PNI > 50).

Body Mass Index (obese when BMI > 27)

$$\frac{\text{Weight in kg}}{(\text{height in m})^2}$$

Basal Calorie Requirement (Harris–Benedict's)

665 + (9.6 × weight in kg) + (1.7 × height in cm) − (4.7 × age in years).

Note: A simpler estimation for calorie requirement is about 25 to 30 kcal/kg.

Miscellaneous

Body Surface Area (BSA in m^2)

$$\sqrt{\frac{\text{Height in cm} \times \text{weight in kg}}{3600}}$$

Ideal or Lean Body Weight Determination (gives ± 10% of ideal body weight)

Allow 100 lbs for the first 5 feet, then add 5 lbs per additional inch. Then multiply to the conversion factor of 2.2 lb/kg.

D | Performance Status

GOG[a]	Karnofsky scale	Performance
0	90–100	Fully active
1	70–80	Restricted strenuous physical activity, but ambulatory
2	50–60	Ambulatory; self-care, unable to work up to 50% of waking hours
3	30–40	Limited self-care; confined to bed/chair up to 50% of waking hours
4	10–20	Completely disabled, no self-care

[a]GOG = Gynecologic Oncology Group scale.

E | Pulmonary Function Test

A. Forced expiratory volume in 1 second (FEV_1):
  1. After maximum inspiration, FEV_1 is the volume of a single, maximally fast expiration in the first second. A normal range is 3 to 5 L.
  2. FEV_1 is expressed in two ways:
     a. As a percentage of the expected FEV_1 for a normal individual of the same age, height, and sex.
     b. As a percentage of the individual's own total forced expiratory volume (vital capacity); that is, (FEV_1) × 100/FVC; this value is usually greater than 75%. *Note:* forced vital capacity (FVC) has a normal value of 4 to 6 L.
B. Interpretation of FEV_1: a measure of flow early in expiration and is effort-dependent. It is decreased in obstructive or restrictive disease. In obstructive diseases, FEV_1 and FVC are decreased and the ratio of FEV_1 to FVC is diminished. In restrictive airway diseases, the FVC is diminished, but the ratio of FEV_1 to FVC is normal.

F | ACLS Algorithms

Figure F-1. Universal Algorithm for
Adults—Emergency Cardiac Care

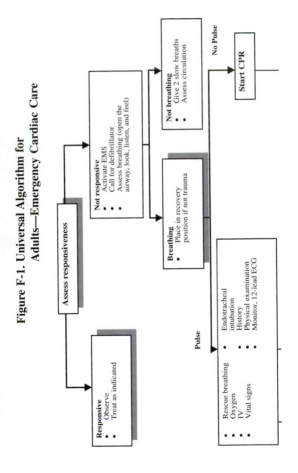

Assess responsiveness

Responsive
- Observe
- Treat as indicated

Not responsive
- Activate EMS
- Call for defibrillator
- Assess breathing (open the airway, look, listen, and feel)

Breathing
- Place in recovery position if not trauma

Not breathing
- Give 2 slow breaths
- Assess circulation

Pulse
- Rescue breathing
- Oxygen
- IV
- Vital signs
- Endotracheal intubation
- History
- Physical examination
- Monitor, 12-lead ECG

No Pulse

Start CPR

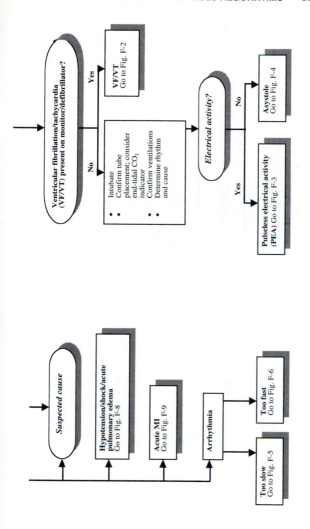

Figure F-2. Ventricular Fibrillation/Pulseless Ventricular Tachycardia (VF/VT) Algorithm

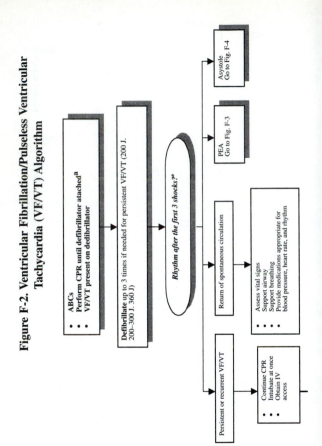

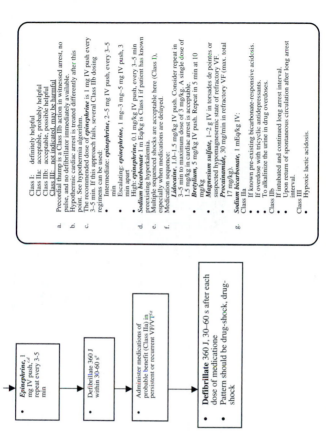

Class I: definitely helpful
Class IIa: acceptable, probably helpful
Class IIb: acceptable, possible helpful
Class III: not indicated, may be harmful

a. Precordial thump is a Class IIb action in witnessed arrest, no pulse, and no defibrillator immediately available.

b. Hypothermic cardiac arrest is treated differently after this point. See hypothermia algorithm.

c. The recommended dose of *epinephrine* is 1 mg IV push every 3–5 min. If this approach fails, several Class IIb dosing regimens can be used:

- Intermediate: *epinephrine*, 2–5 mg IV push, every 3–5 min

- Escalating: *epinephrine*, 1 mg–3 mg–5 mg IV push, 3 min apart

- High: *epinephrine*, 0.1 mg/kg IV push, every 3–5 min

d. *Sodium bicarbonate* 1 m Eq/kg is Class I if patient has known preexisting hyperkalemia.

e. Multiple sequenced shocks are acceptable here (Class I), especially when medications are delayed.

f. Medication sequence:

- *Lidocaine*, 1.0–1.5 mg/kg IV push. Consider repeat in 3–5 min to maximum dose of 3 mg/kg. A single dose of 1.5 mg/kg in cardiac arrest is acceptable.

- *Bretylium*, 5 mg/kg IV push. Repeat in 5 min at 10 mg/kg

- *Magnesium sulfate*, 1–2 g IV in torsades de pointes or suspected hypomagnesemic state of refractory VF.

- *Procainamide*, 30 mg/min in refractory VF (max. total 17 mg/kg).

g. *Sodium bicarbonate*, 1 mEq/kg IV:

Class IIa
- If known pre-existing bicarbonate-responsive acidosis.
- If overdose with tricyclic antidepressants.
- To alkalinize the urine in drug overdoses.

Class IIb
- If intubated and continued long arrest interval.
- Upon return of spontaneous circulation after long arrest interval.

Class III
- Hypoxic lactic acidosis.

- *Epinephrine*, 1 mg IV push,[c,d] repeat every 3–5 min

- Defibrillate 360 J within 30–60 s[e]

- Administer medications of probable benefit (Class IIa) in persistent or recurrent VF/VT[f,g]

- **Defibrillate** 360 J, 30–60 s after each dose of medication[e]
- Pattern should be drug-shock, drug-shock

Figure F-3. Pulseless Electrical Activity (PEA) Algorithm (Electromechanical Dissociation [EMD])

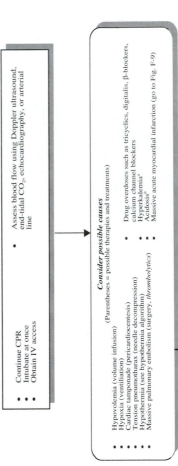

Includes:

- Electromechanical dissociation (EMD)
- Pseudo-EMD
- Idioventricular rhythms
- Ventricular escape rhythms
- Bradyasystolic rhythms
- Postdefibrillation idioventricular rhythms

- Continue CPR
- Intubate at once
- Obtain IV access

- Assess blood flow using Doppler ultrasound, end-tidal CO_2, echocardiography, or arterial line

Consider possible causes
(Parentheses = possible therapies and treatments)

- Hypovolemia (volume infusion)
- Hypoxia (ventilation)
- Cardiac tamponade (pericardiocentesis)
- Tension pneumothorax (needle decompression)
- Hypothermia (see hypothermia algorithm)
- Massive pulmonary embolism (surgery, *thrombolytics*)

- Drug overdoses such as tricyclics, digitalis, β-blockers, calcium channel blockers
- Hyperkalemia[a]
- Acidosis[b]
- Massive acute myocardial infarction (go to Fig. F-9)

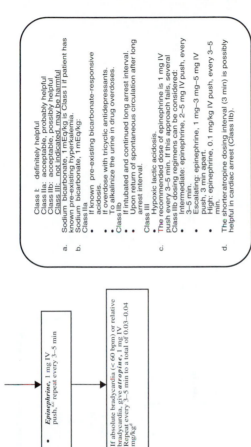

Class I: definitely helpful
Class IIa: acceptable, probably helpful
Class IIb: acceptable, possibly helpful
Class III: not indicated, may be harmful

a. Sodium bicarbonate, 1 mEq/kg is Class I if patient has known pre-existing hyperkalemia.

b. Sodium bicarbonate, 1 mEq/kg:

Class IIa
- If known pre-existing bicarbonate-responsive acidosis.
- If overdose with tricyclic antidepressants.
- To alkalinize the urine in drug overdoses.

Class IIb
- If intubated and continued long arrest interval.
- Upon return of spontaneous circulation after long arrest interval.

Class III
- Hypoxic lactic acidosis.

c. The recommended dose of epinephrine is 1 mg IV push every 3–5 min. If this approach fails, several Class IIb dosing regimens can be considered:
- Intermediate: epinephrine, 2–5 mg IV push, every 3–5 min.
- Escalating: epinephrine, 1 mg–3 mg–5 mg IV push, 3 min apart.
- High: epinephrine, 0.1 mg/kg IV push, every 3–5 min.

d. The shorter atropine dosing interval (3 min) is possibly helpful in cardiac arrest (Class IIb).

- *Epinephrine*, 1 mg IV push,[a,c] repeat every 3–5 min

If absolute bradycardia (< 60 bpm) or relative bradycardia, give *atropine*, 1 mg IV
- Repeat every 3–5 min to a total of 0.03–0.04 mg/kg[d]

Figure F-4. Asystole Treatment Algorithm

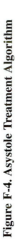

- **Continue CPR**
- **Intubate at once**
- **Obtain IV access**
- **Confirm asystole in more than one lead**

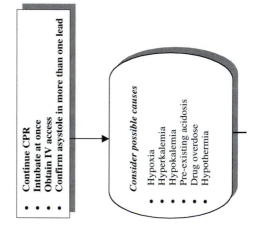

Consider possible causes

- Hypoxia
- Hyperkalemia
- Hypokalemia
- Pre-existing acidosis
- Drug overdose
- Hypothermia

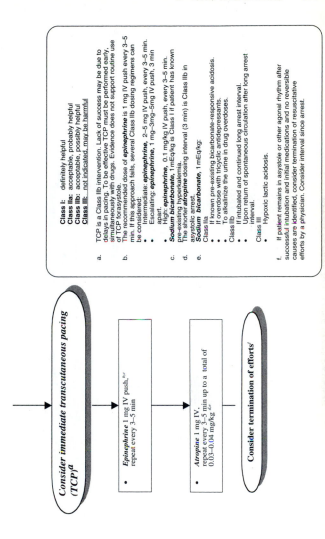

Consider immediate transcutaneous pacing (TCP)[a]

- **Epinephrine** 1 mg IV push,[b,c] repeat every 3–5 min

- **Atropine** 1 mg IV, repeat every 3–5 min up to a total of 0.03–0.04 mg/kg[d,e]

Consider termination of efforts[f]

Class I: definitely helpful
Class IIa: acceptable, probably helpful
Class IIb: acceptable, possibly helpful
Class III: not indicated, may be harmful

a. TCP is a Class IIb intervention. Lack of success may be due to delays in pacing. To be effective TCP must be performed early, simultaneously with drugs. Evidence does not support routine use of TCP for asystole.

b. The recommended dose of *epinephrine* is 1 mg IV push every 3–5 min. If this approach fails, several Class IIb dosing regimens can be considered:
   - Intermediate: *epinephrine*, 2–5 mg IV push, every 3–5 min.
   - Escalating: *epinephrine*, 1 mg–3mg–5mg IV push, 3 min apart.
   - High: *epinephrine*, 0.1 mg/kg IV push, every 3–5 min.

c. *Sodium bicarbonate*, 1mEq/kg is Class I if patient has known pre-existing hyperkalemia.

d. The shorter *atropine* dosing interval (3 min) is Class IIb in asystolic arrest.

e. *Sodium bicarbonate*, 1 mEq/kg:
   Class IIa
   - If known pre-existing bicarbonate-responsive acidosis.
   - If overdose with tricyclic antidepressants.
   - To alkalinize the urine in drug overdoses.
   Class IIb
   - If intubated and continued long arrest interval.
   - Upon return of spontaneous circulation after long arrest interval.
   Class III
   - Hypoxic lactic acidosis.

f. If patient remains in asystole or other agonal rhythm after successful intubation and initial medications and no reversible causes are identified, consider termination of resuscitative efforts by a physician. Consider interval since arrest.

Figure F-5. Bradycardia Algorithm (Patient Not in Cardiac Arrest)

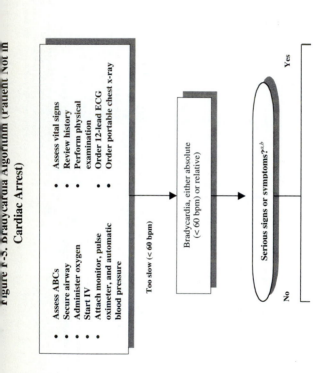

- Assess ABCs
- Secure airway
- Administer oxygen
- Start IV
- Attach monitor, pulse oximeter, and automatic blood pressure

- Assess vital signs
- Review history
- Perform physical examination
- Order 12-lead ECG
- Order portable chest x-ray

Too slow (< 60 bpm)

Bradycardia, either absolute (< 60 bpm) or relative

Serious signs or symptoms?[a,b]

No   Yes

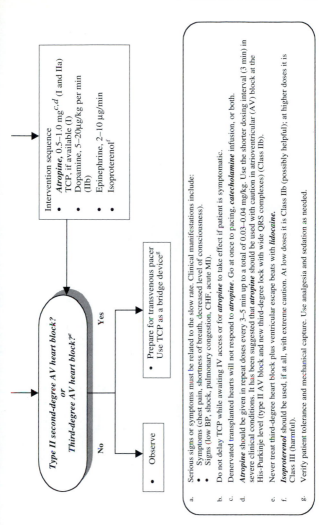

Intervention sequence

- **Atropine**, 0.5–1.0 mg[c,d] (I and IIa)
- TCP, if available (I)
- Dopamine, 5–20μg/kg per min (IIb)
- Epinephrine, 2–10 μg/min[f]
- Isoproterenol[f]

Type II second-degree AV heart block?
or
Third-degree AV heart block?[a,e]

No → • Observe

Yes → • Prepare for transvenous pacer
  Use TCP as a bridge device[g]

a. Serious signs or symptoms must be related to the slow rate. Clinical manifestations include:
  - Symptoms (chest pain, shortness of breath, decreased level of consciousness).
  - Signs (low BP, shock, pulmonary congestion, CHF; acute MI).

b. Do not delay TCP while awaiting IV access or for *atropine* to take effect if patient is symptomatic.

c. Denervated transplanted hearts will not respond to *atropine*. Go at once to pacing, *catecholamine* infusion, or both.

d. *Atropine* should be given in repeat doses every 3–5 min up to a total of 0.03–0.04 mg/kg. Use the shorter dosing interval (3 min) in severe clinical conditions. It has been suggested that *atropine* should be used with caution in atrioventricular (AV) block at the His-Purkinje level (type II AV block and new third-degree block with wide QRS complexes) (Class IIb).

e. Never treat third-degree heart block plus ventricular escape beats with *lidocaine*.

f. *Isoproterenol* should be used, if at all, with extreme caution. At low doses it is Class IIb (possibly helpful); at higher doses it is Class III (harmful).

g. Verify patient tolerance and mechanical capture. Use analgesia and sedation as needed.

Figure F-6. Tachycardia Algorithm

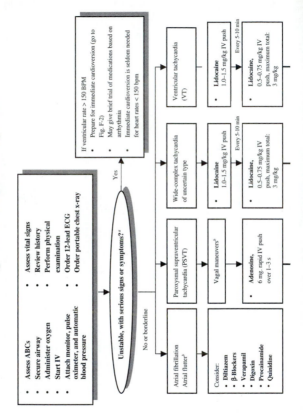

- Assess ABCs
- Secure airway
- Administer oxygen
- Start IV
- Attach monitor, pulse oximeter, and automatic blood pressure

- Assess vital signs
- Review history
- Perform physical examination
- Order 12-lead ECG
- Order portable chest x-ray

Unstable, with serious signs or symptoms?[a]

No or borderline

Yes

If ventricular rate > 150 BPM
- Prepare for immediate cardioversion (go to Fig. F-2)
- May give brief trial of medications based on arrhythmia
- Immediate cardioversion is seldom needed for heart rates < 150 bpm

Atrial fibrillation
Atrial flutter[c]

Consider:
- Diltiazem
- β-Blockers
- Verapamil
- Digoxin
- Procainamide
- Quinidine

Paroxysmal supraventricular tachycardia (PSVT)

Vagal maneuvers[b]

Adenosine, 6 mg rapid IV push over 1–3 s

Wide-complex tachycardia of uncertain type

Lidocaine 1.0–1.5 mg/kg IV push

Every 5–10 min

Lidocaine, 0.5–0.75 mg/kg IV push, maximum total: 3 mg/kg

Ventricular tachycardia (VT)

Lidocaine 1.0–1.5 mg/kg IV push

Every 5–10 min

Lidocaine, 0.5–0.75 mg/kg IV push, maximum total: 3 mg/kg

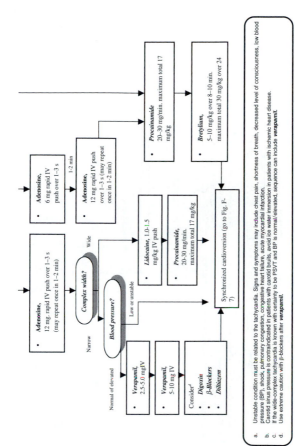

- **Adenosine,**
  12 mg. rapid IV push over 1–3 s
  (may repeat once in 1–2 min)

- **Adenosine,**
  6 mg IV
  push over 1–3 s

  1–2 min

- **Adenosine,**
  12 mg rapid IV push
  over 1–3 s (may repeat
  once in 1–2 min)

Complex width?

Narrow — Wide

Blood pressure?

Normal or elevated

Low or unstable

- **Verapamil,**
  2.5–5.0 mg IV

- **Verapamil,**
  5–10 mg IV

- Consider[d]
  - **Digoxin**
  - **β-Blockers**
  - **Diltiazem**

- **Lidocaine,** 1.0–1.5
  mg/kg IV push

- **Procainamide,**
  20–30 mg/min.
  maximum total 17 mg/kg

- **Procainamide**
  20–30 mg/min. maximum total 17 mg/kg

- **Bretylium,**
  5–10 mg/kg over 8–10 min.
  maximum total 30 mg/kg over 24

Synchronized cardioversion (go to Fig. F-7)

a. Unstable condition must be related to the tachycardia. Signs and symptoms may include chest pain, shortness of breath, decreased level of consciousness, low blood pressure (BP), shock, pulmonary congestion, congestive heart failure, acute myocardial infarction.

b. Carotid sinus pressure is contraindicated in patients with carotid bruits, avoid ice water immersion in patients with ischemic heart disease.

c. If the wide-complex tachycardia is known with certainty to be PSVT and BP is normal/elevated, sequence can include **verapamil.**

d. Use extreme caution with β-blockers after **verapamil.**

Figure F-7. The Tachycardia Overview Algorithm

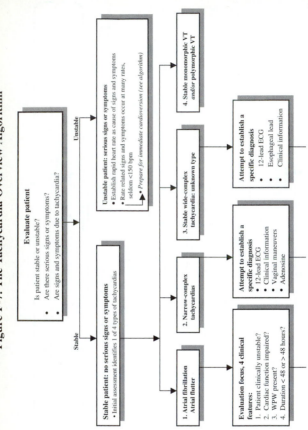

Evaluate patient

Is patient stable or unstable?
- Are there serious signs or symptoms?
- Are signs and symptoms due to tachycardia?

Stable

Unstable

Stable patient: no serious signs or symptoms
- Initial assessment identifies 1 of 4 types of tachycardias

Unstable patient: serious signs or symptoms
- Establish rapid heart rate as cause of signs and symptoms
- Rate related signs and symptoms occur at many rates, seldom <150 bpm
- *Prepare for immediate cardioversion (see algorithm)*

1. Atrial fibrillation
Atrial flutter

2. Narrow-complex tachycardias

3. Stable wide-complex tachycardia: unknown type

4. Stable monomorphic VT *and/or* polymorphic VT

Evaluation focus, 4 clinical features:
1. Patient clinically unstable?
2. Cardiac function impaired?
3. WPW present?
4. Duration < 48 or > 48 hours?

Attempt to establish a specific diagnosis
- 12-lead ECG
- Clinical information
- Vaginal maneuvers
- Adenosine

Attempt to establish a specific diagnosis
- 12-lead ECG
- Esophageal lead
- Clinical information

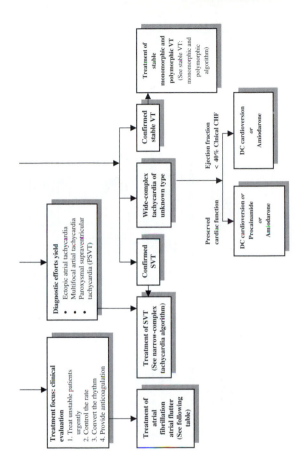

Figure F-8. Acute Pulmonary Edema/Hypotension/Shock Algorithm

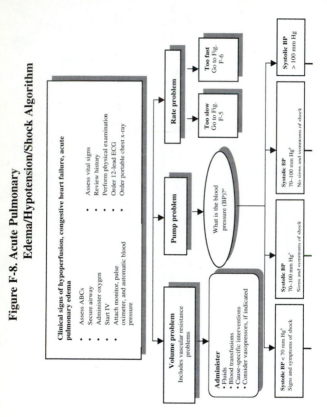

Clinical signs of hypoperfusion, congestive heart failure, acute pulmonary edema

- Assess ABCs
- Secure airway
- Administer oxygen
- Start IV
- Attach monitor, pulse oximeter, and automatic blood pressure

- Assess vital signs
- Review history
- Perform physical examination
- Order 12-lead ECG
- Order portable chest x-ray

Rate problem

Too slow Go to Fig. F-5

Too fast Go to Fig. F-6

Pump problem

What is the blood pressure (BP)?[a]

Volume problem
Includes vascular resistance problems

Administer
- Fluids
- Blood transfusions
- Cause-specific interventions
- Consider vasopressors, if indicated

Systolic BP < 70 mm Hg[a]
Signs and symptoms of shock

Systolic BP 70–100 mm Hg[a]
Signs and symptoms of shock

Systolic BP 70–100 mm Hg[a]
No signs and symptoms of shock

Systolic BP > 100 mm Hg

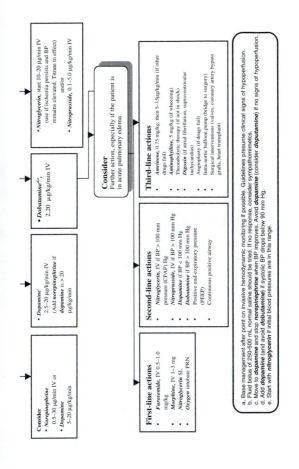

Consider
- *Norepinephrine*
  0.5–30 µg/kg/min IV or
- *Dopamine*
  5–20 µg/kg/min

- *Dopamine*[f]
  2.5–20 µg/kg/min IV
  (Add *norepinephrine* if
  dopamine is > 20
  µg/kg/min

- *Dobutamine*[d,e],
  2.20 µg/kg/min IV

- *Nitroglycerin,* start 10–20 µg/min IV
  (use if ischemia persists and BP
  remains elevated. Titrate to effect)
  and/or
- *Nitroprusside,* 0.1–5.0 µg/kg/min IV

Consider
Further action, especially if the patient is
in acute pulmonary edema

First-line actions
- *Furosemide,* IV 0.5–1.0
  mg/kg
- *Morphine,* IV 1–3 mg
- *Nitroglycerin* SL
- *Oxygen* intubate PRN

Second-line actions
- *Nitroglycerin,* IV if BP > 100 mm
  pressure (CPAP) Hg
- *Nitroprusside,* IV if BP > 100 mm Hg
- *Dopamine* if BP < 100 mm Hg
- *Dobutamine* if BP > 100 mm Hg
- Positive end-expiratory pressure
  (PEEP)
- Continuous positive airway

Third-line actions
- *Amrinone,* 0.75 mg/kg; then 5–15µg/kg/min (if other
  drugs fail)
- *Aminophylline,* 5 mg/kg (if wheezing)
- Thrombolytic therapy (if not in shock)
- *Digoxin* (if atrial fibrillation, supraventricular
  tachycardias)
- Angioplasty (if drugs fail)
- Intra-aortic balloon pump (bridge to surgery)
- Surgical interventions (valves, coronary artery bypass
  grafts, heart transplant)

a. Base management after point on invasive hemodynamic monitoring if possible. Guidelines presume clinical signs of hypoperfusion.
b. Fluid bolus of 250–500 mL normal saline should be tried. If no response, consider sympathomimetics.
c. Move to *dopamine* and stop *norepinephrine* when BP improves. Avoid *dopamine* (consider *dobutamine*) if no signs of hypoperfusion.
d. Add *dopamine* (and avoid *dobutamine*) if systolic BP drops below 90 mm Hg.
e. Start with *nitroglycerin* if initial blood pressures are in this range.

Figure F-9. Stable Ventricular Tachycardia (Monomorphic or Polymorphic) Algorithm

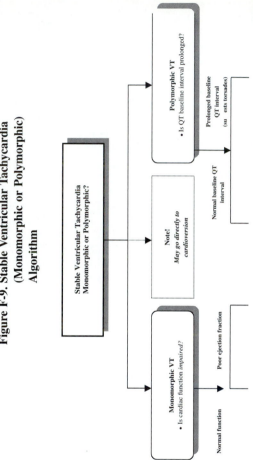

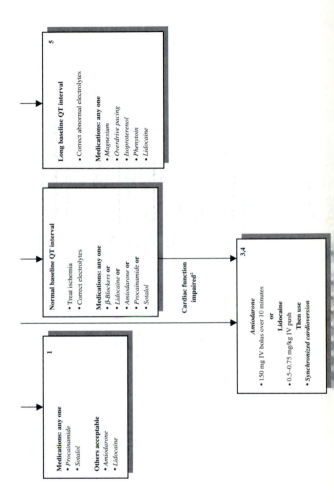

5

Long baseline QT interval

• Correct abnormal electrolytes

Medications: any one

• *Magnesium*
• *Overdrive pacing*
• *Isoproterenol*
• *Phenytoin*
• *Lidocaine*

Normal baseline QT interval

• Treat ischemia
• Correct electrolytes

Medications: any one

• *β-Blockers or*
• *Lidocaine or*
• *Amiodarone or*
• *Procainamide or*
• *Sotalol*

Cardiac function impaired²

1

Medications: any one

• *Procainamide*
• *Sotalol*

Others acceptable

• *Amiodarone*
• *Lidocaine*

3,4

Amiodarone

• 150 mg IV bolus over 10 minutes

or

Lidocaine

• 0.5–0.75 mg/kg IV push

Then use

• *Synchronized cardioversion*

Figure F-10. Chest Pain Algorithm

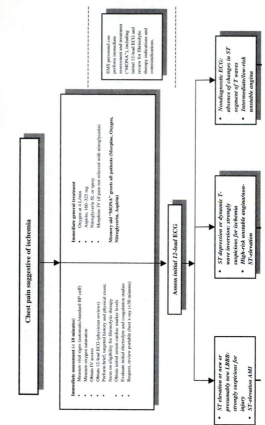

Chest pain suggestive of ischemia

Immediate assessment (< 10 minutes)
- Measure vital signs (automatic/standard BP cuff)
- Measure oxygen saturation
- Obtain IV access
- Obtain 12-lead ECG (physician reviews)
- Perform brief, targeted history and physical exam; focus on eligibility for fibrinolytic therapy
- Obtain initial serum cardiac marker levels
- Evaluate initial electrolyte and coagulation studies
- Request, review portable chest x-ray (<30 minutes)

Immediate general treatment
- Oxygen at 4 L/min
- Aspirin, 160–325 mg
- Nitroglycerin SL or spray
- Morphine IV (if pain not relieved with nitroglycerin)

Memory aid "MONA" greets all patients (Morphine, Oxygen, Nitroglycerin, Aspirin)

EMS personnel can perform immediate assessment and treatment ("MONA"), including initial 12-lead ECG and review for fibrinolytic therapy indications and contraindications.

Assess initial 12-lead ECG

- ST elevation or new or presumably new LBBB: strongly suspicious for injury
  - **ST-elevation AMI**

- ST depression or dynamic T-wave inversion: strongly suspicious for ischemia
  - **High-risk unstable angina/non–ST-elevation**

- Nondiagnostic ECG: absence of changes in ST segment or T waves
  - **Intermediate/low-risk unstable angina**

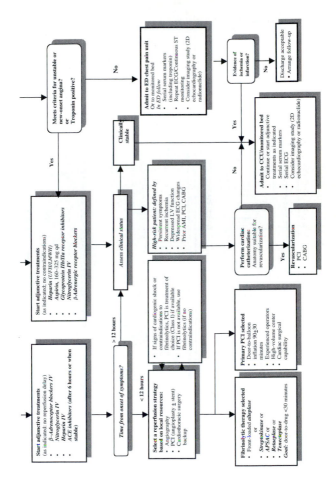

Start adjunctive treatments
(as indicated; no reperfusion delay)
- β-*adrenoceptor blockers IV*
- *Nitroglycerin IV*
- *Heparin IV*
- ACE inhibitors (after 6 hours or when stable)

Time from onset of symptoms?

< 12 hours

> 12 hours

Select a reperfusion strategy based on local resources:
- Angiography
- PCI (angioplasty ± stent)
- Cardiothoracic surgery backup

- If signs of cardiogenic shock or contraindications to fibrinolytics, PCI is treatment of choice (Class I) if available
- If PCI is not available, use fibrinolytics (if no contraindications)

Fibrinolytic therapy selected
- Front-loaded *alteplase* or
- *Streptokinase* or
- *APSAC* or
- *Retaplase* or
- *Tenecteplase*
- Goal: door-to-drug <30 minutes

Primary PCI selected
- Door-to-balloon inflation 90±30 minutes
- Experienced operators
- High-volume center
- Cardiac surgical capability

Assess clinical status

High-risk patient: *defined by*
- Persistent symptoms
- Recurrent ischemia
- Depressed LV function
- Widespread ECG changes
- Prior AMI, PCI, CABG

Clinically stable

Perform cardiac catheterization:
Anatomy suitable for revascularization?

Yes

Revascularization:
- PCI
- CABG

Meets criteria for unstable or new-onset angina?
or
Troponin positive?

Yes

Start adjunctive treatments
(as indicated, no contraindications)
- *Heparin (UFH/LMWH)*
- Aspirin, 160–325 mg qd
- *Glycoprotein IIb/IIa receptor inhibitors*
- *Nitroglycerin IV*
- β-*Adrenergic receptor blockers*

No

Admit to ED chest pain unit
Or to monitored bed
In follow
- Serial serum markers (including troponin)
- Repeat ECG/Continuous ST monitoring
- Consider imaging study (2D echocardiography or radionuclide)

No

Yes

Evidence of ischemia or infarction?

No

Discharge acceptable
- Arrange follow-up

Admit to CCU/monitored bed
- Continue or start adjunctive treatments as indicated
- Serial serum markers
- Serial ECG
- Consider imaging study (2D echocardiography or radionuclide)

Figure F-11. Suspected Stroke Algorithm

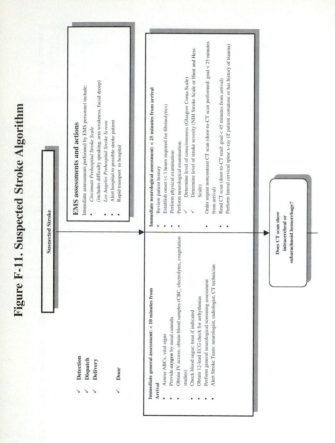

Suspected Stroke

> ✓ **Detection**
> ✓ **Dispatch**
> ✓ **Delivery**
>
> ✓ **Door**

EMS assessments and actions

Immediate assessments performed by EMS personnel include:

- *Cincinnati Prehospital Stroke Scale*
  (includes difficulty speaking, arm weakness, facial droop)
- *Los Angeles Prehospital Stroke Screen*
- Alert hospital to possible stroke patient
- Rapid transport to hospital

Immediate general assessment: < 10 minutes from Arrival

- Assess ABCs, vital signs
- Provide **oxygen** by nasal cannula
- Obtain IV access, obtain blood samples (CBC, electrolytes, coagulation studies)
- Check blood sugar; treat if indicated
- Obtain 12-lead ECG check for arrhythmias
- Perform general neurological screening assessment
- Alert Stroke Team: neurologist, radiologist, CT technician

Immediate neurological assessment: < 25 minutes from arrival

- Review patient history
- Establish onset (< 3 hours required for fibrinolytics)
- Perform physical examination
- Perform neurological examination:
  - ✓ Determine level of consciousness (Glasgow Coma Scale)
  - ✓ Determine level of stroke severity (NIH Stroke Scale or Hunt and Hess Scale)
- Order urgent noncontrast CT scan (door-to-CT scan performed: goal < 25 minutes from arrival)
- Read CT scan (door-to-CT read: goal < 45 minutes from arrival)
- Perform lateral cervical spine x-ray (if patient comatose or has history of trauma)

Does CT scan show intracerebral or subarachnoid hemorrhage?

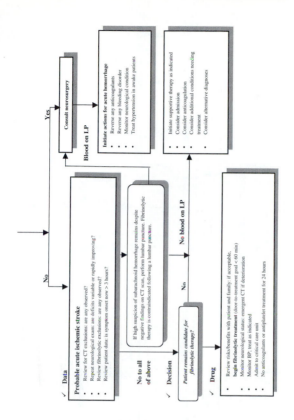

✓ **Data**

Probable acute ischemic stroke
- Review for CT exclusions: are any observed?
- Repeat neurological exam: are deficits variable or rapidly improving?
- Review fibrinolytic exclusions: are any observed?
- Review patient data: is symptom onset now > 3 hours?

No to all of above

If high suspicion of subarachnoid hemorrhage remains despite negative findings on CT scan, perform lumbar puncture. Fibrinolytic therapy is contraindicated following a lumbar puncture.

Blood on LP → **Consult neurosurgery** (Yes)

(No)

No blood on LP

✓ **Decision**

Patient remains candidate for fibrinolytic therapy?

No →

✓ **Drug**

- Review risks/benefits with patient and family: if acceptable, **begin fibrinolytic treatment** (door-to-treatment goal < 60 min)
- Monitor neurological status: emergent CT if deterioration
- Monitor BP: treat as indicated
- Admit to critical care unit
- No anticoagulants or antiplatelet treatment for 24 hours

Initiate actions for acute hemorrhage
- Reverse any anticoagulants
- Reverse any bleeding disorder
- Monitor neurological condition
- Treat hypertension in awake patients

- Initiate supportive therapy as indicated
- Consider admission
- Consider anticoagulation
- Consider additional conditions needing treatment
- Consider alternative diagnoses

Figure F-12. The Acute Pulmonary Edema, Hypotension, and Shock Algorithm

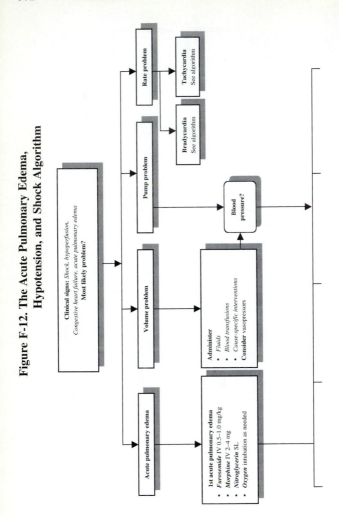

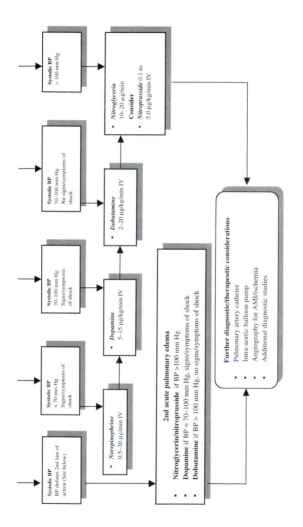

Systolic BP > 100 mm Hg

Systolic BP 70–100 mm Hg No signs/symptoms of shock

Systolic BP 70–100 mm Hg Signs/symptoms of shock

Systolic BP < 70 mm Hg Signs/symptoms of shock

Systolic BP BP defines 2nd line of action (See below)

- *Nitroglycerin* 10–20 µg/min **Consider**
- *Nitroprusside* 0.1 to 5.0 µg/kg/min IV

- *Dobutamine* 2–20 µg/kg/min IV

- *Dopamine* 5–15 µg/kg/min IV

- *Norepinephrine* 0.5–30 µg/min IV

2nd acute pulmonary edema

Nitroglycerin/nitroprusside if BP >100 mm Hg
Dopamine if BP = 70–100 mm Hg, signs/symptoms of shock
Dobutamine if BP > 100 mm Hg, no signs/symptoms of shock

-
-
-

Further diagnostic/therapeutic considerations

- Pulmonary artery catheter
- Intra-aortic balloon pump
- Angiography for AMI/ischemia
- Additional diagnostic studies

INDEX

Page numbers followed by the letters *t* or *f* indicate tables or figures respectively.